Epidemiology and Prevention of Gallstone Disease

Epidemiology and Prevention of Gallstone Disease

Edited by

L. Capocaccia, G. Ricci, F. Angelico, M. Angelico and A. F. Attili

Proceedings of an International Workshop on the Epidemiology and Prevention of Gallstone Disease, held in Rome, December 16–17, 1983

MTP PRESS LIMITED
a member of the KLUWER ACADEMIC PUBLISHERS GROUP
LANCASTER / BOSTON / THE HAGUE / DORDRECHT

Acknowledgement

The Editors wish to express their deep gratitude to Professor Jeremiah Stamler and Professor R. Hermon Dowling for their enthusiastic cooperation and continuous scientific support in the organization of the Workshop.
The Workshop was financially supported by Gipharmex S.p.A., Milan.

Published in the UK and Europe by
MTP Press Limited
Falcon House
Lancaster, England

British Library Cataloguing in Publication Data

Epidemiology and prevention of gallstone disease.
1. Gallstones 2. Cholesterol
3. Epidemiology
I. Capocaccia, L.
616.3'65 RC850

ISBN-13:978-94-010-8972-2 e-ISBN-13:978-94-009-5606-3
DOI: 10.1007/978-94-009-5606-3

Published in the USA by
MTP Press
A division of Kluwer Boston Inc
190 Old Derby Street
Hingham, MA 02043, USA

Library of Congress Cataloging in Publication Data

International Workshop on the Epidemiology and Prevention of Gallstone Disease (1983:Rome, Italy)
Epidemiology and prevention of gallstone disease.

"Proceedings of an International Workshop on the Epidemiology and Prevention of Gallstone Disease, held in Rome, December 16–17, 1983."
Bibliography: p.
Includes index.
1. Calculi, Biliary—Congresses. 2. Calculi, Biliary—Prevention—Congresses. 3. Epidemiology—Congresses. I. Capocaccia, L. II. Title. [DNLM: 1. Cholelithiasis—occurrence—congresses. 2. Cholelithiasis—prevention & control—congresses. WI 755 1593e 1983]
RC850.157 1983 616.6'22 84-12600

Typeset by Cotswold Typesetting Ltd, Gloucester

Contents

List of Contributors

L. BARBARA
Cattedra di Clinica Medica III dell' Università
Bologna
Italy

P. H. BENNETT
Epidemiology and Field Studies Branch
National Institute of Arthritis, Diabetes and Digestive and Kidney Diseases
1550 E. Indian School Road
Phoenix, AZ 85014
USA

M. C. CARRAHER
Southwestern Field Studies Section
National Institute of Arthritis, Diabetes and Digestive and Kidney Diseases
1550 E. Indian School Road
Phoenix, AZ 85014
USA

N. CARULLI
Instituto di Clinica Medica I
Policlinico, Via del Pozzo 71
41100 Modena
Italy

C. COVARRUBIAS
Department of Gastroenterology
Pontificia Universidad Católica de Chile
Casilla 114-D, Santiago
Chile

R. H. DOWLING
Gastroenterology Unit, Department of Medicine
Guy's Hospital and Medical School
London Bridge
London SE1 9RT
United Kingdom

G. D. FRIEDMAN
Department of Medical Methods Research
Kaiser-Permanente Medical Care Program
3451 Piedmont Avenue
Oakland, CA 94611
USA

G. GIUNCHI
III Department of Internal Medicine
University of Rome, "La Sapienza"
00161 Rome
Italy

S. M. GRUNDY
Centre for Human Nutrition
University of Texas Health Science Center at Dallas
5323 Harry Hines
Dallas 75235
USA

K. W. HEATON
Department of Medicine
University of Bristol
Bristol Royal Infirmary
Bristol BS2 8HW
United Kingdom

T. JØRGENSEN
Department of Surgical Gastroenterology
Herlev Hospital, University of Copenhagen
DK-2730 Herlev
Denmark

P. LORIA
Istituto di Clinica Medica I
Policlinico, Via del Pozzo 71
41100 Modena
Italy

R. LUGLI
Ospedale Estense
Viale Vittorio Veneto 9
41100 Modena
Italy

W. C. KNOWLER
Southwestern Field Studies Section
National Institute of Arthritis, Diabetes and Digestive and Kidney Diseases
1550 East Indian School Road
Phoenix, AZ 85014
USA

P. F. MALET
Gastrointestinal Section
University of Pennsylvania School of Medicine
Hospital of the University of Pennsylvania
3400 Spruce Street
Philadelphia, PA 19104
USA

D. MENOZZI
Istituto di Clinica Medica I
Policlinico, Via del Pozzo 71
41100 Modena
Italy

F. MONTIEL
Department of Internal Medicine
Pontificia Universidad Católica de Chile
Casilla 114-D, Santiago
Chile

F. NERVI
Department of Gastroenterology
Pontifica Universidad Católica de Chile
Casilla 114-D, Santiago
Chile

B. PAZ
Department of Gastroenterology
Pontifica Universidad Católica de Chile
Casilla 114-D, Santiago
Chile

D. B. PETITTI
Division of Family and Community Medicine
University of California at San Francisco
School of Medicine, AC-9
San Francisco, CA 94143
USA

D. J. PETTITT
Southwestern Field Studies Section
National Institute of Arthritis, Diabetes and Digestive and Kidney Diseases
1550 E. Indian School Road
Phoenix, AZ 85014
USA

J. M. PRADELLI
Ospedale Estense
Viale Vittorio Veneto 9
41100 Modena
Italy

D. F. RANSOHOFF
Department of Medicine
University Hospitals of Cleveland
Case Western Reserve University School of Medicine
2074 Abington Road
Cleveland, OH 44106
USA

E. RODA
Servizio di Gastroenterologia
Cattedra di Clinica Medica II dell' Università
Bologna
Italy

G. SALVIOLI
Insegnamento di Semeiotica Medica
Istituto di Clinica Medica
University of Modena
41100 Modena
Italy

R. D. SOLOWAY
Gastrointestinal Section
University of Pennsylvania School of Medicine
Hospital of the University of Pennsylvania
3400 Spruce Street
Philadelphia, PA 19104
USA

V. SPERANZA
VI Clinica Chirurgica
Policlinico Umberto I
Viale del Policlinico
00161 Rome
Italy

B. L. STROM
Clinical Epidemiology Unit
University of Pennsylvania
225L NEB/S2
Philadelphia, PA 19104
USA

C. N. WILLIAMS
Division of Gastroenterology
Department of Medicine
Dalhousie University
5849 University Avenue
Halifax, Nova Scotia
Canada B3H1 W2

Composition of the Rome Group for Epidemiology and Prevention of Cholelithiasis (GREPCO)

POLICY BOARD: L. Capocaccia[a] (1979–84), G. Giunchi[a] (1979–84), F. Pocchiari[d] (1979–84), G. Ricci[b] (1979–84)

STEERING COMMITTEE: F. Angelico[b] (1979–84), M. Angelico[a] (1979–84), A. F. Attili[c] (1979–84)

COORDINATION: A. Calvieri[b] (1979–84), P. Clemente[b] (1980–83), A. De Santis[a] (1983–84), L. Lalloni[b] (1979–84), G. Morisi[d] (1979–84), G. C. Urbinati[b] (1982–83)

CLINICAL STAFF: D. Alvaro[a] (1979–83), L. Antonaci[b] (1983–84), S. Cocca[b] (1981–84), M. Colzi[a] (1982–84), S. Ginanni Corradini[a] (1984), A. De Santis[a] (1979–84), P. Guccione[b] (1979–81), M. Marin[a] (1982–84), P. Monini[b] (1979–82), L. Massa[b] (1983–84), C. Stefanutti[b] (1982), E. Scafato[a] (1982-84)

ECHOGRAPHIC AND RADIOLOGIC STAFF: R. Conti[b] (1982–84), L. Lalloni[b] (1979–84), F. Mariucci (1980-81), D. Minasi (1984)

BIOCHEMICAL STAFF: D. Alvaro[a] (1984), M. Arca[b] (1980–84), A. Buongiorno[d] (1980–83), S. Ciocca[a] (1981–84), S. Fazio[a] (1983–84), A. Montali[b] (1980–84), G. Morisi[d] (1980–84), U. Pièche[b] (1980–84), A. Zucca[d] (1981–82)

BIOSTATISTICAL STAFF: Fa. Angelico (1980–82), A. Calvieri[b] (1979–83), R. Capocaccia[d] (1981–84), A. Menotti[d] (1981–84), R. Scipione[d] (1983–84)

EDITORIAL BOARD: F. Angelico[b] (1979–84), M. Angelico[a] (1979–84), M. Arca[b] (1984), A. F. Attili[c] (1979–84), L. Capocaccia[a] (1979–84), G. Ricci[b] (1979–84)

[a] Cattedra di Gastroenterologia II e Istituto di Clinica Medica Generale e Terapia Medica III, Università di Roma "La Sapienza", Rome
[b] Istituto di Terapia Medica Sistematica, Centro per la Lotta alle Malattie Metaboliche e all'Arteriosclerosi, Università di Roma "La Sapienza", Rome
[c] Cattedra di Fisiopatologia Digestiva, Università de l'Aquila, L'Aquila
[d] Istituto Superiore di Sanità, Laboratori di Tecnologie Biomediche e di Epidemiologia e Biostatistica, Rome

Part I
EPIDEMIOLOGY OF GALLSTONE DISEASE TODAY

Chairmen: W. P. CASTELLI and A. MENOTTI

1
Why talk about epidemiology of gallstone disease?

A. MENOTTI

The aims of epidemiological research conducted for scientific purposes are basically three: (1) the definition of the size of the problem (prevalence, incidence, mortality, fatality); (2) the search for 'causes', better called in epidemiology 'risk factors'; (3) the demonstration of the feasibility of primary prevention through preventive trials.

An epidemiological survey has a number of requirements among which are the identification of a specific question, the availability of a denominator representing a 'population', and the adoption of a strictly standardized methodology. The same type of approach and needs are to be considered when dealing with the epidemiology of gallstone disease, which has attracted so much interest during the last few years.

There are at least four good reasons for the rise in this spread of interest. First of all, many clinicians have opened their mind to epidemiology, and have recognized the need to look outside the walls of their clinical wards, outpatient clinics and laboratories, and to approach population studies with a view to answering precise questions, mainly concerning aetiology, natural history and prevention. Second, during the past 20 years comprehensive and standardized procedures have become available for the conducting of population field studies directed at the investigation of chronic non-communicable diseases. Although most of the work in this field has been developed for cardiovascular diseases it is relatively easy to transfer and adapt such procedures to the study of the other conditions. Then echography has appeared, showing its fundamental role in the diagnosis of gallstone disease. It is reported to provide a high sensitivity and specificity compared with traditional X-ray procedures, and some other fundamental prerequisites of tests being employed in epidemiology, i.e. safety, non-invasiveness and relatively simple performance.

Finally the possible interrelationship between gallstone disease and atherosclerosis is another source of interest. In fact some possible partially common metabolic channels, such as those involving lipid metabolism, are apparently involved in both conditions, favouring the merging of interest of those dealing with liver diseases and those dealing with cardiovascular diseases.

From this point of view it is worth recalling one of the early reports when the two conditions were connected. At the beginning of this century De Langen, a Dutch physician working in Indonesia, found the Javanese to be characterized by much lower levels of blood cholesterol than was the rule in the Netherlands, and he associated that difference with a substantial difference in the frequency of disorders which he believed were related to cholesterol metabolism, i.e. atherosclerosis, gallstones and phlebothrombosis[1]. Later he noted that Javanese stewards on Dutch passenger ships who ate Dutch food had similar blood cholesterol levels to Dutchmen, and he advocated a low-cholesterol diet (similar to the Javanese diet) for the prevention of atherosclerosis and gallstones.

The convergence of those elements mentioned above has stimulated several groups even in Italy, such as those in Bologna and Rome, to start important field operations for the epidemiological study of gallstone disease. A number of questions can be answered by such studies and some of them are listed below:

(1) What is the true prevalence of gallstone disease?
(2) What is the proportion of asymptomatic cases?
(3) Is there a different prevalence between sexes?
(4) Which individual characteristics are associated with the presence of the disease?
(5) Which is the metabolic profile associated with the presence of the disease?
(6) What is the incidence of the disease?
(7) Does the incidence differ between sexes?
(8) Which are the risk factors of the disease?
(9) Are there different risk factors for symptomatic vs. asymptomatic cases?
(10) Are risk factors different for the two sexes?
(11) What is the metabolic profile preceding the occurrence of the disease?
(12) Are there similarities or differences between the metabolic disorders preceding atherosclerosis and those preceding gallstone disease?
(13) What is the natural history of asymptomatic cases?
(14) Is there a procedure for preventing the disease?
(15) Is such a procedure, if any, feasible on a large scale?
(16) Is such a procedure compatible with the prevention of other chronic diseases involving lipid metabolism?

There are many theoretical bases indicating that the studies started in Italy and elsewhere can provide interesting results, as suggested by some of those already reported.

References

1. De Langen, C. D. (1933). Significance of geographic pathology in race problems in medicine. *Geneesk Tydschr. Nederl. Indie*, **73**, 1026

2
Findings on gallstone disease in the ISTAT* investigation

G. GIUNCHI

A sample survey on the health conditions of the Italian population was planned by the Central Institute of Statistics. Screening operations were performed between 10 and 15 November 1980 through a questionnaire interview in 75 397 subjects (i.e. 0.134 % of the Italian population) belonging to all Italian regions. Details of the protocol have been published elsewhere[1].

As far as concerns cholelithiasis, each subject was asked whether he was aware of having gallstones.

Prevalence of subjects aware of having gallstones and prospective evaluation of the total number of cases is shown in Table 1. Overall prevalence of cholelithiasis in the Italian population is 1.93 %. Prevalence increases with age, reaching a peak in the 60–69-year age group. The female/male ratio is higher during the women's fertile period. Prospective evaluation of the data acquired from the investigation reveals that the total number of subjects aware of having gallstones in Italy should be 1 087 000, of which 314 000 are males and 773 000 females. It has been reported, however, that awareness of having gallstones is present in only one-third to one-half of all gallstone subjects. It can thus be roughly calculated that the total number of gallstone subjects in Italy should be between 2 and 3 million people.

The distribution of already discovered gallstone disease in different Italian regions is shown in Table 2. Prevalence of the disease varies from 1.16 % in Sicily to 2.98 % in Marche. These regional differences could be explained, at least in part, by differences in hygienic and sanitary conditions and in diagnostic procedures in different areas. It should be remembered that great differences exist also in ethnic and environmental situations.

Prevalence of gallstone disease, with respect to civil status, increases from the unmarried to the married or 'other civil status' (widowed, separated or divorced) (Table 3). Sex and age standardization, performed by the indirect method, tends to lead to a uniform prevalence of the disease between the

*Istituto Centrale di Statistica, Rome

Table 1 Prevalence of gallstones in Italy according to age

Age (years)	*Total*		*Females*		*Males*		F/M Ratio
	n	*Percentage*	*n*	*Percentage*	*n*	*Percentage*	
13	4 000	0.04	1 000	0.02	3 000	0.05	0.4
14–29	27 000	0.21	16 000	0.25	11 000	0.17	1.47
30–39	118 000	1.55	94 000	2.44	24 000	0.64	3.8
40–49	222 000	2.92	158 000	4.05	64 000	1.73	2.34
50–59	298 000	4.00	202 000	5.30	96 000	2.64	2.0
60–70	251 000	4.45	172 000	5.72	79 000	2.99	1.91
71	167 000	4.02	130 000	5.29	37 000	2.18	2.42
Total	1 087 000	1.93	773 000	2.68	314 000	1.14	2.46

Table 2 Distribution of gallstone subjects in different Italian regions

Region	*Males*	*Females*	*Total*	*Prevalence (%)*
Piemonte/Valle Aosta	27 518	62 539	90 057	1.98
Lombardia	47 694	122 755	170 449	1.93
Trentino	3 068	13 077	16 145	1.87
Veneto	16 662	44 417	61 079	1.42
Friuli-Venezia Giulia	6 345	27 249	33 594	2.74
Liguria	15 697	25 590	41 287	2.28
Emilia-Romagna	25 840	72 640	98 480	2.51
Toscana	22 105	55 343	77 448	2.17
Umbria	5 072	12 623	17 695	2.21
Marche	13 679	28 200	41 879	2.98
Lazio	34 624	84 154	118 778	2.37
Abruzzi	10 273	18 297	28 570	2.32
Molise	1 994	3 637	5 631	1.69
Campania	22 575	57 561	80 136	1.47
Puglia	19 301	47 595	66 896	1.71
Basilicata	3 549	9 498	13 047	2.12
Calabria	7 838	31 501	39 339	1.90
Sicilia	23 665	34 318	57 983	1.16
Sardegna	6 583	22 254	28 837	1.81
Italy	314 082	773 248	1 087 330	1.93

Table 3 Cholelithiasis in Italy, prevalence according to civil status

	Civil status			
	Unmarried	*Married*	*Other civil status*	*Total*
Number of cases	72 000	819 000	193 000	1 084 000
Prevalence (%)	0.58	2.84	4.71	2.39
Age and sex standardized prevalence (%)	1.53	2.49	2.48	2.39

married subjects and those with 'other civil status', while the low prevalence in the unmarried group could be partly explained by a possible lower number of pregnancies in females belonging to this group.

Prevalence of gallstones with respect to educational status is reported in Table 4. Prevalence of gallstones is higher in subjects with low level of education (primary school) than in those who reached the secondary or high school level. Age and sex standardization do not greatly modify this trend, which could again be explained by a higher number of pregnancies in females with a low level of education.

In conclusion, although this study recorded only already diagnosed cases of gallstone disease, it shows that the total number of gallstone subjects in Italy should be 1 087 000. Taking into account also the undiscovered cases, prospective evaluation shows figures between 2 and 3 million Italians. A higher prevalence exists in females than in males, especially during the women's fertile period. The observed differences between the different Italian areas suggest that more objective epidemiological studies should be undertaken in different Italian regions.

Table 4 Cholelithiasis in Italy, prevalence according to educational degree

	Educational degree			
	Primary school	*Secondary school*	*High school*	*Total*
Number of cases	873 000	126 000	83 000	1 082 000
Prevalance (%)	3.39	1.03	1.12	2.39
Age and sex standardized prevalence (%)	2.35	1.99	1.69	2.39

Reference

1. Instituto Centrale di Statistica. (1982). Una indagine campionaria sulle condizioni della salute della popolazione e sul ricorso ai servizi sanitari. *Bollettino dell'Istituto Centrale di Statistica,* Suppl. 12

3
The GREPCO research programmes: aims and prevalence data

G. RICCI and the GREPCO Group*

The epidemiological approach to aetiopathogenetic problems, i.e. the study of pathological phenomena in population groups, proved to be extremely fruitful for some diseases. A classical example is coronary heart disease.

As far as gallstone disease is concerned, a careful examination of the literature reveals the rather modest size of the epidemiological approach, at least in those studies designed primarily for this disease. The main reason lies in the fact that a simple and ethically acceptable diagnostic technique applicable to large population samples has not been available so far.

Today, the advent of ultrasonography, which represents a non-invasive diagnostic tool applicable on a large scale, permits a new approach to the epidemiological study of gallstone disease.

On the basis of these considerations, and taking into account the knowledge which may accrue to research in a field of wide social concern such as biliary diseases, the Rome Group for Epidemiology and Prevention of Cholelithiasis (GREPCO) was created in 1980, through the cooperation of the Institute of Systematic Medical Therapy Centre for Metabolic Diseases and Atherosclerosis of the University of Rome 'La Sapienza', the 3rd Institute of Internal Medicine – 2nd Chair of Gastroenterology of the University of Rome 'La Sapienza', and the National Health Institute.

From the start of its activities GREPCO was faced with several open questions: the size of the problem or, in other words, the real prevalence of the disease; its natural history – particularly of silent gallstones – and the three subsequent lines of approach: wait-and-see policy, active medical treatment, or prophylactic cholecystectomy; the identification of risk factors for preventive purposes.

The aims of the Research Group are to establish the prevalence of gallstone disease in different population samples and identify its associated factors; to study its incidence and natural history; to identify risk factors; to design and

* For the composition of the Group see p. xi

carry out primary and secondary prevention programmes; and to organize meetings, workshops and seminars to increase the present knowledge in this field.

The first of such programmes started in 1980, and was aimed at establishing the prevalence of gallstone disease in a sample of female civil servants (1439), aged 20–64 years at entry into the trial. The approach of the study was to assess the prevalence of symptomatic and asymptomatic gallstone disease in Roman women, to ascertain whether they were aware of their condition, and to identify the factors associated with the disease[1–3].

The sample consisted of the entire female working population of a Government Department; the overall participation (75.1 %) can be considered satisfactory; in older age groups, age distribution was similar to that of the general population; the women were invited to participate in a prevention programme not specifically devoted to gallstone disease. The concurrence of these four elements confirms the validity of our sample. It must be added that gallstone disease represents a morbid condition unknown to the majority of its carriers.

The screening procedures included administration of a questionnaire, a clinical examination, the ultrasound examination of the biliary tract, and the collection of a blood sample.

The questionnaire concerned family and personal history, with particular reference to physical activity, dietary habits, slimming diets, tobacco and alcohol consumption, drug consumption, and abdominal symptoms. The physical examination included weight and height, abdomen, and measurement of arterial blood pressure according to the procedures of the London School of Hygiene. Laboratory examinations included determination of fasting blood glucose levels, total and HDL-cholesterol, triglycerides, total and HDL-phospholipids, total serum bile acids (RIA), SGPT, and erythrocyte fatty acids (gas–liquid chromatography). Linear array ALOKA equipment, with a 3 MHz probe, was used for real-time ultrasonography. A standard oral cholecystography was performed when the ultrasound examination was 'inconclusive' – i.e. in case of unclear or non-visualized gallbladder, and in the presence of meteorism or doubtful images – in all echographies positive for gallstones, and in a negative random sample.

Gallstone disease was diagnosed under the following conditions: (1) presence of gallstones at echography and cholecystography; (2) presence of gallstones at echography, but non-visualization of the gallbladder after a double dose of contrast medium at cholecystography; (3) presence of gallstones at oral cholecystography; (4) previous cholecystectomy.

More details on screening procedures, laboratory techniques, and diagnostic criteria are reported elsewhere (see Chapters 12, 16, 20, 23, 24 in this volume).

Table 1 shows the number of women invited, examined, and with a conclusive gallbladder examination, divided into age groups. Altogether, 1081 women had conclusive gallbladder examination. Prevalence data have been analysed on the basis of this final figure.

Prevalence of gallstone disease (presence of gallstones and/or history of cholecystectomy) increases with age from 2.5 % in the 20–29-year-old age

Table 1 Number of women invited, examined, and with conclusive gallbladder examination (figures in parentheses refer to percentage of subjects invited)

Age	*Age (years)*					
	20–29	*30–39*	*40–49*	*50–59*	*60–64*	*20–64*
Subjects invited	204	584	408	198	45	1439
Subjects examined	160 (78.4)	406 (69.5)	314 (76.9)	172 (86.9)	40 (88.8)	1092 (75.9)
Subjects with conclusive gallbladder examination	158 (77.4)	404 (69.1)	311 (76.2)	168 (84.8)	40 (88.8)	1082 (75.1)

group to 25.0 % in the 60–69-year-old age group (Fig. 1). Figure 2 shows the regression curve gallbladder disease/age (gallbladder disease meaning presence of gallstones), using the age coefficient of a multiple logistic function taking into account 19 variables (see Chapter 29, this volume).

How many of the subjects are unaware of having gallstones, as compared to those aware of their condition? How deep does the iceberg 'cholelithiasis' go? In our study, the prevalence of women with gallstone disease was 9.4 %: 35 % had been cholecystectomized, 22 % had gallstones and were aware of their condition, 43 % had gallstones but did not know it. Therefore, about two-thirds of women were unaware of the presence of gallstones.

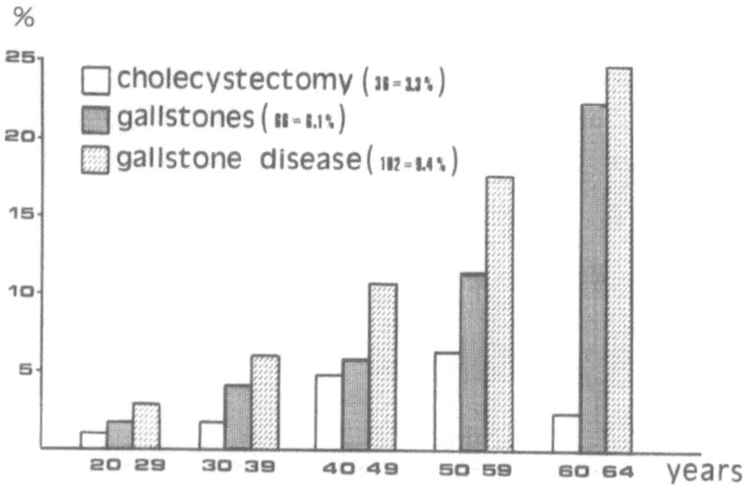

Figure 1 Prevalence of gallstone disease (gallstones + cholecystectomy) in the female population examined by GREPCO, divided by age groups

The second study performed by GREPCO was carried out on two groups of male civil servants aged 49–68 years, who had already participated as control and treatment groups ($n = 358$ and 367 respectively) in the Rome Project of Coronary Heart Disease Prevention (PPCC), a 6-year controlled trial of primary prevention of ischaemic heart disease[4–6]. Men were screened by ultrasounds 3 years after completion of this preventive trial (age at entry: 40–59 years). It must be borne in mind that our investigation on male subjects was aimed at establishing the possible lithogenic effects of both lipid-lowering diets and drugs (see Chapter 25), this volume). Details on the structure and results of PPCC, as well as the preliminary results on the prevalence of gallstone disease in both groups, are reported in Chapter 25 of this volume.

So far, we have also examined, in the site of the treatment group, a sample of 412 male subjects who had not been enrolled in the initial group, due to their younger age or for other reasons. It seemed to us incorrect to obtain prevalence data by grouping together all untreated individuals (358 + 412).

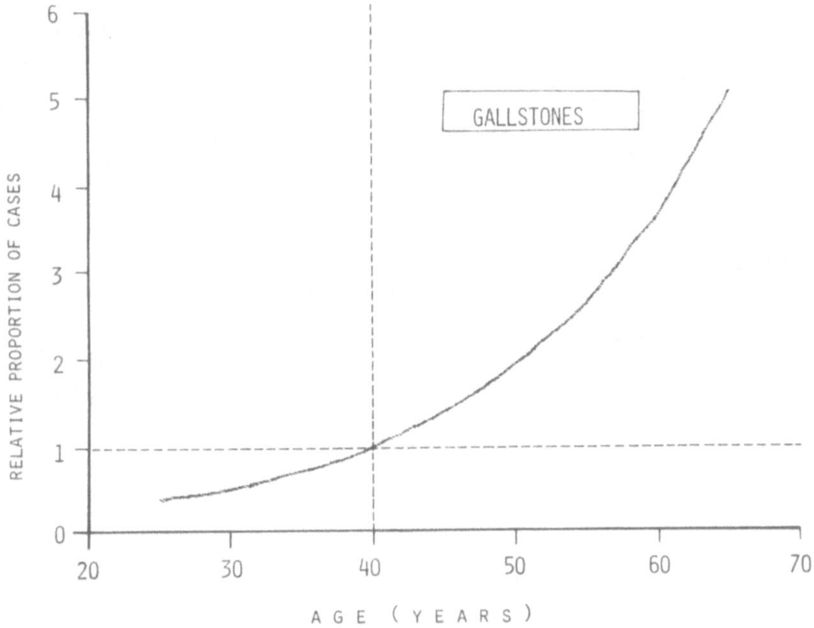

Figure 2 Regression curve gallbladder disease/age (age coefficient of a multiple logistic function) in women with conclusive gallbladder examination

A fairly reliable comparison, limited to three 5-year age groups, is reported in Table 2, which shows the prevalence of gallstone disease (gallstones + cholecystectomy) in the Roman female population, compared to the findings in the male control group enrolled in PPCC. It is evident from this very preliminary table that the prevalence of gallstone disease in the Rome population is rather high in men also, at least in these age groups.

On the basis of our prevalence data, and a women/men ratio of about 1.5, the percentage incidence/year of gallstone disease in our Rome population can be estimated at 0.4 in men and 0.6 in women.

Table 2 Prevalence of gallstone disease (gallstones + cholecystectomy) in male and female civil servants, divided into three 5-year age groups

Age	*Men*		*Women*	
	n	%	*n*	%
49–53	63	7.9	91	14.3
54–58	74	16.2	81	18.5
59–63	141	12.8	48	22.9

References

1. Rome Group for Epidemiology and Prevention of Cholelithiasis (GREPCO) (1982). Prevalenza della colelitiasi: osservazioni preliminari su un campione di popolazione lavorativa femminile. *Epatologia*, **28**, 79–88
2. Rome Group for Epidemiology and Prevention of Cholelithiasis (GREPCO) (1981). Epidemiological study on the prevalence of gallbladder disease: design of the study and preliminary results. *It. J. Gastroenterol.*, **13**, 261 (abstract)
3. Rome Group for Epidemiology and Prevention of Cholelithiasis (GREPCO) (1984). Prevalence of gallstone disease in an Italian adult female population. *Am. J. Epidemiol.*, **119**, 5
4. Research Group of the Rome Project of Coronary Heart Disease Prevention (PPCC) (1976). The Rome Project of Coronary Heart Disease Prevention. *Ann. Ist. Sup. Sanità*, **12**, 316–330
5. The Research Group of the Rome Project of Coronary Heart Disease Prevention (PPCC) (1983). An Italian Preventive Trial of Coronary Heart Disease: The Rome Project of Coronary Heart Disease Prevention. *Proc. Biochem. Pharmacol.*, **19**, 230
6. Gruppo di Ricerca del Progetto Romano di Prevenzione della Cardiopatia Coronarica (1982). Il Progetto Romano di Prevenzione della Cardiopatia Coronarica. Risultati finali. *G. Ital. Cardiol.*, **12**, 541–554

4
Epidemiology of cholelithiasis in the Pima Indians

W. C. KNOWLER, M. J. CARRAHER, D. J. PETTITT and P. H. BENNETT

The Pima Indians of Arizona, USA have participated with the National Institutes of Health in studies of the epidemiology and physiology of several chronic diseases since 1965. Cholelithiasis, diabetes mellitus, and some types of arthritis and eye diseases are extremely common in this population. Gallstones, affecting about 75 % of adult women and 45 % of adult men, are the subject of this paper.

PREVALENCE OF GALLSTONE DISEASE

In the late 1960s a study was undertaken to determine the prevalence of gallbladder disease[1]. A random sample of 50 subjects in each sex, and in each of the decades of age from 15 to 74 years, was selected, and the prevalence of clinically diagnosed gallbladder disease was assessed through a review of medical records. Clinical diagnoses were accepted if the record showed evidence of gallstones by surgery or cholecystography (either by showing stones or by non-visualization of the gallbladder).

The prevalence of symptomatic, or clinically diagnosed, gallbladder disease is shown in Table 1. The Pima findings are compared with the prevalence of gallbladder disease in Framingham, Massachusetts, also estimated from a review of medical records[2]. The Pima rates were much higher, especially in the women.

After the initial ascertainment of clinically diagnosed cases, further cases were detected by performing oral cholecystograms on those without a clinical diagnosis of gallstones[3]. Autopsies of a few subjects who died during the study period supplemented the number of diagnoses. Table 2 shows age–sex-specific prevalence rates of cholelithiasis by previous clinical diagnoses and the total prevalence including cases diagnosed by cholecystography or autopsy. Only about one-third of the cases in men, and half in women, were diagnosed clinically. In the women the prevalence was very high by age 35 years, and it

Table 1 Prevalence of clinically diagnosed gallbladder disease in Pima Indians and in Framingham, Massachusetts (from Ref. 1)

		Pima Indians		*Framingham*	
Sex	*Age (years)*	*No. subjects*	*Prevalence (%)*	*No. subjects*	*Prevalence (%)*
Male	30–39	51	2.0	832	0.1
	40–49	45	2.2	779	0.9
	50–62	57	12.3	725	3.2
Females	30–39	45	35.6	1037	2.3
	40–49	51	39.2	963	6.0
	50–62	62	33.8	873	10.1

Table 2 Prevalence of gallbladder disease in Pima Indians: clinical diagnoses alone and clinical plus cholecystographic diagnoses (from Ref. 3)

Sex	*Age (years)*	*Previous clinical diagnoses (%)*	*Total prevalence (%)*
Male	15–24	0	0
	25–34	4	4
	35–44	0	11
	45–54	4	32
	55–64	19	66
	65–74	9	68
Females	15–24	2	13
	25–34	26	73
	35–44	42	71
	45–54	43	76
	55–64	24	62
	65–74	40	89

varied little above that age. In this study the prevalence of gallstones, as diagnosed clinically or by oral cholecystography, was not associated with obesity, serum cholesterol, diabetes, or parity.

A longitudinal study of chronic diseases in the community has continued to the present[4]. The study includes the systematic review of medical records for diagnosed gallstones, but further cholecystographic surveys have not been performed. The following results apply to clinical diagnoses based on X-ray or surgical evidence of gallstones in subjects of at least half Pima ancestry. Clinical disease appears to be even more frequent now than in the late 1960s. Table 3 shows the age–sex-specific prevalence of diagnosed gallstone disease in those subjects whose records were reviewed between 1965 and 1970, on the left, and those whose records were reviewed between 1978 and 1983, on the right. Diagnosed disease was more common in the more recent period, especially at the older ages. The prevalence rates were statistically significantly higher in the more recent period ($p < 0.001$, controlling for age and sex by the method of Mantel and Haenszel[5]). Because these data are based on reviews of medical records rather than direct examination of the gallbladder, we do not know whether there has been a true increase in the prevalence of gallstones or only an increase in the proportion of cases which are diagnosed

Table 3 Increasing prevalence of clinically diagnosed gallstone disease in Pima Indians

		1965–70		*1978–83*	
Sex	*Age (years)*	*No. subjects*	*Prevalence (%)*	*No. subjects*	*Prevalence (%)*
Male	5–14	570	0.0	435	0.0
	15–24	351	0.3	398	0.3
	25–34	170	1.2	200	1.0
	35–44	152	4.6	127	7.1
	45–54	113	9.7	98	9.2
	55–64	99	10.1	65	20.0
	65–74	96	12.5	45	33.3
	≥75	53	5.7	23	34.8
Females	5–14	597	0.0	426	0.2
	15–24	417	3.1	536	5.2
	25–34	203	20.2	331	18.1
	35–44	206	33.5	186	40.3
	45–54	126	28.6	186	50.5
	55–64	98	36.7	119	52.1
	65–74	89	41.6	60	60.0
	≥75	28	14.3	29	51.7

and documented in the medical record. A systematic survey by cholecystography or ultrasound will be needed to explain this increase.

PREGNANCY AND GALLSTONE DISEASE

The most recent data from each subject's medical record have been examined for relationships with clinically diagnosed gallstones. Among Pima women, diagnosed gallstones are significantly related to gravidity (number of previous pregnancies according to the history given by the woman). Table 4 shows that age-specific disease prevalence increased with gravidity. Even women who had never been pregnant had higher prevalence rates than men, so pregnancy cannot entirely account for the increased prevalence in women. Although parity was not related to disease prevalence in the earlier cholecystographic study[3], the relationship is now apparent with clinically diagnosed disease, in agreement with several other studies[2,6–8]. It must be emphasized again that these are prevalence rates of diagnosed disease only. Thus we do not know if the true prevalence of gallstones is related to the number of pregnancies, or whether pregnancy makes existing gallstones more symptomatic and more likely to be diagnosed.

Associations of cholelithiasis with diabetes mellitus and obesity are discussed elsewhere in this volume (Chapter 13).

GENETIC BASIS OF GALLSTONE DISEASE

Because gallstone disease is so common in this population a genetic basis must be suspected. If so, a relationship with the amount of Indian heritage should be seen. The Indian community contains some people of only partial Indian

Table 4 Prevalence of clinically diagnosed gallbladder disease in Pima Indian women by gravidity

	Number of previous pregnancies					
	0		*1–4*		*≥5*	
Age (years)	*No. subjects*	*Prevalence (%)*	*No. subjects*	*Prevalence (%)*	*No. subjects*	*Prevalence (1 %)*
5–14	600	0.2	2	0	0	—
15–24	409	2	351	7	4	25
25–34	69	12	303	17	85	26
35–44	29	21	110	39	136	44
45–54	15	53	64	47	167	50
55–64	12	17	51	43	110	54
65–74	11	27	48	52	87	64
≥75	6	50	18	44	41	39

heritage, the remaining heritage being mostly Caucasian. The prevalence of diagnosed gallstones in community residents at least 35 years old varied directly with the fraction of Indian heritage, being most common in women who were at least half Indian (Table 5). No gallstone disease was diagnosed in the 41 men of less than 6/8 Indian heritage.

Despite this suggestion of inheritance of the disease, familial aggregation has not been demonstrated. Familial aggregation was studied in 316 Pima women aged 35 to 84 years who belonged to 144 sibships[9]. They represented 116 families with two sisters in this age range and 28 families with three. Table 6 shows the numbers of families having 0, 1, and 2 sisters with gallstones among families with two sisters (on the left), and 0, 1, 2, and 3 affected sisters in families of three (on the right). The observed frequency distribution was very close to expectation under a random distribution of the disease in the population (test for departure from a random distribution, $\chi^2 = 3.92$, d.f. $= 5$, $p = 0.6$). However, the distribution was incompatible with a simple dominant or recessive mode of inheritance. Thus if clinically diagnosed cholelithiasis is an inherited disease in the Pimas, most Pimas may have the necessary gene or genes, with major factors distinguishing Pimas with and without the disease being non-familial.

BILIARY CANCER AND MORTALITY

It has been about 15 years since the cholecystography survey described above. What has happened to these subjects with and without gallstones discovered

Table 5 Prevalence of clinically diagnosed gallbladder disease by degree of Indian heritage in residents of the Pima community, ages ≥ 35 years

Sex	*Eighths Indian heritage*	*No. subjects*	*Prevalence (%)*
Male	0	18	0
	1–3	5	0
	4–5	18	0
	6–7	18	6
	8	902	13
Female	0	7	0
	1–3	13	31
	4–5	23	43
	6–7	40	35
	8	1035	45

Table 6 Distribution of numbers of sisters with gallstones in families with two or three sisters 35–84 years old; expected numbers were derived under the assumption of a random distribution of the disease in the population (from Ref. 9)

	Families with 2 sisters				*Families with 3 sisters*				
No. affected	*0*	*1*	*2*	*Sum*	*0*	*1*	*2*	*3*	*Sum*
Observed	35	57	24	115	6	11	6	5	28
Expected	34.8	57.5	23.8	116	4.6	11.4	9.4	2.6	28

in the survey? Although the follow-up study is not yet complete, preliminary findings suggest an increased incidence of biliary cancer in those who had gallstones. In the 1968 survey 307 Pima subjects had oral cholecystograms, of which 116 were abnormal (43 with stones and 73 with non-visualization). Medical records of 294 of the subjects were reviewed in 1983. Three cases of biliary carcinoma (ICD 8/9 codes 156.1, 156.1, and 156.9) were found in 107 people with abnormal cholecystograms, and none were found in 160 with normal nor in 27 with uncertain cholecystographic findings. These findings are consistent with the hypothesis that gallstones increase the risk of biliary cancer[10], but with this small number of cases a statistically significant difference in cancer incidence between those with and without gallstones cannot be demonstrated.

Although the number of cases of biliary cancer was small, mortality from all causes was about 68 % higher in those with abnormal than in those with normal cholecystograms. Age-adjusted 15-year cumulative mortality rates are shown for those with normal and abnormal X-rays in Table 7. The difference was statistically significant after adjusting[5] for differences in age and sex of the two groups ($p<0.01$). We have not yet determined causes of death or contributions of cholecystectomy or other factors to this mortality difference, important questions for further investigation.

Table 7 Fifteen-year mortality in Pima Indians, age-adjusted to the US White Census, 1970, ages 35–74 (percentage)

Cholecystogram	*Males*	*Females*	*Total*
Normal	34	30	32
Abnormal*	54	53	54

*Abnormal includes readings of gallstones or non-visualization.

NATURAL HISTORY OF GALLSTONE DISEASE

In a search for early physiological abnormalities leading to gallstone disease, studies of biliary secretion have also been performed in the Pima Indians[11-14]. These studies are not discussed here in detail, as the metabolic basis of gallstone production is well covered by other papers in this volume. It has been shown, however, that the bile of many Pima Indians, especially females, becomes lithogenic, or saturated with cholesterol, during adolescence. Figure 1 summarizes some of the epidemiological and physiological studies in Pima girls and women[14]. The prevalence of lithogenic bile, of gallstones diagnosed clinically or by survey X-ray, and of non-visualization of the gallbladder at the survey X-ray – probably a sign of more advanced gallbladder disease – are shown by age. Although these curves represent different cross-sectional studies, the figure suggests a chronology of gallstone formation. Pima women develop lithogenic bile during puberty. About 8 years later X-ray-detectable gallstones develop, and still later the gallbladder becomes non-functional. Finally, those with gallstones have higher mortality rates than those without. Thus efforts to prevent gallstone disease and associated morbidity and

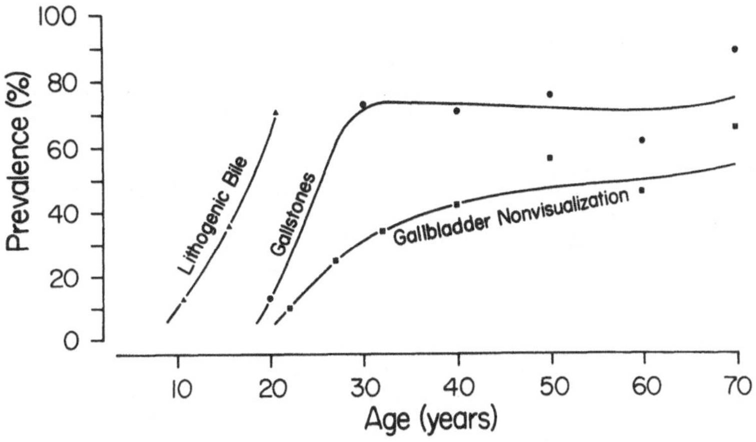

Figure 1 Natural history of cholesterol-saturated bile in Pima women. The age-specific prevalence of bile exceeding the limits of metastable supersaturation with cholesterol is superimposed on cholecystographic data on gallstone prevalence in the same population. Bile first becomes highly saturated during pubertal development. The onset of gallstones occurs during early adulthood. (Used with permission – Ref. 14)

mortality, at least in the Pima Indians, may need to begin in adolescence, when abnormalities of the biliary system are first evident.

Acknowledgments

We thank the members of the Gila River Indian Community for their participation in these studies; the staff of the National Institute of Arthritis, Diabetes, and Digestive and Kidney Diseases in Arizona for conducting the Pima Indian studies; and E. Begay for secretarial assistance.

References

1. Comess, L. J., Bennett, P. H. and Burch, T. A. (1967). Clinical gallbladder disease in Pima Indians: its high prevalence in contrast to Framingham, Massachusetts. *N. Engl. J. Med.*, **277**, 894–898
2. Friedman, G. D., Kannel, W. B. and Dawber, T. R. (1966). The epidemiology of gallbladder disease: observations in the Framingham study. *J. Chron. Dis.*, **19**, 273–292.
3. Sampliner, R. E., Bennett, P. H., Comess, L. J., Rose, F. A., and Burch, T. A. (1970). Gallbladder disease in Pima Indians: demonstration of high prevalence and early onset by cholecystography. *N. Engl. J. Med.*, **283**, 1358–1364
4. Knowler, W. C., Bennett, P. H., Hamman, R. F. and Miller, M. (1978). Diabetes incidence and prevalence in Pima Indians: a 19-fold greater incidence than in Rochester, Minnesota. *Am. J. Epidemiol.*, **108**, 497–505
5. Mantel, N. and Haenszel, W. (1959). Statistical aspects of the analysis of data from retrospective studies of disease. *J. Natl. Cancer Inst.*, **22**, 719–748
6. Thistle, J. L., Eckhart, K. L., Jr., Nensel, R. E., Nobrega, F. T., Poehling, G. G., Reimer, M. and Schoenfield, L. J. (1971). Prevalence of gallbladder disease among Chippewa Indians. *Mayo Clin. Proc.*, **46**, 603–608
7. Williams, C. N., Johnston, J. L. and Weldon, K. L. M. (1977). Prevalence of gallstones and gallbladder disease in Canadian Micmac Indian women. *Can. Med. Assoc. J.*, **117**, 758–760

8. Honoré, L. H. (1980). Cholesterol cholelithiasis in adolescent females: its connection with obesity, parity, and oral contraceptive use – a retrospective study of 31 cases. *Arch. Surg.*, **115**, 62–64.
9. Bennion, L. J. and Knowler, W. C. (1980). Epidemiology of gallstones. In Rotter, J. I., Samloff, I. M. and Rimoin, D. L. (eds.) *Genetics and Heterogeneity of Common Gastrointestinal Disorders*. pp. 297–312. (New York: Academic Press)
10. Way, L. W. and Sleisenger, M. H. (1978). Neoplasms of the gallbladder and bile ducts. In Sleisenger, M. H. and Fordtran, J. S. (eds.) *Gastrointestinal Disease: Pathophysiology, Diagnosis, Management*. pp. 1327–1333. (Philadelphia: W. B. Saunders)
11. Adler, R. D., Metzger, A. L. and Grundy, S. M. (1974). Biliary lipid secretion before and after cholecystectomy in American Indians with cholesterol gallstones. *Gastroenterology*, **66**, 1212–1217
12. Bennion, L. J. and Grundy, S. M. (1975). Effects of obesity and caloric intake on biliary lipid metabolism in man. *J. Clin. Invest.*, **56**, 996–1011
13. Bennion, L. J., Drobny, E., Knowler, W. C., Ginsberg, R. L., Garnick, M. B., Adler, R. D. and Duane, W. C. (1978). Sex differences in the size of bile acid pools. *Metabolism*, **27**, 961–969
14. Bennion, L. J., Knowler, W. C., Mott, D. M., Spagnola, A. M. and Bennett, P. H. (1979). Development of lithogenic bile during puberty in Pima Indians. *N. Engl. J. Med.*, **300**, 873–876

5
Epidemiology of gallstone disease: The 'Sirmione Study'

L. BARBARA for the 'Progetto Sirmione'*

There is convincing evidence in the literature indicating that gallstone disease has become one of the commoner diseases, at least in the Western world. In fact, reports from the USA indicate that about 15 million people have stones in the gallbladder[1]. Unfortunately there is little statistical evidence to support this impression and none in Italy. This is due to the type of epidemiological studies that have been performed so far. These studies are, in fact, mainly based on autoptic findings or surgical records, and do not give a real definition of the prevalence of the disease.

Gallstone disease can be ignored for years, or for ever, because the percentage of symptomatic patients is very low[2]. For this reason only studies based on large population samples can be considered a correct epidemiological approach[3]. We therefore decided to perform a cohort study on the incidence and risk factors of gallstone disease in the town of Sirmione. We will report on the first step of the study concerning the prevalence of the disease.

ABOUT THE TOWN

The town of Sirmione lies on a small peninsula on the southern side of the Garda lake. For its particular geographical location Sirmione has been a well-known tourist area since the times of the Roman poet Catullo. In the surrounding of the town there is also flourishing agriculture (mainly vineyards). The main activity of the population living in the four quarters of Sirmione is therefore, related to tourism (hotels, shops, restaurants) or to agriculture.

Progetto Sirmione:
D. Festi, A. M. Morselli Labate, E. Roda, A. G. Rusticali, C. Sama, C. Sapio, F. Taroni (Clinica Medica III – Università di Bologna).

C. Banterle, S. Colasanti, G. Formentini, F. Nardin, G. Panzolato, A. Puci (Divisione di Medicina Generale – Ospedale di Desenzano).

MATERIALS AND METHODS

The total population of Sirmione amounts to 4520 inhabitants, living in four main quarters: Center, Lugana, Rovizza and Colombare. Out of them a target population of 2732 subjects, aged 18–65 years, was selected. A standard letter, summarizing the purpose of the study and inviting selected subjects for examination on a fixed day was sent. The study protocol included:

(1) an ultrasonographic examination of the upper abdomen;
(2) a questionnaire including demographic and social data, medical and family history and dietary habits;
(3) measures of height, weight and blood pressure;
(4) blood tests for glucose, urea nitrogen, total and HDL cholesterol, triglycerides, GOT, GPT and GGT.

Out of the selected population, 1930 subjects (70.6 %) attended the study. A personal letter was first sent to non-attenders (40 %), and then a telephone call to those who did not come after the second invitation.

Of the 1930 subjects participating in the study 883 were men and 1047 were women. No significant differences in the attendance to the study was found between men and women and age groups, although there was a slight over-representation of women and older age groups in the studied population (Table 1).

Table 1 Percentages of attendance in the study, by sex and age

Age (years)	*Males*	*Females*	*Total*
18–29	56.3	64.0	60.4
30–39	68.6	71.6	70.1
40–49	73.6	79.5	76.6
50–65	75.0	76.6	75.9
Total	68.2	72.9	70.6

'Cases' were defined as subjects who had gallstones at the time of the study revealed by ultrasonography, and those who had undergone previous cholecystectomy (as assessed by positive history and absence of gallbladder at ultrasonography and presence of post-surgery scar). The prevalence of gallstone disease in population accounted for 11 %; 132 subjects (6.9 %) had gallstones at the time of the study, while 78 (4.1 %) were cholecystectomized. The prevalence of disease in females (14.6 %) was double that in males (6.7 %). This trend was maintained both in subjects who had gallstone disease (cholelithiasis plus cholecystectomy) and in subjects who had actually cholelithiasis. According to previous results[3] we also found that the frequency of gallstone disease increases significantly with age (Table 2), being relatively infrequent in the younger population (18–29 years).

When examining our group of 132 subjects who had cholelithiasis, we found that only 24 (18%) already knew that they had gallstones, while 108 (82 %) were unaware of the disease. The questionnaire has inquired on the symptoms the attenders had experienced. We defined 'specific biliary

Table 2 Prevalence of gallstone disease by sex and age (percentages)

Age (years)	*Males*	*Females*	*Total*
18–29	1.1	2.9	2.1
30–39	4.4	9.5	7.0
40–49	9.2	16.1	12.9
50–59	11.0	27.0	19.8
Total	6.7	14.6	11.0

symptoms' as biliary pain or colic (pain in the right upper quadrant with or without nausea and vomiting, which lasted for more than $\frac{1}{2}$ h). Other symptoms that have been related in the past to cholelithiasis[4], such as nausea, vomiting, belching, abdominal discomfort and constipation, have been defined as non-specific biliary symptoms. In our studied population 70 subjects (3.8 %) stated they suffered from specific biliary symptoms. Of those 29 had gallstones, while 103 (78 %) gallstone subjects denied biliary symptoms.

CONCLUSIONS

The purpose of our study was to obtain a better understanding of the epidemiology of gallstone disease. We have so far completed only the first part of the project, dealing with the prevalence of the disease in a sample population living in the north of Italy. Our results have confirmed some of the findings coming from previous studies. In 5 years, when data on the incidence of the disease will be available, we will hopefully be able to have a better understanding of the natural history of this disease.

References

1. Ingelfinger, F. J. (1968). Digestive disease as a national problem. *Gastroenterology*, **55**, 102–104
2. Gracie, W. A. and Ransohoff, D. F. (1982). The natural history of silent gallstones. *N. Engl. J. Med.*, **307**, 798–800
3. Friedman, G. D., Kannel, W. B. and Dawber, T. R. (1966). The epidemiology of gallbladder disease: observations in the Framingham study. *J. Chron. Dis.*, **19**, 273–292
4. Price, W. H. (1963). Gall-bladder dyspepsia. *Br. Med. J.*, **2**, 138–141

6
Epidemiology of gallstone disease in Chile

C. COVARRUBIAS, V. VALDIVIESO AND F. NERVI

Knowledge of the prevalence of gallstones in Chile is derived from several autopsy studies[1–3]. In one of them, of 4355 autopsies performed from 1960 to 1969, the prevalence of gallbladder disease (cholelithiasis and cholecystectomies) was 20 % in men and 50 % in women[1]. Chemical analysis of 138 cases with gallstones demonstrated that 84 % of them had a cholesterol content higher than 50 % of their dry weight. This study demonstrated that the frequency of gallstones increased with age in both sexes, and that they were significantly associated with obesity and gallbladder cancer.

When age-adjusted gallstone prevalences are compared between different countries, it is apparent that the prevalence in Chilean women is almost double that found in Czechoslovakia, Sweden, England and West Germany[4]. On the basis of data provided by Marinović's autopsy study[1], it can be estimated that there are a total of 1.7 million subjects with gallstones from a total population of 12 million Chileans.

The impact of gallstone disease in the Chilean health system is reflected by the 40 000 cholecystectomies performed each year. Approximately 33 % of the total annual surgical procedures correspond to cholecystectomies. Although the surgical morbity and mortality rates for gallstones disease are similar in Chile compared to figures from Europe and the United States[5], the overall mortality rate of gallstone disease[6] is 6.2 per 100 000, one of the highest in the world, as shown in Fig. 1.

With the aim of obtaining a better knowledge of the epidemiology of gallstone disease in Chile, we performed a prospective study in a living population from a suburban area of Santiago. We wanted to know the prevalence of gallstones assessed by cholecystography, and to have the chance to follow up these subjects. In this manner we would be able to know the incidence of the disease and some characteristics of the natural history of gallstone disease in Chile.

PREVALENCE OF GALLSTONES IN AN ACTIVE POPULATION

This study was initiated in 1972, selecting randomly 250 homes in the

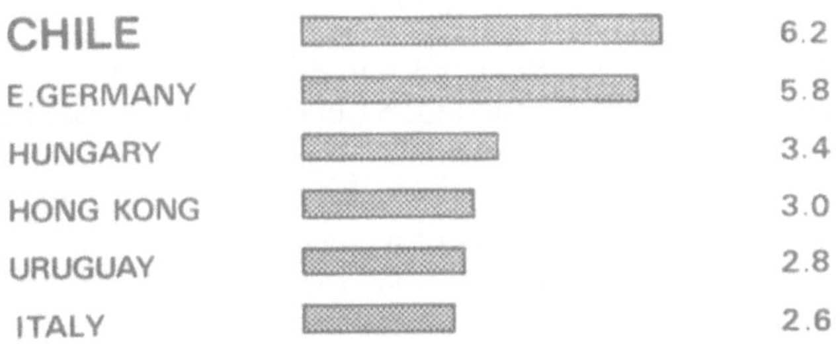

Figure 1 Mortality rates (per 100 000) of gallbladder disease in different countries, age-adjusted (from Ref. 6)

suburb of San Gregorio, Santiago. Their inhabitants were informed of the nature of the project and volunteered to participate. A total of 625 subjects were studied with oral cholecystograms over a period of 4 years, using iopanoic acid as contrast medium; 433 of them were under 30 years of age; in this young group, 46 % were men. On the other hand, only 37 % of the 192 subjects older than 30 years were men, reflecting our difficulties in recruiting adult male volunteers because of their reluctance to lose work.

We considered as gallstone disease the cases with a functioning gallbladder harbouring stones, those with double radiological exclusion and those that had been cholecystectomized. The results are shown in Fig. 2: 51 % of the women and 17 % of the men over 20 years of age had gallstones. These figures are similar to those obtained in previous autopsy studies[1-3]. The early appearance of the disease in women is remarkable: 6.5 % of the female teenagers had gallstones and 3.5 % of them had already been cholecystectomized.

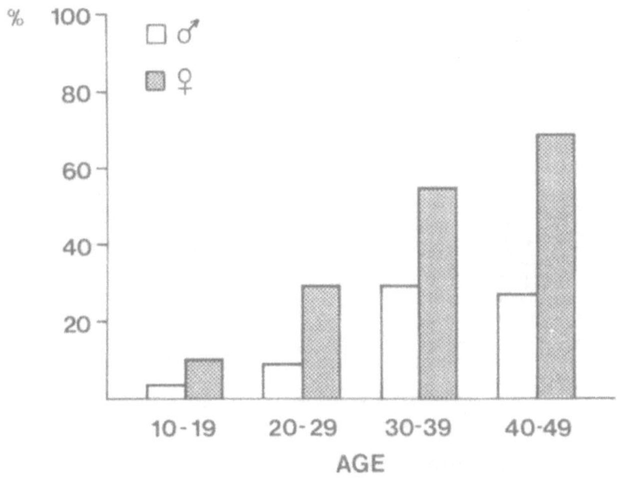

Figure 2 Prevalence of gallstones estimated in 625 subjects older than 10 years. Sixty-eight per cent of these subjects were under 30 years

INCIDENCE OF GALLSTONES IN A YOUNG POPULATION

The incidence of the disease was studied in 75 subjects under 30 years of age having a first normal cholecystogram: 51 of them were women and 24 men, with an average age of 20 years and an age range of 15–30. The second radiological study was performed 5 years later. An incidence of 6% of gallstones was found in the group of women, while no cases were detected among men. This finding confirms that the main risk factors apparent in young people are sex-related.

NATURAL HISTORY OF GALLSTONE DISEASE

From 1972 to 1975, 77 subjects with gallstones were identified by cholecystography. According to the blind nature of the study, they remained unaware of the results of their X-ray studies. In 1981, 6–10 years after their diagnosis, 25 of them were not living in the area and were lost to follow-up, and five had died from causes unrelated to their biliary tract disease (Fig. 3). The remaining 47 cases were subjected to a clinical interview and, if not yet operated, to a new cholecystogram. The clinical follow-up of these patients is shown in Fig. 4. Only 21 of them (45%) remained asymptomatic, meaning that true 'silent stones' constitute a minority of our gallstone population. Of the 26 symptomatic patients, 11 had been operated, seven of them electively. The other four went to surgery because of acute complications of the disease: one case of acute cholecystitis and three cases of common duct stone.

The distinguishing feature of this follow-up study is the blind nature of its prospective design. The population studied was unselected and therefore not necessarily asymptomatic at the beginning of the study. These characteristics do not permit a comparison with other published studies related with the natural history of gallstone disease. Gracie and Ransohoff, for example, studied a selected population of totally asymptomatic subjects, the majority of whom

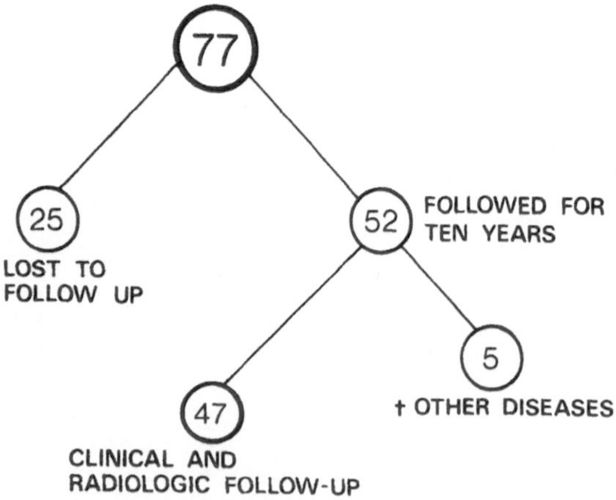

Figure 3 Follow-up of 77 subjects with gallstones, 10 years after diagnosis. Eighty per cent of them were women

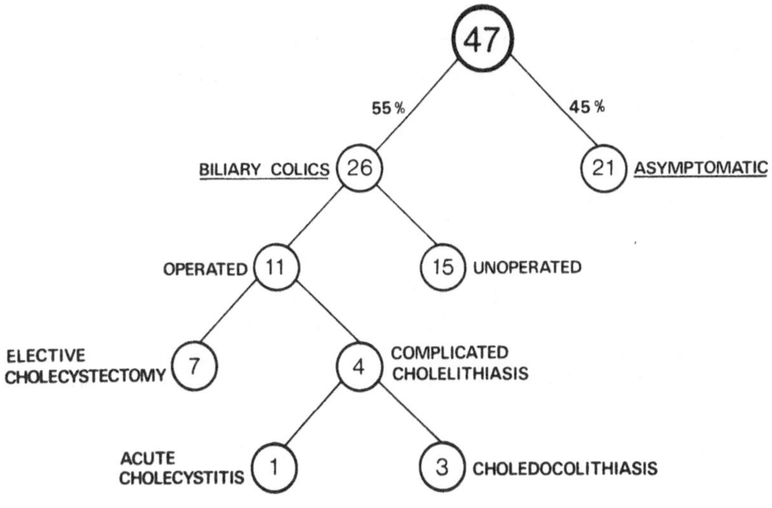

Figure 4 Clinical follow-up

were men[7]. Other studies were performed in patients subjected to cholecystography, presumably because of gastrointestinal symptoms[8,9].

The relatively high frequency of symptoms clearly attributable to gallstone disease, in this population sample, is similar to the frequency reported by Wenckert and Robertson[8]. However, their study was performed in previously symptomatic patients; therefore it is not strictly comparable with the present investigation.

We also followed the radiological evolution of these 47 patients, repeating their cholecystograms, as shown in Fig. 5. In 25 of them the first radiological examinations revealed a functioning gallbladder harbouring stones; 6–10 years later six of them had been operated, eleven still had a functioning gallbladder and eight had evolved to a radiological exclusion. Six of these latter subjects had had biliary colics; on the other hand, only one patient with functioning gallbladder in the second cholecystogram developed symptoms.

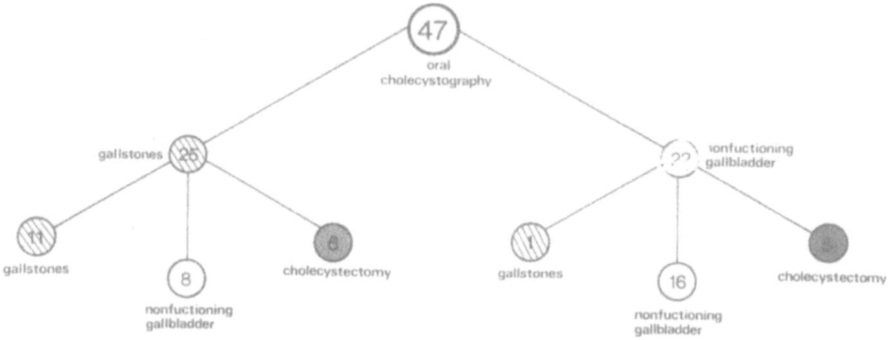

Figure 5 Radiological follow-up

This suggests that the radiological exclusion could be a consequence of repeated bouts of cystic occlusion and gallbladder inflammation.

The first cholecystography revealed a radiological exclusion in 22 patients. Six to 10 years later, five of them had been operated, three because of acute complication. Sixteen patients persisted with their radiological exclusion and only one showed a weak contrast. This suggests that complications of gallstone disease are commoner in the group of patients having a radiological exclusion.

In summary, this study confirms the high prevalence of gallstones previously estimated through autopsy studies in Chile. Although our population was relatively small, and the proportion of men was disproportionally lower than expected (because of the inherent difficulties of studying men during working hours), it is apparent that gallstone disease appears very early in life. It is also apparent that the natural course of gallstone disease is frequently symptomatic in Chile, including a high incidence of acute surgical complications.

References

1. Marinović, I., Guerra, C. and Larach, A. (1972). Incidencia de litiasis biliar en material de autopsias y análisis de la composición de cálculos. *Rev. Med. Chile*, **100**, 1320–1327
2. Medina, E., Irarrázaval, M., Kaempffer, A., De Croizet, V. and Toporowicz, M. (1972). Epidemiología de las colecistopatías en Chile. *Rev. Med. Chile*, **100**, 1376–1381
3. Medina, E., Pascual, J. and Medina, R. (1983). Frecuencia de la litiasis biliar en Chile. *Rev. Med. Chile*, **111**, 668–675
4. Lowenfels, A. B. (1980). Gallstones and the risk of cancer. *Gut*, **21**, 1090–1092
5. Llanos, O., Jasen, A., San Martín, S., Sanhueza, S. and Tocornal, J. (1979). Morbilidad y mortalidad de la cirugía de la litiasis biliar. *Rev. Med. Chile*, **107**, 400–405
6. W.H.O. *World Health Statistics Annual* (1977) (Geneva: World Health Organization)
7. Gracie, W. A. and Ransohoff, D. F. (1982). The natural history of silent gallstones. *N. Engl. J. Med.*, **307**, 798–800
8. Wenckert, A. and Robertson, B. (1966). The natural course of gallstone disease. *Gastroenterology*, **50**, 376–381
9. Lund, J. (1960). Surgical indications in cholelithiasis: prophylactic cholecystectomy elucidated on the basis of long-term follow-up on 526 nonoperated cases. *Ann. Surg.*, **151**, 153–162

7
Cholecystolithiasis in a Danish community: design of a cross-sectional and longitudinal survey

T. JØRGENSEN

ABSTRACT

An age- and sex-stratified random sample of 4808 persons is obtained in 11 municipalities. The gallbladder is evaluated by real-time ultrasonography, the body mass index is registered, and fasting serum cholesterol measured. A questionnaire regarding gastrointestinal symptoms, diseases, life habits, weight history, socioeconomic factors, and gynaecological and obstetric history, is completed. After 5 years the procedure is repeated in the same cohort. The morbidity and mortality of the cohort is followed through central registers.

INTRODUCTION

The aim of the present cross-sectional and longitudinal survey is to elucidate the following problems related to gallstone disease:

(1) What is the prevalence and incidence of gallstones in a Danish community?
(2) What gastrointestinal symptoms may be ascribed to gallstones?
(3) What are the risk factors for development of gallstones?
(4) What therapeutic approach should be used, with persons having asymptomatic gallstones?

As the cross-sectional survey is not yet finished, this is only a description of the study design with some methodological considerations.

MATERIAL AND METHODS

An age- and sex-stratified random sample of 4808 persons, aged 30, 40, 50, and 60 years, is obtained from the 'Central Person Register'. The study population covers 11 municipalities in the western part of Copenhagen County. The overall population is reasonably representative of the total Danish population as regards age, sex, education, occupation, income and housing. The most important differences are under-representation of agriculture, horticulture and fishery[1]. At the same time, the study population is used in an international cardiovascular project – MONICA[2].

All persons are invited for a general health examination. It is indicated that the data collected are to be used in a research project on chronic diseases. Persons not attending are invited a second time. When necessary a third invitation is made by telephone – or by another letter. The morbidity and occupation of non-participants are compared with that of the participants by data from telephone interview and central registers.

If any diseases are discovered the participants are informed and referred to their general practitioner. As it is a debatable issue whether or not asymptomatic gallstones necessitate surgery, we are unable to give rational advice for this condition. We therefore decided not to inform the participants about the findings. The ethical committee for Copenhagen County approved this decision.

Information is obtained through questionnaires (Table 1) and paraclinical data (Table 2). The upper abdomen is examined by ultrasonography using a Toshiba SAL 20A real-time, linear array scanner with a 2.4 MHz probe. The participants have been fasting for 12 h, and are, by routine, examined in supine, left lateral decubitus, and erect positions. The findings are classified according to Table 3.

Table 1 Information from questionnaires

Gastrointestinal symptoms
Diseases
Weight history
Life habits (including physical activity and dietary habits)
Gynaecological and obstetric history
Socioeconomic status

Table 2 Paraclinical data

Occurrence of gallstones and other gallbladder pathology
Height and weight
Fasting total serum-cholesterol and high-density lipoprotein cholesterol (HDL)
Cardiovascular status

In the longitudinal survey the cohort will be followed through life, as regards:

(1) morbidity, through the 'Central Patient Register of Hospital Admittance', where all hospital admissions in Denmark currently are registered;
(2) mortality and immigration, through the 'Person Number Register'.

Table 3 Ultrasonic classification in fasting persons

(1)	Gallbladder lumen without echoes (*no gallstones*)
(2)	Shadowing echoes in the gallbladder lumen. The echoes move with gravity, except when obviously impeded by anatomical conditions, or wedged into the infundibulum (*gallstones*)
(3)	Non-visualization of the gallbladder lumen with high-density echoes and acoustic shadow in the gallbladder fossa (*gallstones*)
(4)	Gallbladder lumen with non-shadowing echoes moving with gravity (*possible gallstones*)
(5)	Gallbladder lumen with echoes attached to the inside of the wall ('polypoid lesions') (*possible gallstones*)
(6)	Non-visualization of the gallbladder lumen without high-density echoes and acoustic shadow in the gallbladder fossa (*cholecystectomized persons* or *agenesis of the gallbladder*)

At least one incidence survey is planned, as the cohort after 5 years will have a new ultrasonic examination performed.

DISCUSSION

This study should elucidate the problems mentioned. The *prevalence* and *incidence* of gallstones in Denmark is not known. Upper abdominal *dyspepsia* cannot be ascribed to the presence of gallstones[3,4]. Bainton[4] even found no significant relation to upper *abdominal pain*. There has been a tradition in clinical medicine that gallstone patients are characterized by different well-known entities. The persistence of this tradition can, however, be ascribed far more to the catchy slogan by which it has been popularized than to the strength of arguments arising from accurate scientific work.

Risk factors to gallstone disease have predominantly been evaluated from hospital material, which comprises only a smaller part of the total occurrence of gallstones[4,5]. The danger of both admission rate bias and diagnostic suspicion bias is obvious[6]. The postulate of, for example, higher parity among gallstone patients has only been confirmed in one prevalence survey[7], but not in three others[3,5,8]. We therefore need more prevalence – or rather, incidence – surveys in assessing the different hypotheses of risk factors to gallstones.

The fear of later complications with increased operation mortality, has led to advocation of early *cholecystectomy*[9,10]. But we do not know the probability that surgery will, in fact, be required for subsequent disease. We therefore need a description of the natural history of the asymptomatic gallstones managed expectantly. The recent work of Gracie and Ransohoff[11], who followed 123 persons with asymptomatic gallstones, has, besides its unrepresentativeness, the shortcoming that the persons were aware of their gallstones. Such a group will not necessarily experience the same course as persons not aware of their diagnosis – the latter situation being the condition for most people with asymptomatic gallstones.

Acknowledgments

The survey was supported by the Danish Medical Research Council (12-7173); the Danish Hospital Foundation for Medical Research; Region of Copenhagen, the Faroë Islands and Greenland (23/81, 37/83); the Danish Health Insurance Foundation (H 11/12-82, H 11/37-83); Leo Pharmaceutical Products (1982) and the Foundation of 1870 (AG 120/81).

References

1. Hollnagel, H. (1980). The health structure of 40-year-old men and women in the Glostrup area, Denmark. General design, sampling results, and referrals for further medical care. *Dan. Med. Bull.*, **27**, 121–130
2. Kirchhoff, M., Schroll, M., Kirkby, H., Hansen, B. S., Sanders, S., Sjφl, A., Jφrgensen, T. and Hansen, P. F. (1983). Screening I, Danmonica, Part of the MONICA Project (Multinational Monitoring of Trends and Determinants in CVD). *CVD Epidemiology Newsletter*, **34**, 32
3. Price, W. H. (1963). Gallbladder dyspepsia. *Br. Med. J.*, **2**, 138–141
4. Bainton, D., Davies, G. T., Evans, K. T. and Gravelle, I. H. (1976). Gallbladder disease. Prevalence in a South Wales industrial town. *N. Engl. J. Med.*, **294**, 1147–1149
5. Sampliner, R. E., Bennett, P. H., Comess, L. J., Rose, F. A. and Burch, T. A. (1970). Gallbladder disease in Pima Indians. Demonstration of high prevalence and early onset by cholecystography. *N. Engl. J. Med.*, **283**, 1358–1364.
6. van der Linden, W. (1961). Some biological traits in female gallstone-disease patients. *Acta Chir. Scand.*, Suppl. 269.
7. Williams, C. N., Johnston, J. L. and Weldon, K. L. M. (1977). Prevalence of gallstones and gallbladder disease in Canadian Micmac Indian women. *Can. Med. Assoc. J.*, **117**, 758–760
8. Williams, C. N. and Johnston, J. L. (1980). Prevalence of gallstones and risk factors in Caucasian women in a rural Canadian community. *Can. Med. Assoc. J.*, **120**, 664–668
9. Glenn, F. (1981). Biliary tract disease. *Surg. Gynecol. Obstet.*, **153**, 401–402
10. Glenn, F. (1981). Silent gallstones. *Ann. Surg.*, **193**, 251–252
11. Gracie, W. A. and Ransohoff, D. F. (1982). The natural history of silent gallstones. *N. Engl. J. Med.*, **307**, 798–800

Part 2
METABOLIC ASPECTS OF GALLSTONE DISEASE AND LESSONS FROM EPIDEMIOLOGY

Chairmen: L. CAPOCACCIA and S. M. GRUNDY

8
Physicochemical aspects of cholesterol gallstone formation

G. SALVIOLI, R. LUGLI and J. M. PRADELLI

LIPID COMPONENTS OF BILE AND CHOLESTEROL CRYSTAL PRECIPITATION

Formation of cholesterol gallstones is a non-biological event caused by changes in the chemical and physical properties of bile which lead to formation of a normally absent solid phase[1].

Cholesterol (Ch) is the major component of gallstones found in western man[2]. In healthy subjects bile is a single-phase isotropic liquid made up of bile salts (BS), phospholipids (95 % lecithin, Lec), lipopigments and cholesterol. These compounds are dissolved in mixed micellar form completely saturated with cholesterol and 50 % saturated with lecithin[3].

Maximum Ch solubility in artificial mixtures resembling human bile has been determined[1,4,5]; this value depends on total lipid concentration, ionic strength, etc. The presence of bile salts (such as ursodeoxycholic acid) having a low cholesterol solubilization capacity[6] seems to reduce the cholesterol solubilizing capacity of the artificial mixtures.

Bile may be defined as abnormal in terms of lipid composition (molar percentages of Ch, Lec, and BS) and/or microscopic morphology (polarized light microscopy can reveal Ch crystals or liquid crystals)[7,8]. The chemico-physical composition of bile can be predicted by plotting molar percentages of the three lipid components on triangular coordinates; values of maximum Ch solubility and the limits of the metastable area are indicated in Fig. 1[3]. The area above the latter contains two phases: Ch crystals plus saturated micelles. The most important parameters influencing the maximum Ch solubility are total lipid concentration, BS/Lec molar ratio, and BS type (for example the presence of ursodeoxycholic acid in the biliary pool)[3,6]. When biliary Ch percentage exceeds maximum cholesterol solubility the solution is metastable and Ch crystal precipitation can occur.

Metastability is a state of incomplete and unstable crystallinity, detectable by X-ray diffraction, which reaches a lower free energy with the formation of

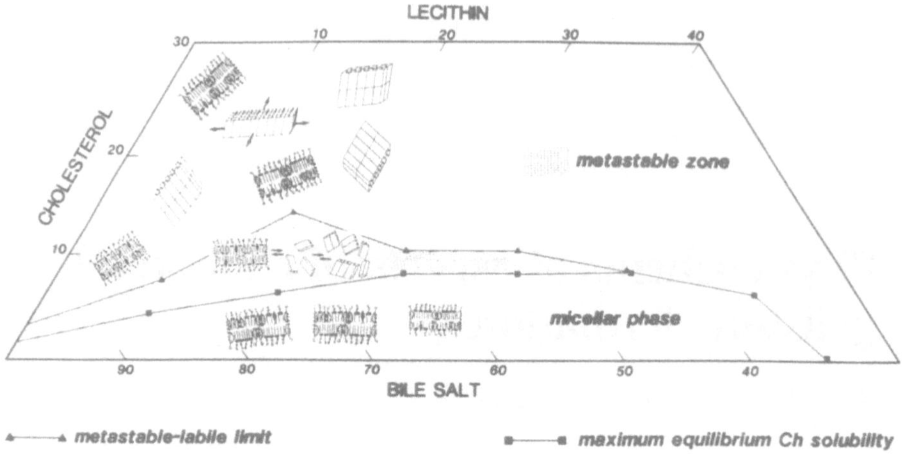

Figure 1 In this phase diagram each point represents the molar percentage of the three biliary lipids (Ch, Lec and BS) and also the physical phases present. The three lipids mixed in different molar proportions can produce different phases at equilibrium, that is when the system reaches a constant energy[13]. The formation of Ch crystals is due to a change of the chemicophysical properties of bile with formation of a solid phase, consequent to variation of total free energy of the system. For further explanation see text

solid and ordered crystals. The maximum degree and duration of the metastable state of human bile is not well known. The metastable region of bile is much larger than that found in the artificial bile system[3,5], thus suggesting a high resistance of human bile to precipitation in spite of high Ch supersaturation. This property and its variations are probably a key factor in formation of Ch gallstones.

In humans, fasting bile is frequently supersaturated with Ch (above all hepatic bile)[3,9]; Ch monohydrate crystals are detectable in gallbladder biles of the majority of cholesterol gallstone patients[3,7,10], but are absent in normal subjects in spite of cholesterol supersaturation[3,9,10]. Even though metastable Ch supersaturation is frequent in humans, a correlation between supersaturation and Ch stone formation is not the rule. Another important point is that the appearance of Ch liquid crystals[8] can precede solid crystal precipitation[11,12], and that high amounts of Ch can be solubilized in vesicle form[12].

The process of Ch precipitation in crystalline form is termed nucleation; nucleation rate is incompletely understood and is influenced by a balance between nucleating and antinucleating factors. The first appearance of crystals is followed by their growth, and stone formation is induced. Unfortunately results obtained *in vitro* using mixtures resembling human bile are not always indicative of *in vivo* processes. Figure 2 depicts the natural history of Ch stone formation with three stages: the first is characterized by supersaturated bile which can form crystals under particular conditions (bile stasis, inflammation, etc.) (second stage); the third phase is the clinical form of gallstones disease.

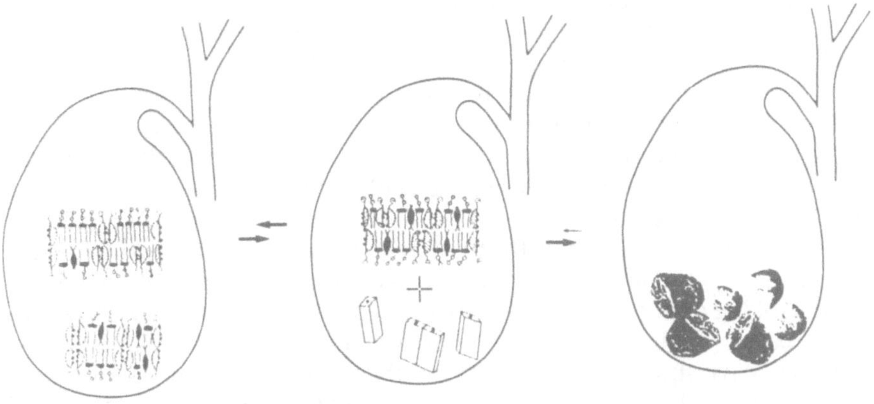

Figure 2 Steps of cholesterol gallstone formation. To date only the last stage has been used for epidemiological studies

FACTORS INFLUENCING THE NUCLEATION PROCESS

Cholesterol monohydrate molecules form flat parallelogram-shaped crystals which intersect at angles of 79.2° and 100.8°[14] and consist of a tilted bilayer of Ch molecules hydrogen-bonded to water and packed side-to-side along their long axis. Their growth occurs faster on these planes, whereas it is slower on the surfaces perpendicular to the molecular axis[14,15].

When and how does the formation of Ch crystals occur? Different possible mechanisms of nucleation exist, as suggested in Fig. 3. Biliary supersaturation of Ch seems to be an important prerequisite. At low supersaturation, induction times can be so long, and growth so slow, that only a small fraction of solubilized Ch precipitates; the importance of this slow nucleation and

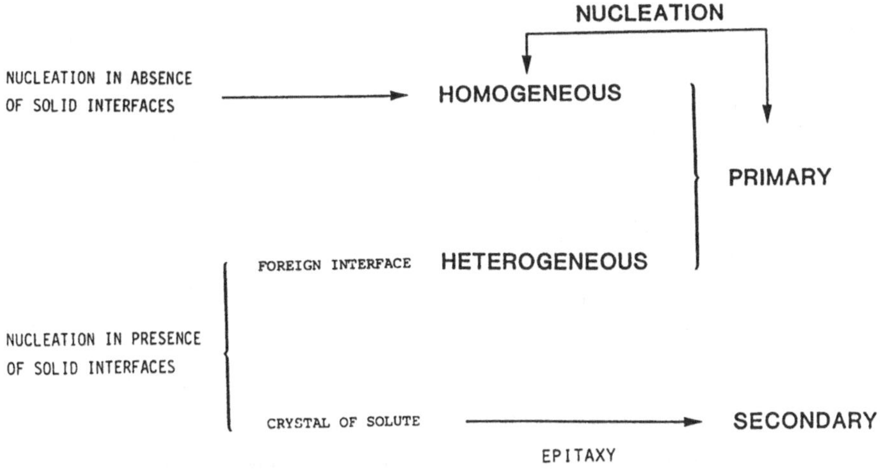

Figure 3 Nucleation phenomena. For further explanation see text

growth is thus small from a physiological standpoint[16]. High supersaturation occurs during fasting, such as during the overnight period when the gallbladder does not contract; nucleation would be favoured under these conditions, but dissolution may be faster than nucleation[3, 16].

Supersaturation of Ch in bile is not always a necessary cause for crystal precipitation[3], and saturation index does not always clearly distinguish normal and Ch gallstone biles. On the contrary nucleation time values can provide a good distinction between biles of normal subjects and Ch gallstone patients[17]. The composition of the two biles is the same regarding the amounts and percentages of lipids; the only observed difference is lower total proteins content of the abnormal bile[17]. In normal bile samples, an inverse correlation exists between biliary Ch saturation and nucleation time[17]. Model bile solutions have shorter nucleation times than true bile; this value, however, increases when biliary protein fractions are added to the tube contents[17]. It has been proposed that factors usually present in biliary proteins might inhibit nucleation[15,17].

Homogeneous and heterogeneous nucleation

Figure 4 presents a schematic representation of the nucleation process. Homogeneous nucleation occurs only at high supersaturation levels (about 300%), but this condition is unlikely in human bile[15]. In contrast, the presence of nucleating factors induces a more rapid nucleation.

Nucleus formation rate *in vitro* is dependent on supersaturation degree[16]: two different nucleation models are possible. At low supersaturation values

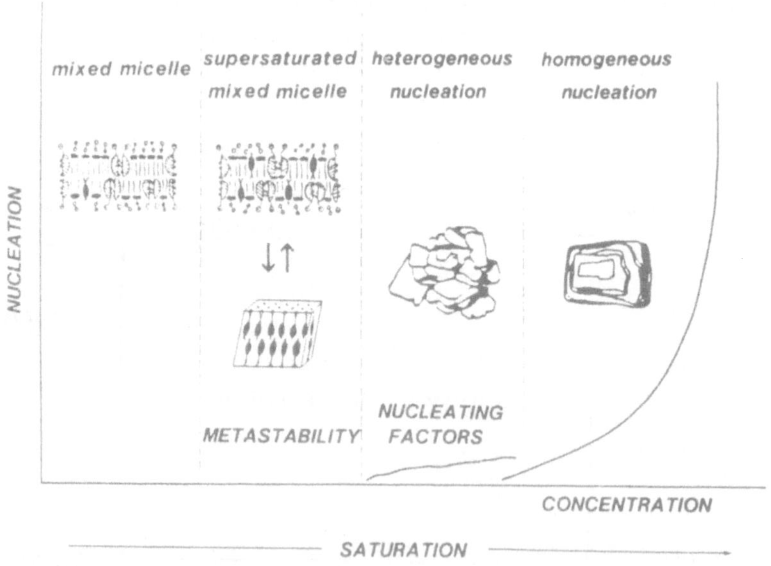

Figure 4 Different phases and modalities of the nucleation process of cholesterol in bile. See text for explanation

the system follows a spiral-steps model, but at high supersaturation values a faster process, termed surface nucleation model, is active on the two-dimensional surface nuclei[16].

Figure 5 shows the relationships between supersaturation of a solution and critical nucleus size. Critical cluster size can be defined as the smallest cluster which decreases its free energy by growing and not by dissolving[18]. For a given supersaturation the clusters falling below the curve dissolve, whereas those above it are stable and can grow. As solution supersaturation increases, the number of molecules required to form a cluster of critical size decreases. Higher activation energy (E_3) is required to form a stable crystal at low supersaturation values than at high supersaturation.

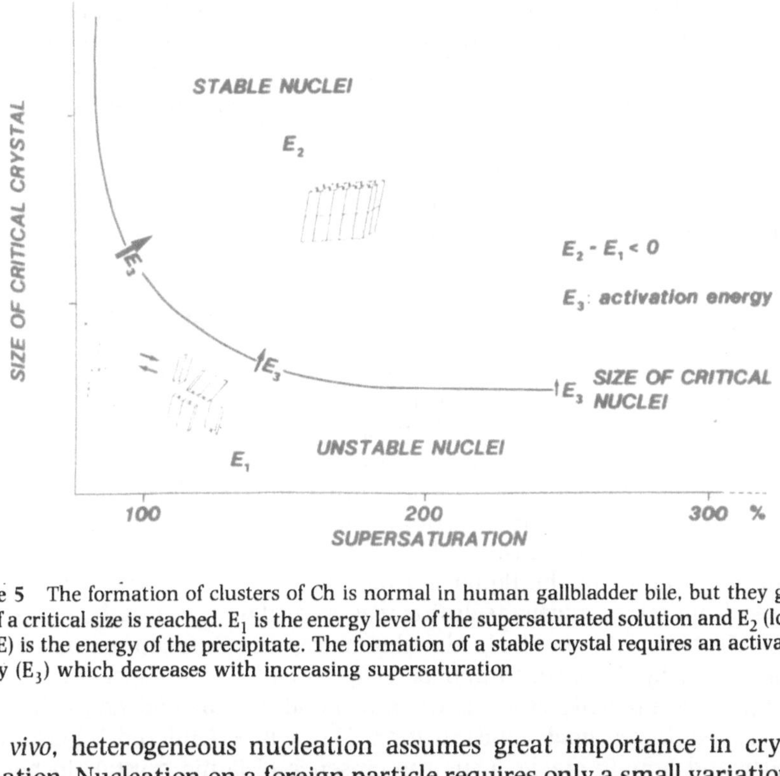

Figure 5 The formation of clusters of Ch is normal in human gallbladder bile, but they grow only if a critical size is reached. E_1 is the energy level of the supersaturated solution and E_2 (lower than E) is the energy of the precipitate. The formation of a stable crystal requires an activation energy (E_3) which decreases with increasing supersaturation

In vivo, heterogeneous nucleation assumes great importance in crystal formation. Nucleation on a foreign particle requires only a small variation of free energy in comparison to that inducing nucleation in the bulk solution[18]. The catalytic effect of heteronuclei reduces the critical supersaturation at which a rapid increase of nucleation occurs and the metastable zone ends.

At low supersaturation values nucleation can be induced by the presence of 10–100 nm diameter particles. Possible crystallization-inducing nuclei are bacteria, calcium soaps, calcium bilirubinate, calcium carbonate, bile pigment (e.g. calcium bilirubinate), and probably some bile salts; these interact at the interface and reduce the free energy required to form a critical nucleus. It is noteworthy that epitaxy (secondary nucleation) may occur in which crystals of either hydroxyapatite (or other inorganic crystals) or Ch monohydrate serve as a nucleus for growth of the other[14].

Nucleation rates of both processes are diffusion-dependent and the diffusion coefficients of the bile solutions are important.

Methods for measuring nucleation

Nucleation of Ch has been studied in artificial mixtures resembling bile (containing physiological proportions and concentration of Ch, Lec and BS), and in true gallbladder or hepatic bile at 37 °C obtained at surgery and in sterile conditions. Holan *et al.*[17] used ultracentrifugation and microscopic examination to evaluate crystal morphology; the observation was stopped with the appearance of Ch crystals. Toor *et al.*[16] used model bile solutions (containing labelled Ch) prepared by the co-precipitation method; after 10 days incubation to reach equilibrium the number of particles was counted in a Coulter Counter (to evaluate the number and diameter of the crystals) and filtered through 0.22 μm polycarbonate filter (to determine cholesterol mass). Large aggregate formation ($>70\ \mu$m) can alter the accuracy of this measurement; recently a radiochemical assay of Ch crystal has been proposed[19]: bile-like solutions are filtered on glass micro-fibre filters and washed before determination of retained Ch.

Problems regarding cholesterol crystal formation in bile

Bile taken from experimental prairie dogs fed a Ch-enriched diet shows the presence of Ch in liquid crystal form. Nucleation-initiating events seem to be related to mesophase formation[11], which is also able to retard Ch crystal formation in the metastable supersaturated system and can contribute to Ch dissolution[20]. The sequence supersaturated micelle→liquid crystal→solid microcrystals may operate *in vivo* and its importance is probably largely dependent on Lec concentration[11,12].

The importance of the liquid crystal state in the formation of solid Ch crystals from mixed micellar solution was studied by Mazer and Carey[12], who demonstrated *in vitro* that large globular microprecipitates appear in solutions having total lipid concentration of 10 g/100 ml and a supersaturation of 160 %; these precipitates coalesce into liquid crystal and hence form Ch crystals. At lower lipid concentration (3 g/100 ml) microprecipitates are smaller and remain stable. Thus the presence of liquid crystals in bile can either inhibit or induce Ch crystal formation. *In vitro* studies on nucleation time suggest that defective gallbladder function may contribute to the production of rapid nucleation[21]; gallbladder bile nucleates faster than hepatic bile even though the latter is more saturated in cholesterol. Hence a nucleation defect exists in cholesterol cholelithiasis independent of cholesterol saturation[21]. Moreover bile from subjects without gallstones does not develop crystals even though most have supersaturated bile[10].

Another important point is that low concentrations of gallbladder bile (10 %) added to hepatic bile can induce Ch nucleation; the variations are not attributable to changes of Ch saturation, but seem to be due to a factor present even when bile is pre-filtered through an XM-300 Amicon filter to eliminate residual microcrystals (size of less than 300 000 dalton)[22].

In summary the events influencing nucleation kinetic processes are: (1) biliary Ch supersaturation; (2) time; (3) presence of nucleating agents. Surprisingly, in spite of high supersaturation (> 200 %) and metastability of hepatic bile, Ch crystals have not been detected microscopically[3,10], but this does not rule out the fact that they could be found by more sophisticated methods.

Antinucleating factors are probably present; these are possibly active at the surface and may also act to retard the dissolution process. The nature of the liquid/solid interface enclosing the system can be important. The properties of the gallbladder lining are not well known; it has been shown, however, that urothelial containers elevate the metastable limit of nucleation in comparison to glass containers[23]. Similar conditions could also prevail in the gallbladder–bile system.

GROWTH OF CHOLESTEROL CRYSTALS

This phase of stone formation follows the nucleation and depends (like the dissolution process) on surface area, adsorption and diffusion rate, degree of supersaturation, temperature, and total lipid concentration. In the absence of liquid flow, molecular transport to the newly formed crystal surface is diffusion controlled[24]; the high viscosity of bile renders the intervention of a convective mechanism unlikely.

Spiral-type dislocation induces a growth in which new crystal deposition occurs at the screw edge; this model can be applied to slowly growing crystals. At higher supersaturation values, growth is faster and occurs on crystal sides[16].

Growth rates for Ch crystals are much lower than those for ionic crystals[25]. Diameters of the formed particles are greater when the system is highly supersaturated with cholesterol and when a higher lipid concentration is present[12,16]. Growth rate is of crucial importance (as is the dissolution rate) since it determines the time required to obtain crystals of sufficient size for retention in the gallbladder; the rate of these processes is more important than the equilibrium solubility in determining gallstone formation.

Growth rate is enhanced by cations such as calcium and magnesium[16], both of which are found as components of Ch stones[26,27]; KCl has an inhibitory effect on crystal formation[16].

NON-CHOLESTEROL COMPONENTS OF BILE AND THEIR PRESENCE IN CHOLESTEROL GALLSTONES

The composition of Ch gallstones is of course characterized by large amounts of Ch; minor components can be present inside the stone and may play a key role in the nucleation process. For example, acidic phospholipids promote

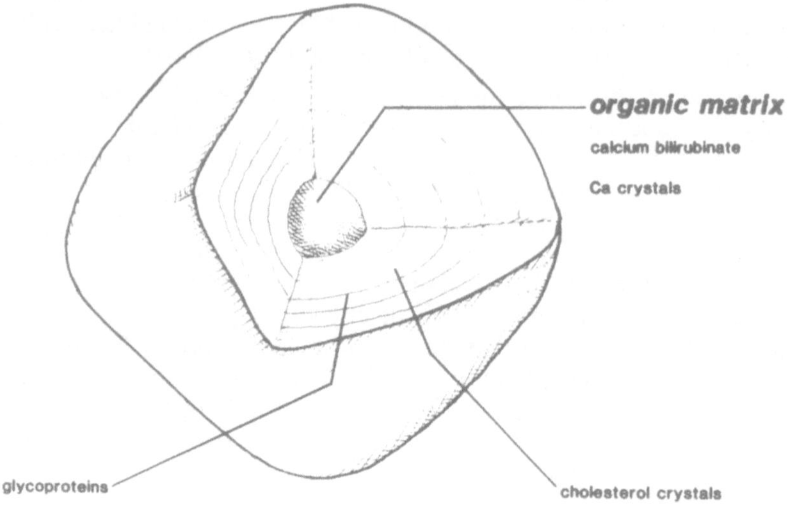

Figure 6 Schematic structure of cholesterol gallstone. See text for explanation

deposition of hydroxyapatite[28]. Figure 6 shows the schematic structure of a Ch gallstone.

Pigments (e.g. calcium bilirubinate) have been found in gallstone cores [29]; calcite, aragonite and vaterite may also be present[26,27]. Layers of calcium bilirubinate and Ch can be detected as an expression of alternative depositions. Increasing percentages of gallstone opacification (11.2–24.1 %) have been found in patients taking ursodeoxycholic acid (UDCA) for extended periods[30,31]; glycoursodeoxycholic acid (GUDC), the predominant biliary bile salt in patients taking UDCA, may have a different affinity for Ca and induce its precipitation on gallstones. Appreciable amounts of sulphated glycoproteins have been found in gallstones[32,33] and these are also able to bind calcium[34]. The calcium content in bile is around 7–20 mg/100 ml and is in part present in ionized form[35]. The micellar binding of Ca accounts for 75 % of non-ionized calcium; this binding decreases the tendency of calcium to form insoluble salts in bile which could induce secondary nucleation of cholesterol. The presence of calcium salt crystals is not easily detectable in bile; their minute size (700–2000 Å) requires the use of complicated techniques. Calcium salts, such as apatite, can probably act as heterogeneous nuclei but their concentration in normal gallbladder bile is similar to that of gallstone patient bile (0.19 vs. 0.23 % of total solid)[17]. Free fatty acids (insoluble at pH 7) are present in bile[36] and could induce Ch precipitation, as could unconjugated bilirubin (2 mg/dl in gallbladder bile)[37], which is insoluble and capable of binding calcium to form insoluble calcium bilirubinate. Proteins are also present in bile in very low concentrations (20 mg/ml). Apo B and apo AI can also be found (60 and 35 μg/ml respectively); they may represent lipoprotein components excreted into bile, though their physiological importance is not known[38]. The problem of protein–lipid complexes in bile is still unresolved even though these complexes have been demonstrated by the use of Biogel A5 or CsCl gradient ultracentrifugation.

ROLE OF GALLBLADDER IN CHOLESTEROL GALLSTONE FORMATION

The gallbladder plays an important role in Ch crystal formation via increased mucin secretion and reduced emptying rates; these two variations can occur together[39]. The properties of gallbladder mucus are not completely known (Fig. 7); it does, however, have a polymeric structure due to hydrophobic and disulphide bonds[40].

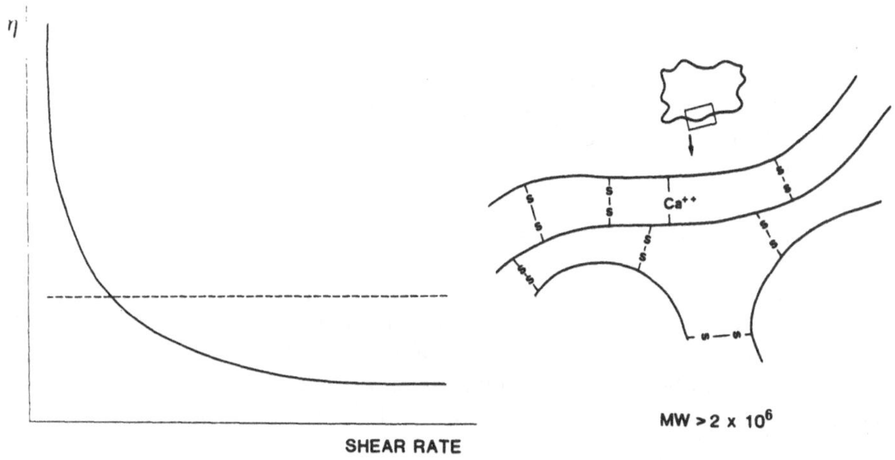

Figure 7 Structure and properties of mucus. Mucus is a viscoelastic gel having MW $> 2 \times 10^6$ with viscosity which decreases with increasing shear rate owing to its thyxotropic behaviour[39]. It represents a barrier preventing damage of the gallbladder mucosa—which has phospholipases—and acts as a hydrodynamic lubricant

High molecular weight mucus-glycoproteins are secreted in increased concentration in patients with lithogenic bile[41] and in experimental cholesterol-fed prairie dogs[42].

Stones grow gradually by sedimentation around an initial nucleus. In the Syrian hamster Ch stone formation occurs by precipitation of Ch around a fibrillar mucus network[43]. Mucoid material is visible in several layers of stones[42] and mucin and bilirubin have been recognized in the central core of cholesterol gallstones[27] (see Fig. 6).

Mucus can associate with bilirubin[34] and calcium[32], and these complexes can then act as initiating factors for heterogeneous Ch nucleation of supersaturated bile[44]. Increased production and viscosity of gallbladder mucus may predispose to the formation of sludge[45,46] in the gallbladder (fine particulate matter similar to the core material of Ch gallstones and made of a suspension of pigment precipitates) during biliary stasis, such as during long-term total parenteral feeding.

Experiments with cholesterol-fed prairie dogs show alterations of biliary flow (increased intragallbladder pressure and increased resistance in the cystic duct) due to high bile viscosity[47,48]; sphincterotomy prevents the formation of cholesterol gallstones, an effect reversed by atropine administration[49]. Therefore increased viscosity of mucus can retard gallbladder emptying, and bile acids can reduce mucus viscosity[50].

Another relevant problem is the possible formation of lysolecithin in bile consequent to hydrolysis of biliary Lec by the action of gallbladder wall phospholipases[51]. Large amounts of Ch can be solubilized by lysolecithin and its formation is contemporaneous to the formation of free fatty acids and possibly of prostaglandins which mediate increased mucus secretion[42].

CONCLUSIONS

Nucleation and growth rates of Ch crystals, and the presence of particles accelerating these processes, are the most important factors leading to Ch gallstone formation in humans. *In vitro* experiments provide results which at times differ from those obtained using true bile; in particular induction time of Ch crystals is longer *in vivo* than *in vitro*. The time required to obtain crystals of sufficient size for retention by the gallbladder during its emptying is very long, and consequently other incompletely understood factors (such as a delayed emptying of the gallbladder) can determine the retention of small Ch crystals during normal cyclic activity of the gallbladder. Thus, the process of Ch precipitation in the gallbladder is profoundly influenced not only by Ch supersaturation, but also by gallbladder motility, by biliary flow, and by the minor components of bile which will require more in-depth study.

References

1. Admirand, W. H. and Small, D. M. (1968). The physical–chemical basis of cholesterol gallstone formation in man. *J. Clin. Invest.*, **47**, 1043–1052
2. Been, J. M., Bills, P. M. and Lewis, D. (1974). Microstructure of gallstones. *Gastroenterology*,**76**, 548–555
3. Carey, M. C. and Small, D. M. (1978). The physical chemistry of cholesterol solubility in bile. Relationship to gallstone formation and dissolution in man. *J. Clin. Invest.*, **61**, 998–1026
4. Hegardt, F. G. and Dam, H. (1974). The solubility of cholesterol in aqueous solution of bile salts and lecithin. *Zeit. Ernaehrungswiss.*, **10**, 228–33
5. Holzbach, R. T., Marsh, M., Olszewski, M. and Holan, K. (1973). Cholesterol solubility in bile. Evidence that supersaturated bile is frequent in healthy man. *J. Clin. Invest.*, **52**, 1467–79
6. Carey, M. C. (1978). Critical tables for calculating the cholesterol saturation of native bile. *J. Lipid Res.*, **19**, 945–955
7. Van der Linden, W. and Nakayama, F. (1974). Occurrence of cholesterol crystals in human bile. *Gut*, **15**, 630–635
8. Olszewski, M. F., Holzbach, R. T., Saupe, A. and Brown, G. H. (1973). Liquid crystals in human bile. *Nature*, **242**, 336–37
9. Somjen, G. J. and Gilat, T. (1983). A non-micellar mode of cholesterol transport in human bile. *FEBS Lett.*, **156**, 265–68
10. Sedaghat, A. and Grundy, S. M. (1980). Cholesterol crystals and the formation of cholesterol gallstones. *N. Engl. J. Med.*, **302**, 1224–27

11. Holzbach, R. T. and Corbusier, C. (1978). Liquid crystals and cholesterol nucleation during equilibration in supersaturated bile analogs. *Biochim. Biophys. Acta*, **528**, 436–444
12. Mazer, N. A. and Carey, M. C. (1983). Quasi-elastic light-scattering studies of aqueous biliary lipid systems. Cholesterol solubilization and precipitation in model bile solutions. *Biochemistry*, **22**, 426–442
13. Gibbs, J. W. (1928). *The Collected Works of J. Willard Gibbs*. (New York: Longmans, Green and Co.)
14. Craven, B. M. (1976). Crystal structure of cholesterol monohydrate. *Nature*, **260**, 727–729
15. Small, D. M. (1980). Cholesterol nucleation and growth in gallstone formation. *N. Engl. J. Med.*, **302**, 1305–1307
16. Toor, E. W., Evans, D. F. and Cussler, E. L. (1978). Cholesterol monohydrate growth in model bile solutions. *Proc. Natl. Acad. Sci.*, **75**, 6230–6234
17. Holan, K. R., Holzbach, R. T., Hermann, R. E., Cooperman, A. M. and Claffey, W. J. (1979). Nucleation time: a key factor in the pathogenesis of cholesterol gallstone disease. *Gastroenterology*, **77**, 611–617
18. Garside, J. (1982). Nucleation. In Nancollas, G. H. (ed.) *Biological Mineralization and Demineralization. Dahlem Konferenzen*. pp. 23–35. (Berlin, Heidelberg, New York: Springer–Verlag)
19. Whiting, M. J. and Watts, J. McK. (1983). Cholesterol crystal formation and growth in model bile solutions. *J. Lipid Res.*, **24**, 861–868
20. Salvioli, G., Igimi, H. and Carey, M. C. (1983). Cholesterol gallstone dissolution in bile. Dissolution kinetics of crystalline cholesterol monohydrate by conjugated chenodeoxycholate–lecithin and conjugated urodeoxycholate–lecithin mixtures: dissimilar phase equilibria and dissolution mechanisms. *J. Lipid Res.*, **24**, 701–719
21. Gollish, S. H., Burnstein, M. J., Ilson, R. G., Petrunka, C. N. and Strasberg, S. M. (1983). Nucleation of cholesterol monohydrate crystals from hepatic and gallbladder bile of patients with cholesterol gallstones. *Gut*, **24**, 836–844
22. Burnstein, M. J., Ilson, R. G., Petrunka, C. N., Taylor, R. D. and Strasberg, S. M. (1983). Evidence for a potent nucleating factor in the gallbladder bile of patients with cholesterol gallstones. *Gastroenterology*, **85**, 801–807
23. Gill, W. B., Ruggiero, K. J. and Fromes, M. C. (1980). Elevation of the metastable limits and absence of container surface nucleation for calcium oxalate crystallization in a urothelial-lined system as compared to glass containers. *Invest. Urol.*, **18**, 157–161
24. Higuchi, W. I. and Saad, H. Y. (1965). Cholesterol particles growth and solution rates in aqueous media. *J. Pharm. Sci.*, **54**, 72–78
25. Ohara, M. and Reid, R. C. (1973). *Modeling Crystal Growth Rates from Solutions*. pp. 19–45. (Englewood Cliffs, NJ: Prentice-Hall)
26. Sutor, D. J. and Wooley, S. E. (1973). The nature and incidence of gallstones containing calcium. *Gut*, **14**, 215–20, I
27. Been, J. M., Bills, P. M. and Lewis, D. (1978). Microstructure of gallstones. *Gastroenterology*, **76**, 548–555
28. Boskey, A. L., Boyan Salyers, B. D., Burnstein, L. S. and Mandel, I. D. (1983). Lipids associated with mineralization of human submandibular gland sialoliths. *Arch. Oral Biol.*, **26**, 779–785
29. Bogren, H. and Larsson, K. (1963). Crystalline components of biliary calculi. *Scand. J. Clin. Lab. Invest.*, **15**, 569–572
30. Bateson, M. C., Bouchier, I. A. D. and Trash, D. B. (1981). Calcification of radiolucent gallstones during treatment with ursodeoxycholic acid. *Br. Med. J.*, **283**, 645
31. Gleeson, D., Ruppin, D. C., Murphy, G. M. and Dowling, R. H. (1983). Second look at ursodeoxycholic acid (UDCA): high efficacy for partial but low efficacy for complete gallstone dissolution, and a high rate of acquired stone opacification. *Gut*, **24**, A999 (abstract)
32. Maki, T., Matsushiro, T., Suzuki, N. and Nakamura, N. (1971). Role of sulfated glycoprotein in gallstone formation. *Surg. Gynecol. Obstet.*, **132**, 846–854
33. Womack, N. A. (1971). The development of gallstones. *Surg. Gynecol. Obstet.*, **132**, 37–45
34. Smith, B. F. and LaMont, J. T. (1983). Bovine gallbladder mucin binds bilirubin in vitro. *Gastroenterology*, **85**, 707–712
35. Sutor, D. J. (1980). Ionized-calcium in pathological human bile. *J. Clin. Pathol.*, **33**, 86–88

36. Mingrone, G., Greco, A. V. and Passi, S. (1983). The possible role of free fatty acids in the pathogenesis of cholesterol gallstones in man. *Biochim. Biophys. Acta*, **751**, 138–144
37. Masuda, H. and Nakayama, F. (1979). Composition of bile pigment in gallstones and bile and their etiological significance. *J. Lab. Clin. Med.*, **93**, 353–360
38. Kawamoto, T., Kost, L. J., Sewell, R. B., Mao, S. J. T., Thistle, J. L. and LaRusso, N. F. (1982). Biliary excretion of the protein and lipid components of lipoproteins. *Hepatology*, **2**, 699 (abstract)
39. King, M. (1980). Viscoelastic properties of airway mucus. *Fed. Proc.*, **39**, 3080–3085
40. Pearson, J. P., Kaura, R., Taylor, W. and Allen, A. (1983). The composition and polymeric structure of mucus glycoprotein from human gallbladder. *Biochim. Biophys. Acta*, **706**, 221–228
41. Bouchier, I. A. D., Copperband, S. R. and El Kidsl, B. M. (1965). Mucous substances and viscosity of normal and pathological human bile. *Gastroenterology*, **49**, 343–352
42. Lee, S. P., LaMont, J. T. and Carey, M. C. (1981). Role of gallbladder mucus hypersecretion in the evaluation of cholesterol gallstones. *J. Clin. Invest.*, **67**, 1712–1723
43. Schade, H. (1911). Zur Genese der Gallensteine. *Z. Exp. Pathol. Ther.*, **8**, 92–124
44. Levy, P., Smith, B. F., Atkinson, D. and LaMont, J. T. (1983). Human gallbladder mucin enhances in vitro nucleation of cholesterol monohydrate crystals. *Gastroenterology*, **84**, 1382 (abstract)
45. Allen, B., Bernhoft, R., Blanckaert, N., Svanvik, J., Filly, R., Gooding, G. and Way, L. (1981). Sludge is calcium bilirubinate associated with bile stasis. *Am. J. Surg.*, **141**, 51–54
46. Pitt, H. A., King, W., Mann, L. L., Roslyn, J. J., Bequist, W. E., Ament, M. E. and DenBesten, L. (1983). Increased risk of cholelithiasis with prolonged total parenteral nutrition. *Am. J. Surg.*, **145**, 106–112
47. Doty, J. E., Pitt, H. A., Kuchenbecker, S. L. and DenBesten, L. (1983). Impaired gallbladder emptying before gallstone formation in the prairie dog. *Gastroenterology*, **85**, 168–174
48. Doty, J. E., Pitt, H. A., Kuchenbecker, S. L., Porter-Fink, V. and DenBesten, L. (1983). The role of gallbladder mucus in the pathogenesis of cholesterol gallstones. *Am. J. Surg.*, **145**, 54–61
49. Hutton, S. W., Siewert, C. E. Jr., Vennes, J. A. and Duane, W. C. (1982). Inhibition of gallstone formation by sphincterotomy in the prairie dog: reversal by atropine. *Gastroenterology*, **82**, 1308–1313
50. Martin, G. P., Marriott, C. and Kellaway, I. W. (1978). Direct effect of bile salts and phospholipids on the physical properties of mucus. *Gut*, **19**, 103–107
51. Tagesson, C., Norrby, S. and Sjödahl, R. (1979). The prerequisites for local lysolecithin formation in the human gallbladder. III: Demonstration of two different phospholipase A activities. *Scand. J. Gastroenterol.*, **14**, 379–84

9
Metabolic factors in pathogenesis of cholesterol gallstones: implications for gallstone prevention

S. M. GRUNDY

CONCEPT OF GALLSTONE PREVENTION

Current treatment of clinical gallstone disease is generally successful. Cholecystectomy carries a low mortality and usually effects a complete cure. The recent introduction of pharmacological dissolution of cholesterol gallstones with oral administration of bile acids (chenodeoxycholic acid and ursodeoxycholic acid) appears to be an important addition to therapy of gallstones[1]. Despite these good therapeutic modalities for treatment of existing cholelithiasis, gallstones remain an important cause of morbidity and mortality. The prevalence of gallstones in many populations is enormous. Cholecystitis and obstructive jaundice are common clinical problems throughout the world. Although the risks for mortality from gallbladder disease and cholecystectomy are relatively lower in young and middle-aged adults, the risk increases greatly with advancing years. Gallstone disease is also costly both in financial terms and in time lost from work. For these reasons consideration must be given to whether gallstones can be prevented. If prevention is both possible and practical, the benefits would be great. The purpose of this review is to examine the question of gallstone prevention in the light of current knowledge about the pathogenesis of cholesterol stones. Therefore the mechanisms responsible for gallstone formation will be reviewed first, and the concept of risk factors for gallstone disease will be developed. If risk factors working through known pathogenic mechanisms can be identified and modified, they might provide a foundation upon which to develop a programme of gallstone prevention.

MECHANISMS FOR CHOLESTEROL GALLSTONE FORMATION

Three metabolic defects appear to be necessary for the formation of cholesterol gallstones. These are (a) the development of supersaturated bile, (b) the formation of cholesterol monohydrate crystals, and (c) the growth of cholesterol stones. All three processes are required for the formation of stones, and each can be considered in turn.

Mechanisms for development of supersaturated bile

Cholesterol is completely insoluble in aqueous solutions, and special mechanisms are required for its solubilization and transport in bile. The major transport systems appears to be mixed micelles containing bile acids and lecithin. Both bile acids and lecithin have detergent-like properties; that is, they have a polar head group and a non-polar tail. When these lipids are present in solutions above a critical concentration they self-aggregate to produce mixed micelles. Their hydrophobic tails are directed towards the centre of micelles, and their polar head groups are oriented into the aqueous phase. Cholesterol can be dissolved in the centre of these micelles. The maximum solubility of cholesterol in bile acid–lecithin micelles occurs when the molar ratios of lecithin to bile acids is in the range 0.2–0.3. Solubility also is enhanced when total lipid concentration is high.

Although mixed micelles can solubilize and transport considerable quantities of cholesterol through bile, the amount of cholesterol is sometimes more than can be transported easily. When this occurs the bile becomes supersaturated with cholesterol[2]. Two kinds of supersaturated bile have been defined[3]: metastable bile is only mildly supersaturated; it can hold cholesterol in solutions for prolonged periods, but eventually precipitation of the cholesterol will occur; labile bile is highly supersaturated; the excess cholesterol precipitates rapidly. The degree of supersaturation is therefore crucial; bile with labile supersaturation is much more lithogenic.

The saturation of bile is a function of the metabolism of each of the biliary lipids – cholesterol, bile acids and lecithin – as well as their interaction. Abnormalities in the metabolism of bile acids can lead to depletion of the bile acid pool. When this occurs insufficient bile acids are available for normal cholesterol transport, and supersaturation develops. Disorders in the metabolism of lecithin have also been implicated in supersaturation, but they have not been proven with certainty. Even when the metabolisms of bile acids and lecithin are normal, supersaturation can be present when an excess of cholesterol enters the bile for excretion.

In many species the composition of bile is relatively constant throughout the day and night. In most humans, however, this constancy of composition is not maintained throughout the 24 h cycle[4]. During the day, when the enterohepatic circulation (EHC) of bile acids is stimulated by intake of food, saturation is at its lowest; but at night saturation can increase markedly. The critical causes of the diurnal variation in bile lipid composition appear two-fold: (a) a reduction in output of bile acids, and (b) a rise in the cholesterol/lecithin ratio[5,6]. Outputs of lecithin fall in parallel with those of bile acids during fasting. Although secretion of cholesterol also declines, the fall is not as much as for lecithin, and saturation rises. Thus, a dissociation in outputs of lecithin and cholesterol appears to be an important factor in causation of supersaturated bile.

Alternative systems of biliary cholesterol transport

The bile contains many substances besides the biliary lipids. These other substances could also affect cholesterol solubility in bile, either increasing or decreasing it. For example, specialized proteins might act as an auxiliary mechanism for enhancing the solubility of cholesterol. In other words, these proteins might be analogous to the apoproteins of the plasma lipoproteins. The latter are large molecules with detergent properties not unlike the bile acids. Apoproteins, like bile acids, interact with lecithin, producing a complex with a hydrophobic core. Since the concentrations of proteins in bile are as high as 1 g/dl there is the potential for their playing an important role in cholesterol solubilization. Furthermore, it is possible that a portion of biliary cholesterol is transported in pure phospholipid vesicles. Thus bile may contain a whole array of systems for holding cholesterol in solution – pure bile acid micelles, mixed micelles, phospholipid vesicles and lipid–protein complexes. Although the mixed micelles are probably the most important mechanism, these other systems could play a crucial role in the prevention of cholesterol precipitation and hence gallstone formation.

Mechanisms of cholesterol nucleation (crystallization)

There is increasing evidence that many people have supersaturated bile, at least during part of the 24 h cycle, and yet do not develop gallstones[7,8]. Perhaps their biliary cholesterol is held in solution by one of the auxiliary systems described above. Regardless, the next critical step in the formation of gallstones is the development of cholesterol crystals. Even when supersaturation is present for long periods, if crystallization does not occur gallstones will not develop. We therefore must ask why some patients with supersaturated bile develop gallstones while others do not. Studies in our laboratory have shown that most patients with cholesterol gallstones have crystals of cholesterol monohydrate in their bile[7,8]. A much higher correlation seems to exist between the presence of cholesterol crystals and gallstones than between supersaturated bile and stones. Our data suggest that if a person continuously produces cholesterol crystals, the development of gallstones is highly likely.

What factors lead to crystal formation? The degree of saturation could be one factor. Crystals are seemingly more likely to occur from labile supersaturated bile than from metastable bile. The presence of other factors in bile could also be an important factor. Recently, Burnstein *et al.*[9] have presented evidence for a potent nucleating factor in the gallbladder bile of patients with cholesterol gallstones. Their study was carried out to determine whether the rapid nucleation time of gallbladder bile obtained from patients with gallstones is due to addition of a nucleating agent or removal of an antinucleating agent from bile. Bile from gallstone patients was mixed with normal bile, and the mixtures had rapid nucleating times similar to those of gallbladder bile from gallstone patients, suggesting that a nucleating factor was present in the abnormal bile. Further reduction in amounts of abnormal bile added to normal bile demonstrated that the nucleating factor is potent. Filtration of the abnormal bile through an XM-300 Amicon filter did not eliminate the nucleating potency. Although this work strongly suggests that bile from gallstone patients contains a nucleating factor, instead of normal bile containing an antinucleating factor, the nature of the nucleating factor has not been determined.

Mechanisms responsible for stone growth

Even though cholesterol crystals appear to be the critical link between supersaturated bile and cholesterol stones, a gallstone cannot develop unless crystals aggregate and these aggregations grow. How exactly do stones grow? Once a stone reaches a certain size, does growth occur by direct incorporation of cholesterol molecules on the surface of the stone, or must there be further accretion of cholesterol crystals? When gallstones are subjected to scanning electron microscopy, the cut surfaces appear to contain many distinct cholesterol crystals. The adherence of crystals, however, may not be the only mechanism. Calcium salts are commonly present in gallstones, and these salts might contribute to crystal aggregation and accretion. Clearly, more studies are needed to explain the growth of cholesterol stones.

RISK FACTORS FOR GALLSTONES

Obesity

Cholesterol gallstones are more common in obese patients than in non-obese. The link between obesity and gallstones is supersaturated bile. Obesity raises the saturation of bile by increasing hepatic secretion of cholesterol[10]. A high output of cholesterol in bile is secondary to a heightened synthesis of cholesterol in obese people. Most obese people have supersaturated bile, but all do not develop gallstones[7]. This proves that supersaturation of bile does not invariably cause gallstones. Other factors are required, particularly the formation of cholesterol crystals[7,8]. Those obese people without gallstones also do not have cholesterol crystals in bile.

Sex

Women are more likely to develop gallstones than men. The reasons for this sex difference are not entirely understood. Apparently, bile tends to be more saturated in women[4,11], possibly due to the synthesis of less chenodiol[12]. Oestrogens probably alter the composition of bile; they have been reported to reduce the pool sizes of bile acids and to increase biliary outputs. These hormones may have other actions, such as promoting development of cholesterol crystals or facilitating the growth of stones. Also, progesterone apparently causes relaxation of smooth muscles and delays emptying of the gallbladder[13]; this effect may allow stones to grow faster.

Pregnancy

Pregnancy is thought by many investigators to promote the formation of gallstones. The exact reasons are unknown. Composition of bile may be altered adversely by the hormonal changes of pregnancy. Gallbladder emptying is sluggish to allow stone growth. Marked weight-gain may acutely increase saturation of bile with cholesterol. If small stones are carried in the gallbladder at the time of conception they may grow rapidly and become symptomatic because of the factors listed above.

Genetics

Cholelithiasis appears to cluster in families. While environmental factors, such as obesity, may similarly affect the several members of one family, genetic influences may also be at work. Abnormalities in the metabolism of cholesterol or bile acids could cause supersaturated bile; alternatively, if the bile of some people contains powerful nucleating factors for biliary cholesterol, these too might be inherited.

Race

Gallstones are more common in some races than others. One of the highest incidences of cholesterol gallstones occurs in American Indians[14]. Almost all tribes in the United States are affected. Gallstone disease also seems to have a high prevalence throughout Central and South America. Factors related to the Indian race may be involved in these regions. The basic abnormality in the bile of American Indians appears to be a deficiency of bile acids[11]. These people apparently have a defect in regulation of bile acid synthesis. When bile acids are lost normally through the intestine, there is insufficient compensatory increase in bile acid synthesis to restore a normal pool size of bile acids. A low bile acid pool is especially noticeable in Indian women, in whom prevalence of gallstones exceeds that in Indian men. The major cause of excess gallstones in Indians seems to be related mainly to supersaturated bile. Obesity is a major factor for two reasons. Many Indians are prone to obesity, and the excess biliary cholesterol in the obese compounds the deficiency of bile acids to produce severe supersaturation. Whether Indians have unusual nucleating factors is unknown.

Other populations have a high prevalence of gallstones. Scandinavian women are prone to gallstone disease, and their tendency is not necessarily related to obesity. On the other hand, cholelithiasis in the black population is relatively rare. The differences among these populations – whether due to differences in lipid metabolism or nucleating factors – are not known.

Gastrointestinal disease

Several disorders of the gastrointestinal tract have been reported to predispose to gallstone disease. Ileal disease leads to depletion of the bile acid pool and hence to supersaturated bile[15]. Gallstones are common in cystic fibrosis[16,17]. The abnormal mucus secreted in this disorder could promote crystal formation, but supersaturated bile has also been reported. Coeliac disease is associated with a sluggish gallbladder contraction, apparently caused by lack of cholecystokinin from the intestinal mucosa. Atony of the gallbladder also can be due to diabetic neuropathy.

Rapid weight loss

Certainly the obese state is associated with increased risk for gallstones, but rapid weight loss also may enhance risk, in some people at least[10]. The reason is increased supersaturation of bile, and two factors are responsible. One is a decrease in synthesis and pool sizes of bile acids, and the second is mobilization of cholesterol from adipose tissue stores. The cholesterol lost from adipose tissue enters the bile mainly as cholesterol and not as bile acids. The result is increased saturation of bile.

Hypertriglyceridaemia

Several reports suggest that patients with hypertriglyceridaemia have an increased likelihood of developing cholesterol gallstones. Hypertriglyceridaemic patients have an enhanced synthesis of cholesterol and bile acid, and a high saturation of bile. The major cause of this high saturation appears to be an elevated secretion of cholesterol in bile. Many patients with raised plasma triglycerides are obese, and obesity could be one factor contributing to supersaturation of bile. Still, some forms of hypertriglyceridaemia *per se* seem to cause a high saturation of bile. These forms are probably characterized by overproduction of lipoproteins as well as by a high synthesis of biliary lipids.

Fibric acid derivatives

Clofibrate and related drugs enhance the saturation of bile[18-20]. These agents increase biliary secretion of cholesterol and reduce synthesis of bile acids. In a small percentage of patients treated with the fibric acids, cholesterol gallstones develop.

Other hypolipidaemic agents

Because clofibrate increases chances for gallstones some investigators have speculated that all forms of hypolipidaemic therapy will enhance bile saturation. This is not true, however. Nicotinic acid might cause a slight increase in saturation, but not to a dangerous level. The same can be said for the bile acid sequestrants. Rarely patients treated with sequestrants may have a marked rise in saturation, but most do not. Another hypocholesterolaemic drug, probucol, seemingly has no effect on bile saturation.

PREVENTION OF GALLSTONES BY MODIFICATION OF RISK FACTORS

The best hope for reducing morbidity and mortality from gallstone disease lies in prevention. Bile acid therapy may have a place in treatment of some patients with gallstones, but surgery will probably remain the major approach to this disease. Only through prevention will it be possible to alter the burden of cholelithiasis throughout the world. Consequently, a crucial question is whether gallstones can be prevented. If so, one approach is through modification of risk factors. It stands to reason that avoidance of the risk factors for cholelithiasis should prevent the development of gallstones. However, this conclusion may not be as obvious as it seems. An unresolved question is the relative importance of supersaturated bile vs. the nucleation process. If the development of supersaturated bile is the major factor then prevention of gallstones will be less difficult than if nucleating agents are the determining factor. For this reason we must differentiate the two processes when considering the possible prevention of gallstones. First, we can address the question of whether modification of risk factors affecting bile saturation will prevent gallstones. Second, will it be necessary to interfere with nucleation to prevent stone formation?

Prevention of gallstones by avoidance of obesity

Epidemiological studies suggest that obese people have about twice the risk for gallstones as non-obese people. This enhanced risk extends to both sexes. The sex differential still exists in overweight people, but the doubling of risk occurs for both sexes. This relationship strongly suggests that avoidance of obesity would prevent gallstones. It is true that many obese people never develop cholelithiasis[7]; they seem protected despite supersaturation, possibly because they are lacking in nucleating factors. But will avoidance of obesity prevent cholesterol stones even in susceptible people? Epidemiological data would suggest so, although more investigations are needed to determine whether people with nucleating factors will develop stones regardless of their body weight.

Prevention of gallstones by controlling diet composition

A common observation is that populations consuming high-fat, high-cholesterol diets have a high prevalence of gallstones. However, obesity is common in such populations, and the importance of diet composition in determining rates of cholelithiasis has not been elucidated. A high-cholesterol diet has been implicated in raising bile saturation, but the influence of dietary cholesterol on saturation may not be great. If a high-fat diet is more lithogenic than a low-fat diet, it has not been determined. Polyunsaturated fats have been reported to be lithogenic, but this action may be limited to patients who have an underlying obesity or hypertriglyceridaemia. An important question is thus whether diets rich in total fats and cholesterol increase the risk for gallstones. If so, avoidance of such diets might decrease the likelihood of developing stones.

Avoidance of lithogenic drugs

It was indicated above that fibric acid derivatives raise the saturation of bile and hence the danger of gallstones. The potential lithogenicity of other drugs may yet be detected. For example, we have shown that the antimicrobial rifampin increases the saturation of bile and thus may be lithogenic[21]. More investigations are needed to discover whether other drugs hold the same danger. Considering the large number of drugs used in clinical medicine today, it would not be surprising if at least some of them were to be associated with gallstone formation. By the same token their avoidance could prevent the development of stones.

Low-dose bile acid therapy for gallstone prevention

Bile acids (chenodeoxycholic acid or ursodeoxycholic acid) obviously cannot be used on a large scale. However, in some patients their use might be considered. The ideal patient would be one with recurrent symptoms from small gallstones. These stones could pass into the common bile duct and cause pain or obstruction. Such stones should be dissolved readily by bile acid therapy, and future episodes should be prevented. Obviously, cholecystectomy would eliminate the problem altogether, but some patients might be candidates for medical prophylaxis.

Avoidance of cholesterol crystal formation

The ideal means of gallstone prevention would be the blockage of the nucleation process. When this process is not active gallstones seemingly do not occur even in the presence of supersaturated bile. Since the mechanisms responsible for nucleation are not understood, we are not yet able to develop specific approaches to interfere with crystal formation. Therefore, further research into the control of cholesterol solubilization in bile is needed. Auxiliary systems for holding biliary cholesterol in solution should be explored. Such studies might reveal a simple method for the avoidance of nucleation and thus the prevention of gallstones.

References

1. Schoenfield, L. J. and Lachin, J. M.; The Steering Committee, and the National Cooperative Gallstone Study Group. National Cooperative Gallstone Study (1981). Chenodiol (chenodeoxycholic acid) for dissolution of gallstones: The National Cooperative Gallstone Study. *Ann. Intern. Med.*, **95**, 257–282
2. Admirand, W. H. and Small, D. M. (1968). The physicocochemical basis of cholesterol gallstone formation in man. *J. Clin. Invest.*, **47**, 1043–1052
3. Carey, M. C. and Small, D. M. (1978). The physical chemistry of cholesterol solubility in bile. Relationship to gallstone formation and dissolution in man. *J. Clin. Invest.*, **61**, 998–1026
4. Metzger, A. L., Adler, R. A., Heymsfield, S. and Grundy, S. M. (1973). Diurnal variation in biliary lipid composition: possible role in cholesterol gallstone formation. *N. Engl. J. Med.*, **288**, 333–336
5. Mok, H. Y. I., von Bergmann, K. and Grundy, S. M. (1978). Factors affecting bile saturation at low outputs of bile acids. In Paumgartner, G., Stiehl, A. and Gerok, W. (eds.) *Biological Effects of Bile Acids*. pp. 39–51. (Lancaster: MTP Press)
6. Mok, H. Y. I., von Bergmann, K. and Grundy, S. M. (1978). Effects of interruption of enterohepatic circulation on biliary lipid secretion in man. *Am. J. Dig. Dis.*, **23**, 1067–1075
7. Sedaghat, A. and Grundy, S. M. (1980). Cholesterol crystals and the formation of cholesterol gallstones. *N. Engl. J. Med.*, **302**, 1274–1277
8. Sedaghat, A., Kesaniemi, Y. A. and Grundy, S. M. (1983). Cholesterol crystals – a crucial link in the formation of cholesterol gallstones. In Paumgartner, G. Stiehl, A. and Gerok, W. (eds.) *Bile Acids and Cholesterol in Health and Disease*. (Lancaster: MTP Press)
9. Burnstein, M. J., Ilson, R. G., Petrunka, C. N., Taylor, R. D. and Strasberg, S. M. (1983). Evidence for a potent nucleating factor in the gallbladder bile of patients with cholesterol gallstones. *Gastroenterology*, **85**, 801–807
10. Bennion, L. J. and Grundy, S. M. (1975). Effects of diabetes mellitus on cholesterol metabolism in man. *J. Clin. Invest.*, **56**, 996–1011
11. Grundy, S. M., Metzger, A. I. and Alder, R. D. (1972). Mechanisms of lithogenic bile formation in American Indian women with cholesterol gallstones. *J. Clin. Invest.*, **51**, 3026–3043
12. Bennion, L. J., Ginsberg, R. L., Garnick, M. B. and Bennett, P. H. (1976). Effects of oral contraceptives on the gallbladder bile of normal women. *N. Engl. J. Med.*, **294**, 189–192
13. Nilsson, S. and Stattin, S. (1967). Gallbladder emptying during the normal menstrual cycle: a cholecystographic study. *Acta. Chir. Scand.*, **133**, 648–652
14. Sampliner, R. E., Bennett, P. H., Comess, I. H., Rose, F. A. and Burch, T. A. (1970). Gallbladder disease in Pima Indians. *N. Engl. J. Med.*, **283**, 1358–1364
15. Heaton, K. W. and Read, A. E. (1969). Gallstones in patients with disorders of the terminal ileum and distributed bile salt metabolism. *Br. Med. J.*, **3**, 494–496
16. Rovsing, H. and Sloth, K. (1973). Micro gallbladder and biliary calculi in mucoviscidosis. *Acta Radiol.*, **14**, 588–592
17. Roy, C. C., Weber, A. M. and Morin, C. L. (1977). Abnormal biliary lipid composition in cystic fibrosis: Effects of pancreatic enzymes. *N. Engl. J. Med.*, **297**, 1301–1305
18. Grundy, S. M., Ahrens, E. H. Jr., Salen, G., Schreibman, P. H. and Nestel, P. J. (1972). Mechanisms of action of clofibrate on cholesterol metabolism in patients with hyperlipidemia. *J. Lipid Res.*, **13**, 531–551
19. Grundy, S. M. and Mok, H. Y. I. (1977). Colestipol, clofibrate and phytosterols in combined therapy of hyperlipidemia. *J. Lab. Clin. Med.*, **89**, 354–366
20. Pertsemlidis, D., Panveliwalla, D. and Ahrens, E. H. Jr. (1974). Effects of clofibrate and of an esterogen–progestin combination on fasting biliary lipids and cholic acid kinetics in man. *Gastroenterology*, **66**, 565–573
21. von Bergmann, K., Fierer, J., Mok, H. Y. I. and Grundy, S. M. (1981). Effects of rifampin on biliary lipids in man. *Antimicrobial Agents Chemother.*, **19**, 342–345

10
Classification and pathogenesis of pigment gallstones

R. D. SOLOWAY and P. F. MALET

ABSTRACT

Pigment gallstones contain a variety of insoluble calcium salts. Calcium bilirubinate is usually the major component while cholesterol accounts for less than 50% by weight. There are two types of pigment stones, identifiable by epidemiological, clinical, morphological and compositional features. The pathogenesis of each is conjectural. Black stones have a glass-like featureless appearance on fracturing. They form in the gallbladder and do not recur after cholecystectomy. They are found in 60–80% of patients with haemolysis, but are usually found in the general population in elderly, thin patients without haemolysis. Calcium phosphate and carbonate are frequently also present and may predominate. The remainder consists primarily of a protein network, mostly glycoprotein, which may slowly trap and interdigitate with a network of microcrystalline calcium salts. Brown stones have a rough surface and on cross-section demonstrate alternating brown and tan layers containing predominantly calcium bilirubinate and calcium salts of fatty acids respectively. Glycoproteins are much less prominent. Brown stones are associated with stasis, bacterial infection and parasites, whereas black stones are found in sterile bile. The female:male ratio for both types is 1.25:1. In the West, brown stones usually form in the common duct, more than a year after cholecystectomy for cholesterol or black stones. In the Orient, brown stones form *de novo* anywhere within the biliary tract and are the major cause of intrahepatic stones, cholangiohepatitis and liver failure. They are believed to form by rapid non-crystalline precipitation of calcium salts of bilirubin and fatty acids following enzymatic hydrolysis of bilirubin glucuronide and lecithin. These enzymes could originate from bacteria and/or from damaged biliary epithelium. Thus, aside from being pigmented and containing calcium bilirubinate, there are no common features in the pathogenesis of black and brown pigment stones, and they form in mutually exclusive circumstances.

The epidemiological data presently available support the hypothesis that the conditions under which pigment stones form are not only separate from those for cholesterol stones but prevent the simultaneous formation of cholesterol stones. Similarly the conditions for formation of the two subtypes of pigment stones – black and brown stones – preclude simultaneous formation of the other. This presentation will provide a classification of pigment stones and summarize the available chemical, structural and epidemiological data, all of which support the above hypotheses.

CLASSIFICATION

Pigment stones contain a variety of insoluble calcium salts[1,2]. Calcium bilirubinate is usually the major component but other salts are almost always present and may predominate; these salts include carbonate, phosphate and a variety of fatty acids, predominantly palmitate. Cholesterol accounts for less than 50% and usually less than 20% of stone weight. The two types of pigment stones are identifiable by epidemiological, clinical, morphological and compositional features. The pathogenesis of each type is, at present, conjectural.

Black pigment stones are black to deep brown in colour. The surface is irregular and on fracturing black stones have a glass-like, featureless appearance. They form predominantly in the gallbladder and very rarely recur after cholecystectomy. They were first identified in patients with haemolysis or cirrhosis but are usually found in thin, elderly patients without a predisposing disease. This type of stone contains calcium salts of bilirubinate, carbonate and phosphate. The remainder of the stone consists chiefly of proteins, primarily mucin glycoproteins[3], which may slowly trap and interdigitate with a network of crystalline calcium salts[4].

Brown stones are much softer and have a rough flaky surface. On cross-section they demonstrate alternating brown and tan layers. The brown layers contain non-crystalline calcium bilirubinate while the tan layers contain primarily calcium salts of fatty acids resembling the fatty acid composition of biliary lecithin. The glycoprotein content of these stones is less prominent. Such stones form throughout the biliary tract and recur frequently after cholecystectomy and/or sphincteroplasty. Brown stones are associated with stasis and infection[5] while black stones are found in sterile bile[6]. In Western countries brown stones usually form within the common bile duct more than a year after cholecystectomy[7]. In contrast, in the Orient, brown stones can form anywhere within the biliary tract and are the predominant cause of intrahepatic stones and cholangiohepatitis[8]. They are believed to form by rapid, episodic non-crystalline precipitation of calcium salts following bacterial enzymatic hydrolysis in bile of bilirubin diglucuronide and lecithin.

CHEMICAL FEATURES

Both black and brown stones have a wide variety of composition from patient to patient (Table 1). However, within a set of stones from a single patient the composition and cross-sectional picture is remarkably similar[9], indicating that conditions for stone formation were the same throughout the gallbladder

Table 1 Features of black and brown pigment gallstones[2]

Clinical associations	*Black*	*Brown*
Incidence increases with age	Yes	Yes
Female predominance	Yes	Yes
Haemolysis and/or cirrhosis	Yes	No
Low-protein diet	No	Yes
Bacterial infection in bile	Uncommonly	Nearly 100%
Recurrent stones	Uncommonly	Quite frequently
Location in biliary tree	Usually limited to gallbladder	Intra- and extrahepatic ducts and gallbladder
Morphology	Black to brown, 50% amorphous, remainder crystalline	Brown, laminated
Radiodensity	50% opaque	Lucent
Major stone components (% dry weight = mean (range))		
Calcium bilirubinate	34% (9–80%)	63% (28–79%)
Calcium palmitate	Rarely present	15 (12–67)
Calcium phosphate	6 (0–32)	0.1 (0–0.8)
Calcium carbonate	9 (0–41)	Rarely present
Cholesterol	3 (1–11)	11 (2–28)
Bile salts	1 (0.1–5)	1 (0.1–5)
Unmeasured	39 (10–67)	0 (0–31)

and that conditions for stone formation varied during stone growth but these variations occurred uniformly throughout the gallbladder. In 2–5% of cases cholesterol and brown and black stones can occur in layers[10]; when this occurs all stones in a gallbladder have the same cross-sectional composition. The nidation process for pigment stones is separate from that of cholesterol stones even though the centres of cholesterol stones are darker than the periphery. The centres of most cholesterol stones, when examined using scanning electron microscopy, demonstrated stacks of cholesterol crystals and only three of more than 200 cholesterol stones had a centre resembling the glass-like configuration of the black stones or the microcrystalline rod-like structure of calcium salts. In most cholesterol stones, calcium salts account for less than 10% of stone content in the centre or in pigmented rings seen on cross-section. In these stones the calcium salts appear to be incorporated into the cholesterol crystals since structures seen in pigment stones are not identified.

CLINICAL FEATURES

Black stones have been identified in increased incidence in patients with congenital haemolytic anaemias, alcoholic cirrhosis and following insertion of prosthetic mechanical heart valves. Most black stones occur in elderly patients, who are less than 100 % of ideal body weight and who have no other discernible illness[10]. Since black pigment stones are difficult to identify clinically, epidemiological studies have not been possible, except in retrospective studies of consecutive patients who have undergone biliary tract surgery. In a study in Philadelphia[10], 92 patients were examined and 27 % had pigment stones. There was a slight female predominance, 1.25:1, which has been confirmed in Japanese studies[11]. Patients with black stones were significantly older than those with cholesterol stones, so that between the ages of 70 and 90 more than 50 % of those coming to surgery had black stones. Only two patients in the Philadelphia study[10] had layered stones.

A discriminant analysis based on clinical and radiographic features was developed, which seemed to be quite accurate when prospectively applied to two other groups of patients[12]. The important features of this formula that favoured pigment stones included: (1) calcification of the stone centre, (2) less than 10 stones present within the gallbladder, (3) the presence of an irregular stone surface, (4) the absence of floating stones on oral cholecystography, (5) an average stone diameter equal to or less than 6 mm, (6) the presence of whole stone calcification, (7) the absence of rim calcification and (8) a Caucasian patient. The presence of buoyancy was the only feature absolutely eliminating pigment stones but was present in only 20 % of cholesterol stones. This feature may not apply in areas with a high incidence of brown stones since brown stones may float.

EPIDEMIOLOGICAL FEATURES

Data have been derived exclusively from operative series since there is no non-invasive means of positively identifying pigment stones. The operative incidence of both brown and black stones varies with geographical location and is quite different for the two types. Black stones vary from 27 %[10] to 5 % in the United States and averaged 15 % in the National Cooperative Gallstone Study, if 50 % of the stones had been eliminated by the admission requirement for stone radiolucency[13]. None of these series contained brown gallbladder stones. In India, black stones occur in 33 % and brown stones in 9 %[14]. In Indian populations in the western hemisphere the incidence of non-cholesterol stones is low. In a population containing a high proportion of Indians in La Paz, Bolivia, there were no pigment stones in 132 consecutive patients undergoing cholecystectomy for cholelithiasis[14]. In Japan[11] the operative incidence of black stones is 9 % and of brown stones is 16 %. Black stones show no difference between urban and rural populations but brown stones are more common in rural hospitals (17 %) than in urban hospitals (10 %)[11]. Since the late 1940s in Japan, where repeated surgical series have been collected, the incidence of brown stones has been decreasing while the incidence of cholesterol stones has been increasing. In contrast, the incidence of black stones has been constant.

CHEMICAL–STRUCTURAL FEATURES

Black stones contain calcium salts of bilirubinate, carbonate and phosphate[15]. Despite chemical and physical behaviour that suggests the presence of a bilirubin polymer in these stones[16,17] none has been identified and the only identifiable pigment on stone dissolution using direct diazotization with ethyl anthranilate is the α_0 pigment representing one half of the unconjugated bilirubin molecule[18]. Exposure of these stones to an oxygen plasma (O^-) atmosphere leads to oxidation of the organic components and retention of the calcium salts. Serial scanning electron photomicrographs demonstrate an interconnecting network of crevasses, indicating the location of the glycoprotein network which interdigitates with a network of calcium salts. Fracture sections of stones with exposure of the resultant surface to argon etching have demonstrated rod-like structures in stones containing solely calcium phosphate[4]. These structures can also be examined by point analysis using electron scanning for chemical analysis and have been found to be 400–800 Å microcrystals of calcium bilirubinate (by inference) and calcium phosphate (by identification)[9]. Mucin glycoproteins have recently been demonstrated to account for a large proportion of the protein in black stones[3]. In turn, protein accounts for the majority of the macromolecular components in these stones.

In contrast, brown stones demonstrate no distinct organic network on exposure to an oxygen plasma; instead the stones tend to crumble. The glycoprotein content is much lower than in black stones. Calcium phosphate is present in very small amounts and calcium carbonate cannot be identified. Argon etching with repeated scanning electron photomicrographs fails to demonstrate microcrystalline calcium bilirubinate[4].

Thus, from all aspects, brown and black pigment stones appear to have a separate pathogenesis and pattern of growth. The tendency to form one type of stone excludes simultaneous formation of the other type. Black stones seem to form slowly in the gallbladder where gallbladder mucin serves as a matrix, perhaps within the gallbladder glands, for stone nidation and early growth. The stone is eventually extruded into the gallbladder lumen. Recurrence of these stones is prevented by cholecystectomy despite continuing episodic severe haemolysis such as in patients with sickle cell disease. Brown stones appear to form rapidly, with repeated cyclic layering of calcium bilirubinate or calcium salts of fatty acids produced by hydrolysis of biliary components. Whether the phospholipidases and the β-glucuronidases responsible for formation of these products are of bacterial or of biliary epithelial origin is a question under current debate. Further knowledge of the natural history and pathogenesis of these conditions will lead to more direct management and perhaps prevention.

Acknowledgments

The authors wish to thank Ms Elizabeth Garrett for expert secretarial assistance. This work was supported by NIH grant AM 16549.

References

1. Soloway, R. D., Trotman, B. W. and Ostrow, J. D. (1977). Progress in gastroenterology, pigment gallstones. *Gastroenterology*, **72**, 167–182
2. Trotman, B. W. and Soloway, R. D. (1982). Pigment gallstone disease: summary of the National Institutes of Health International Workshop. *Hepatology*, **2**, 879–884
3. Lamont, J. T., Ventola, A. S., Trotman, B. W. and Soloway, R. D. (1983). Mucin glycoprotein content of human pigment gallstones. *Hepatology*, **3**, 377–382
4. Malet, P. F., Takabayashi, A., Trotman, B. W., Soloway, R. D. and Weston, N. E. (1984). Black and brown pigment gallstones differ in microstructure and microcomposition. *Hepatology*, **4**, 227–234
5. Tabata, M. and Nakayama, F. (1981). Bacteria and gallstone: etiological significance. *Dig. Dis. Sci.*, **26**, 218–224
6. Goodhart, G. L., Levison, M. E., Trotman, B. W. and Soloway, R. D. (1978). Pigment vs cholesterol cholelithiasis. Bacteriology of gallbladder stone, bile and tissue correlated with biliary lipid analysis. *Am. J. Dig. Dis.*, **23**, 877–882
7. Malet, P. F., Huang, G., Long, W. B., Trotman, B. W. and Soloway, R. D. (1982). The post-cholecystectomy interval influences the composition of common bile duct gallstones. *Hepatology*, **2**, 843 (abstract)
8. Nagase, M., Hikasa, Y., Soloway, R. D., Tanimura, H., Setoyama, M. and Kato, H. (1980). Gallstones in Western Japan. Factors affecting the prevalence of intrahepatic gallstones. *Gastroenterology*, **78**, 684–690
9. Trotman, B. W., Ostrow, J. D., Soloway, R. D., Cheong, E. B. and Longyear, R. B. (1974). Pigment vs cholesterol cholelithiasis: comparison of stone and bile composition. *Am. J. Dig. Dis.*, **19**, 585–590
10. Trotman, B. W. and Soloway, R. D. (1975). Pigment vs cholesterol cholelithiasis: clinical and epidemiological aspects. *Am. J. Dig. Dis.*, **20**, 735–740
11. Hikasa, Y., Nagase, M., Soloway, R. D., Tanimura, H., Setoyama, M. and Kato, H. (1981). Gallstones in Western Japan. Epidemiologic factors affecting the type and location of gallstones. *Arch. Jap. Chir.*, **50**, 272–288
12. Dolgin, S. M., Schwartz, J. S., Kressel, H. Y., Soloway, R. D., Miller, W. T., Trotman, B. W., Soloway, A. S. and Good, L. I. (1981). Identification of patients with cholesterol or pigment gallstones using discriminant analysis of radiographic features. *N. Engl. J. Med.*, **304**, 808–811
13. Schoenfield, L. J., Lachin, J. M., and the Steering Committee for the National Cooperative Gallstone Study (1981). Chenodiol (chenodeoxycholic acid) for the dissolution of gallstones: The National Cooperative Gallstone Study. *Ann. Intern. Med.*, **95**, 257–282
14. Soloway, R. D., Takabayashi, A., Rios-Dalenz, J., Nakayama, R., Tandon, R. K., Trotman, B. W. and Henson, D. E. (1981). Geographic differences in the operative incidence and type of pigment gallstones and in the noncholesterol components of cholesterol gallstones. *Hepatol. Rapid Lit. Rev.*, **11**, 1637–1638
15. Trotman, B. W., Morris, T. A. III, Sanchez, H. M., Soloway, R. D. and Ostrow, J. D. (1977). Pigment vs cholesterol cholelithiasis. Identification and quantification by infrared spectroscopy. *Gastroenterology*, **72**, 495–498
16. Black, B. F., Carr, S. H., Ohkubo, H. and Ostrow, J. D. (1982). Equilibrium swelling of pigment gallstones: evidence for a network polymer structure. *Biopolymers*, **21**, 601–610
17. Zilm, K. W., Grant, D. M., Englert, E. E. Jr *et al.* (1980). The use of solid ^{13}C nuclear magnetic resonance for the characterization of cholesterol and bilirubin pigment composition of human gallstones. *Biochem. Biophys. Res. Commun.*, **93**, 857–866
18. Soloway, R. D., Trotman, B. W., Yu, J. M., Malet, P. F. and Falk, H. (1983). Unconjugated bilirubin is quantitatively the predominant pigment in pigment gallstones. *Hepatology*, **3**, 836 (abstract)
19. Malet, P. F., Williamson, C., Trotman, B. W. and Soloway, R. D. (1982). Cross-sectional microstructure and composition of cholesterol gallstones identify the distribution of calcium salts. *Hepatology*, **2**, 743 (abstract)

11
Epidemiological and biochemical aspects of an important sequel to cholelithiasis: gallbladder cancer

B. L. STROM

INTRODUCTION

The clinical presentation of patients with gallbladder cancer is similar to that of those suffering from the more common pancreatic cancer. The prognosis is similarly poor. Cancer of the gallbladder is known to vary widely in incidence[1]. It is more common in certain Latin American countries than in North American countries; more common in the southwest, north central, and Appalachian regions than other regions of the USA; more common in women than in men; and more common in Indians than whites, but lower in blacks than either of the other groups[2]. A recent paper[3] reported the incidence of gallbladder cancer as five times more frequent in La Paz, Bolivia, than in the USA. This higher incidence could not be explained by differences in the age or sex distribution of the two populations, and was only partially explained by differences in racial composition. Inasmuch as gallbladder cancer rarely occurs in the absence of cholelithiasis, some authors have suggested that routine cholecystectomy might be considered when gallstones are discovered, simply as prophylaxis against gallbladder cancer[1,4]. Other papers in this symposium describe, in detail, the epidemiology of cholelithiasis. In this paper the epidemiology of this very serious sequel of cholelithiasis will be discussed, especially as to the degree that it provides clues to the disease's aetiology. The literature on gallbladder carcinoma comprises case reports, case series, descriptive epidemiological studies, analyses of secular trends, and experimental animal studies, all of which are useful in generating hypotheses about disease aetiology. Analytical epidemiological studies are notably lacking. The available data will be reviewed. In addition, some intriguing biochemical clues to its aetiology will be reviewed, as well as the approach currently under way to explore these clues in more detail.

DESCRIPTIVE EPIDEMIOLOGY

The incidence of biliary tract cancer shows enormous world-wide variation[1,5]. In 1978 the disease accounted for 2469 US deaths, representing approximately 0.3 % and 1.0 % of all cancer deaths in men and women, respectively[6]. It was the fifth most common gastrointestinal malignancy in the USA[7,8]. In contrast, Chile has the highest gallbladder cancer mortality rate in the world[9,10]. Cancers of the gallbladder and biliary ducts accounted for 5.25 % of *all* cancer deaths in Chile in 1975, making it that nation's fourth leading cause of cancer mortality. The age-adjusted mortality rate for cancer of the biliary tract in women in Santiago is 9.0 per 100 000 population. As another example, in Mexico City, where it is the fourth most frequently occurring malignancy in women, the corresponding rate is 8.5[11]. These international variations have resulted in many hypotheses as to aetiology.

Geographical variations in biliary tract cancer mortality have also been noted within the USA, with elevated rates clustered in its southwest, Appalachian, and north-central regions[2]. While the Indian/Spanish composition of the southwestern US population is believed to account for that cluster, and the general increased incidence of gallbladder disease in Appalachia may be related to the elevated mortality from gallbladder disease there[12], no explanation has been offered for the north-central clustering. The incidence of malignant neoplasms of the biliary tract has also been noted to vary by age, sex and race.

Marked differences among the epidemiology of cancers of the gallbladder, extrahepatic bile ducts, ampulla of Vater, and other upper gastrointestinal malignancies suggest that these are independent disease entities. The sex and racial distributions of these cancers are different. Whereas gallbladder cancer has a striking female preponderance, ranging from 1.7 to 10:1, the cancers of the ampulla of Vater, pancreas and liver all have a male preponderance (3:1, 1.6–5:1 and 2–4:1, respectively)[7–9,13–30]. Cancer of the extrahepatic bile ducts has a variable sex ratio, but is usually more common in males. Populations which have been identified as having an increased incidence of gallbladder cancer include: American Indian women and Spanish-American women in the southwestern USA and Latin America[1,5,31,32]; Japanese women in Japan[30]; African Rhodesian women[2]; European immigrant women in Israel[29]; and northern Europeans[5]. Gallbladder cancer is the most common gastrointestinal malignancy among the American Indians of the southwest[33]. Low rates have been observed among: South African Bantus[2]; Nigerians[2]; New Zealand Maoris[2]; and Chinese natives and immigrants[30]. In contrast, high rates of pancreatic cancer have been observed in the Maoris of New Zealand, native Hawaiians and black Americans; high rates of liver cancer have been noted in Asia; and high rates of extrahepatic bile duct cancer have been found in Japanese Hawaiians[7,8,11,34–38]. In general, these are all considered to be diseases of the elderly[5,7,8,14,15,18–21,24–28,34,39].

A recently published report based on data from the La Paz, Bolivia Tumor Registry confirmed the female predilection of both gallbladder cancer and cholelithiasis (2:1 and 2.3:1 females:males, respectively). In contrast to some prior findings, cancer of the extrahepatic bile ducts also showed a female preponderance[3]. Compared to the USA, an increased age- and sex-adjusted incidence of gallbladder carcinoma was found for all racial groups, with Indians having the highest rates, mestizos having intermediate rates, and whites having the lowest rates. There was a greater incidence of gallbladder cancer than cancer of the extrahepatic bile ducts within each of the three racial groups. This contrasts with data from other centres which have shown equal incidence rates for these cancers. Yet carcinoma of the gallbladder was most common in women aged 50–59 and men over age 70, and was rarely observed before the age of 40, while surgery for cholelithiasis was most frequently seen in patients aged 30–39. It thus appeared that if gallbladder cancer is related to the presence of gallstones there must be a 20–30-year delay in the clinical onset of cancer. Ninety-two per cent of gallbladder cancer patients also had gallstones. However, because the presence of gallstones in patients with extrahepatic bile duct cancer was not recorded, it was not possible to compare stone frequency among patients with both types of cancer.

As independent diseases, each of these cancers may possess its own set of risk factors. The failure of prior studies to explore these is largely due to the fact that, until recently, the International Classification of Diseases classified these diseases together instead of separately (e.g., as 'cancer of the biliary tract'). In another recent study data on the incidence of cancers of the gallbladder, extrahepatic bile duct and ampulla of the Vater were obtained from ten cancer registries in the USA, Canada, Europe and Asia[40]. Using log–linear modelling the authors confirmed that women are at higher risk of acquiring gallbladder cancer than men, men are at higher risk of acquiring cancer of the ampulla of Vater than women, but that men and women are equally likely to acquire cancer of the extrahepatic biliary tract. The incidence of all three diseases increased dramatically with age. Even after controlling for interactions between age, sex and disease, the risk of acquiring each of the three types of extrahepatic biliary tract cancer varied differently by geographical location. All of these epidemiological differences lend more support to the idea that these are different diseases.

ANALYTICAL EPIDEMIOLOGY

With one exception there is a conspicuous absence of controlled human studies which would enable us to test specific hypotheses and draw causal inferences about presumptive aetiological factors. While the aetiology of gallbladder cancer remains obscure, numerous risk factors have been postulated: advanced age; female sex; ethnicity; cholelithiasis[1,2,16,17,27–29,39,41–45]; pre-existing biliary tract disease[16,42,46]; bile stasis[14,23]; chronic inflammation of the gallbladder[16,25,46]; benign gallbladder neoplasms[1,23,42,47]; occupational exposures[1,48]; chemical carcinogens[48]; diet[31]; radiation[49]; and chronic mechanical irritation[23]. Geographical variation in the distribution of gallbladder cancer may reflect either genetic or cultural differences among populations[1]. A genetic gradient for the disease is suggested by a strikingly high incidence in North and South American Indian populations (e.g. Mexico and Bolivia), an intermediate incidence in racially mixed Latin American populations, and a low incidence among non-Indian populations in the USA and in European populations, including Spain. A cultural gradient for the disease is suggested by its high incidence in Latin American countries with a predominantly European heritage (e.g. Chile).

An excess of both gallbladder and other types of biliary tract cancers has been associated with occupation in the automotive and rubber industries[50], while an excess of gallbladder cancer has been reported in workers in the textile and metal industries[50]. An excess of other types of biliary tract cancer has been associated with occupation in the aircraft, chemical and wood-finishing industries[50]. Chemicals used in these particular occupations may be responsible for the excesses observed.

The possibility of a causal link between cholelithiasis and gallbladder cancer has been noted since 1924[44]. The fact that cholelithiasis has been observed in more than 80% of patients with gallbladder cancer[14,19,21,26,27,29,39,40,43,45,51] has led some investigators to speculate that gallstones may be important in the pathogenesis of gallbladder cancer or, alternatively, that risk factors for gallstones may likewise predispose to carcinoma. The one, very recent, case–control study conducted by a retrospective chart review even noted an association between size of gallstones and risk of gallbladder cancer[52]. However, other researchers have disagreed, feeling that there is no aetiological relationship between the two[53,54]. Attempts to induce gallbladder cancer in the laboratory using animal analogues to gallstones, particularly regarding chemical and/or mechanical irritation as possible aetiologies, have produced intriguing but inconclusive results[55–57]. Methylcholanthrene pellets implanted in cat, hamster and dog gallbladders[56,58,59]; human gallstones implanted in cat gallbladders[44]; and sterile, hard foreign bodies implanted in guinea pig gallbladders[55] have all induced malignant tumours. Similar results have been observed in hamsters implanted with cholesterol pellets and treated with dimethylnitrosamine[57], and dogs fed *o*-amino-azotoluene[60] and toxic levels of the insecticide Aramite, a mixture of 2-(*p*-tert-butylphenoxy)isopropyl-2-choloroethyl sulphite and bis-2-(*p*-tert-butylphenoxy)isopropyl sulphite[61]. However, these data can be considered consistent with a number of the previously mentioned mechanical and/or chemical aetiologies: stones, abnormal bile, etc. In addition, other investigators have been unable to induce cancer in similar animal experiments[62,63]. Finally, extrapolation of these animal data to humans and other animal species is, of course, difficult.

Other data pointing to a relationship between cholelithiasis and gallbladder cancer are that risk factors for cholelithiasis overlap to a certain extent with those for gallbladder and other types of biliary tract cancer. These overlapping risk factors include: advanced age[64]; female sex[64]; increasing parity[64–66]; ethnic predisposition (American Indian being the most susceptible)[12,67–70]; obesity[64,65,71–73]; dietary habits (particularly cholesterol, carbohydrate, fat and fibre intake)[74–76]; exogenous oestrogens[12,71,77–80]; clofibrate (which increases bile saturation while achieving its therapeutic goal of lowering serum cholesterol)[72,79,81,82]; gastrointestinal disorders (regional enteritis, ileal disorders and cystic fibrosis)[71,72,83-85]; immune deficiency[86]; haemolytic disease (sickle cell anaemia)[72]; and family history[87,88].

BIOCHEMICAL EPIDEMIOLOGY

Finally, biochemical factors have also been suggested as playing a role in the aetiology of biliary cancers. The biliary tract is continually exposed to bile, a complex combination of chemicals which have the potential to be quite toxic. Recently, bile and gallstone specimens have been obtained from four groups of Bolivian patients: patients with cancers of the gallbladder, cancers of the extrahepatic bile ducts, cholelithiasis, and normal biliary tracts. The specimens, along with others obtained from US patients, were analysed biochemically. The constituents of specimens from different countries and from patients with different diseases were compared. Biochemical differences were sought which would serve as clues to the aetiology of gallbladder cancer[89].

Twenty-two of the 24 Bolivian patients with gallbladder cancer were found also to have cholelithiasis. The gallstones of these 22 patients, and those of 82 Bolivian patients without cancer, were examined by infrared spectroscopy. Uniformly, their predominant constituent was cholesterol. This was in contrast to the group of US patients, 27% of whom had black pigment stones. In the US samples, bile lipid concentrations were similar in patients with cholelithiasis and normal controls. The mean lipid molar ratio of bile salts and phospholipids to cholesterol was also similar in the cholelithiasis patients and the normal controls (10.6* and 9.7*, respectively). In contrast, the bile from Bolivian patients with cholelithiasis was more dilute than both the bile from Bolivian controls and the US patients with cholelithiasis. The lipid ratio in the Bolivian stone patients was no different from that of Bolivian controls (13.0). However, because the bile was significantly more dilute, the lipid ratio in the Bolivian stone patients was much closer to the edge of the micellar zone and to cholesterol supersaturation than in the Bolivian controls. This is consistent with the predominance of cholesterol stones observed.

To examine other factors in bile which could result in modified cholesterol content, the bile specimens were also analysed for specific bile acid conjugates. Bile acids can be conjugated at the carboxyl group with either glycine or taurine, and can additionally be sulphated at the 3-alpha hydroxyl group. Both conjugations usually improve solubility. Sulphation usually increases solubility even further, although recent physicochemical studies[92] indicate that sodium sulphoglycolithocholate is no more soluble than glycolithocholate at 37 °C. Using high-performance liquid chromatography (HPLC), it was seen that there was an increase in the proportions of glycine and taurine conjugates of lithocholic acid in stones compared to their concentrations in bile. Thus, the precipitation of stones certainly does not seem to be secondary to excessive *de*conjugation. No differences were found

* A ratio of 10 is at the limit of cholesterol saturation in bile of normal concentration, i.e. containing 10% solids[90,91].

among the US study groups and the Bolivian controls in stone or bile concentrations of the conjugates of the major bile acids (cholic, chenodeoxycholic, deoxycholic, ursodeoxycholic and lithocholic acids). Similarly, no differences were found in the ratio of glycine conjugates to taurine conjugates[93]. In contrast, in Bolivian patients with cholelithiasis there was an increase in the secondary bile acids, deoxycholic and lithocholic acids. There were virtually no lithocholic acid conjugates in the biles of US patients, with or without gallstones, or in Bolivian controls, but there were significant concentrations of tauro- and glycolithocholic acids in the biles of Bolivian patients with gallstones and in patients with gallstones and cancer. Levels of glycolithocholic acid were increased in Bolivian patients with cholelithiasis and increased even further in patients with cholelithiasis and cancer. Thus, the large proportion of lithocholic acid in the patients' bile may predispose to gallstone formation, and such patients may have an increased susceptibility to cancer because their bile contains a large proportion of glycolithocholic acid, a known co-carcinogen[94].

Lithocholic acid is formed during the enteric portion of the enterohepatic circulation of chenodeoxycholic acid, by removal of the 7-alpha-hydroxyl group by bacterial 7-alpha-dehydroxylase. It appears in bile following passive reabsorption of a small fraction of lithocholate produced in the colon, which is followed by conjugation in the liver with either glycine or taurine in the liver. Now that chenodeoxycholic acid is commercially available as a pharmaceutical agent for dissolving cholesterol gallstones, this metabolism to lithocholic acid has raised concerns about its potential as a carcinogen, concerns which will be tested in the USA in a long-term post-marketing drug surveillance study[95].

The majority of lithocholic acid in man is present as sulphated lithocholic acid conjugates, rendering it more soluble and less toxic. Sulphation also allows increased excretion of lithocholic acid in the stool, by decreasing intestinal reabsorption. To investigate mechanisms by which large quantities of lithocholic acid might accumulate in the bile of Bolivian patients with cholelithiasis, the proportion of sulphated lithocholic acid conjugates to unsulphated conjugates was also examined[96]. It was found that virtually all of the glyco- and taurolithocholic acid in the bile of US and Bolivian controls and US patients with cholelithiasis was sulphated (96–100%). In contrast, Bolivian patients with cholelithiasis had a similar concentration of sulphates, but a lower proportion of sulphated lithocholic acid conjugates, as they had a higher concentration of glyco- and taurolithocholic acid. Bolivian cancer patients had a much lower concentration of sulphates as well as a lower proportion of sulphated conjugates. Thus, in addition to having more lithocholic acid, a toxic bile acid, Bolivian stone and cancer patients appeared to be less able to sulphate this to a less toxic form.

There are many possible causes for this. Increased colonic production of lithocholic acid is possible but unlikely, as lithocholic and deoxycholic acids are relatively poorly absorbed from the colon, comprising the majority of bile acids recovered from the stool of patients. Direct hepatic formation of lithocholic acid is possible, but has not been described in man. Inadequate hepatic sulphation of lithocholic acid conjugates[97] is also possible, perhaps resulting from a low concentration of the necessary enzyme in Bolivians with cholelithiasis. The alternative is an increased production of lithocholic acid due to bacterial dehydroxylation[98] of chenodeoxycholic acid in infected bile or in the small intestine, which usually does not contribute much to the body's lithocholic acid pool, leading to an increased concentration of lithocholic acid in the small intestine and, thus, increased small intestine reabsorption, even in the presence of large concentrations of other bile acids. It has been demonstrated that lithocholic acid was efficiently absorbed from the small intestine when fed orally to man. Bolivian patients may thus have an increased load of lithocholic acid presented to the liver, which may exceed the liver's sulphation capacity[99] and lead to secretion of unsulphated lithocholic acid in the bile. This would, in turn, continue to be reabsorbed by the small intestine. The proportions of chenodeoxycholic acid in the bile of US controls, US patients with cholelithiasis, and Bolivian controls were $41.7 \pm 4.2\,\%$ (SD), $42.5 \pm 3.6\,\%$ and $35.4 \pm 7.4\,\%$, respectively. The bile of Bolivian patients with cholelithiasis contained $27.4 \pm 5.9\,\%$ chenodeoxycholic acid and that of patients with cholelithiasis and cancer contained $28.7 \pm 5.6\,\%$. This lower concentration of chenodeoxycholic acid supports the hypothesis that, in these patients, an increased proportion of chenodeoxycholic acid in bile is converted to lithocholic acid by bacterial dehydroxylation. Since cholesterol stones were uniformly present, and these stones were not associated with clinically apparent infection[100], it is unlikely that the biles of these patients were infected. It is more likely that there was small intestinal overgrowth of bacteria, as has been noted in many tropical countries[97,101].

However, we must be cautious in drawing conclusions about disease aetiology from these data. First, the patients included may not be representative. Second, stone and bile specimens were obtained from only a minority of patients in the study. This raises the potential for biased patient selection if participation were related to any of the factors measured. Third, samples from the US patients and the Bolivian patients were not collected concurrently. Some of the variations in the findings could be due to other changes in biology and/or laboratory techniques over time. Finally, the sample sizes were small. For example, the authors could not differentiate statistically between the bile constituent concentrations in the Bolivian study groups, even though the mean concentrations differed considerably. Thus, they could not determine whether cancer patients are more like normals or more like cholelithiasis patients in their bile constituents.

Thus, this investigation raises interesting hypotheses, but can only be viewed as a preliminary study. What is needed is a much larger, longer, multicentre trial, more successful and systematic in obtaining specimens, which can look at demographic, environmental, genetic, clinical and biochemical risk factors, individually and in combination.

IMPLICATIONS

Cancers of the biliary tract provide a unique opportunity to combine biochemistry and epidemiology in the search for the aetiology of a cancer.

Different parts of the biliary tract are bathed in the same material, bile: a complex mixture of potentially toxic chemicals. Yet, significant differences in the epidemiology of these cancers have suggested that they are distinctive disease entities, each with its own respective sets of risk factors. Carcinoma of the gallbladder appears to be related to age, sex, race and geographical location, as well as to the presence, and probably the size, of gallstones. Cancers of other parts of the biliary tract differ greatly in their epidemiology. In one country with a high incidence of gallbladder cancer, pilot data reveal that gallstone patients seem to have different gallstone and bile constituents from gallstone patients without cancer, from US gallstone patients without cancer, and from US normals. In addition, those data reveal that gallstone patients have high levels of a toxic bile acid, and do not sulphate it as well to a non-toxic form.

These findings raise a large number of aetiological possibilities: demographic factors such as age and sex; race; diet; geography; environmental exposures, such as radiation and occupational exposures; and medical history (e.g. cholelithiasis, biliary infection). At this time there is insufficient evidence to exclude any of these possibilities.

In addition, these findings lead to a number of different hypotheses about mechanisms of carcinogenesis: genetic differences in the hepatic synthesis of bile constituents and/or in gallbladder concentrating function; dietary influences on different bile acid constituents; other environmental exposure(s) affecting bile acid constituents; bacterial overgrowth in the biliary tract and/or small intestine causing a breakdown or reabsorption of biliary lipids and/or chronic irritation; toxic bile acids creating irritation and a propensity to gallstones and tumour formation; and mechanical irritation from gallstones, especially in the presence of toxic bile acids.

Needless to say, it is not possible to address all of these hypotheses in a single study. Given the many variables which have been proposed as possible aetiologies on the basis of animal data, case reports, case series and analyses of secular trends, a systematic retrospective biochemically oriented case–control study is the next logical step in gallbladder cancer research. This design allows numerous factors to be investigated as potential risk factors and aetiological inferences to be derived on the basis of estimated relative risks. The results of such a study would enable one to more specifically characterize a population at increased risk for gallbladder cancer. The availability of bile and gallstone specimens for biochemical analysis and the development of technology to analyse bile acids and other cancer markers in serum, such as carcinoembryonic antigen, provide an opportunity to combine epidemiology and biochemistry in a collaborative study on these important and fascinating diseases. Such a study is currently under way, involving collaborators in La Paz, Bolivia; Mexico City, Mexico; and Philadelphia, Pennsylvania, USA.

Other studies would, of course, also be useful at this time. There is presently no evidence to support the premise that these diseases are genetically transmitted. Although disease incidence varies according to ethnic group, it is not known how much of this variation is due to genetic influences and how much is due to cultural influences. It would therefore be useful to conduct genetic studies in which detailed family histories could be analysed by a genetic epidemiologist. Detailed studies of familial aggregation of serum and other markers, comparing pedigrees to genetic models of heritability, might be useful later.

Similarly, diet should be investigated as a possible risk factor. Unfortunately, at present, there are no good specific dietary hypotheses towards which one could focus a dietary history. A detailed 24 h or 72 h dietary history would be difficult, expensive, and would be unlikely to be productive. It is likely, in fact, to be misleading, inasmuch as a cancer patient is likely to have changed his diet in the few months before admission to the hospital for surgery, and it is not realistic to expect to get good data on the diet ingested months or years before the date of the questionnaire. Better approaches would be either: (1) to get complete dietary histories on family members, as surrogates for long-term patient dietary histories, or (2) to get dietary histories on patients with incidentally found precursor lesions.

Thus, although a major public health concern in selected populations, little progress has been made on the early diagnosis and treatment of gallbladder cancer. Recent data have suggested that the disease is distinct from tumours of other gastrointestinal sites. With continued work, as outlined, it is hoped that progress can be made on the early diagnosis and, eventually, prevention of this disease. In the process, significant contributions may be made to understanding the process of carcinogenesis, in general.

References

1. Diehl, A. K. (1980). Epidemiology of gallbladder cancer: a synthesis of recent data. *J. Natl. Cancer Inst.*, **65**, 1209–1214
2. Fraumeni, J. F. (1975). Cancers of the pancreas and biliary tract: epidemiological considerations. *Cancer Res.*, **35**, 3437–3446
3. Rios-Dalenz, J., Takabayashi, A., Henson, D. E., Strom, B. L. and Soloway, R. D. (1983). Cancer of the extrahepatic biliary tract in Bolivia: epidemiology. *Int. J. Epidemiol.*, **12**, 156–160
4. Diehl, A. K. and Beral, V. (1981). Cholecystectomy and changing mortality from gallbladder cancer. *Lancet*, **2**, 187–189
5. Waterhouse, J., Muir, C., Correa, P. and Powell, J. (eds.) (1976). *Cancer Incidence in Five Continents*. IARC Scientific Publications No. 15. (Lyon: International Agency for Research on Cancer)
6. Cancer statistics (1978). *Ca-A Cancer Journal for Clinicians*, **20**, 17–32
7. Spiro, H. M. (1970). *Clinical Gastroenterology*. (New York: Macmillan)
8. Robbins, S. L. and Cotran, R. S. (1979). *Pathologic Basis of Disease*. 2nd Edn. (Philadelphia: W. B. Saunders)
9. Armijo, R. (1981). Descriptive epidemiology of cancer in Chile. 1973–1978. Paper presented at 3rd Symposium on Epidemiology and Cancer Registries in the Pacific Basin, 19–23 January
10. Armijo, R. (1978). The epidemiology of cancer in Chile. *National Cancer Institute Monograph*, **53**, 115–118
11. Puffer, R. R. and Griffith, G. W. (1967). *Patterns of Urban Mortality*. Science Publication No. 151. (Washington DC: Pan American Health Organization)
12. Richardson, J. D., Scutchfield, F. D., Proudfoot, W. H. and Benson, A. S. (1973). Epidemiology of gallbladder disease in all Appalachian community. *Health Service Report*, **88**, 241–246
13. Balaroutsos, C., Bastounis, E., Karamanakos, P. and Golematis, B. (1974). Primary carcinoma of the gallbladder: analysis of 22 cases. *Am. J. Surg.*, **40**, 605–608

14. Strauch, G. O. (1960). Primary carcinoma of the gallbladder. *Surgery*, **47**, 368–381
15. Piehler, J. M. and Crichlow, R. W. (1978). Primary carcinoma of the gallbladder. *Surg. Gynecol. Obstet.*, **147**, 929–942
16. Arner, O. and von Schreeb, T. (1959). Carcinoma of the gallbladder. *Acta Chir. Scand.*, **116**, 477–483
17. Bossart, P. A., Patterson, A. H. and Zintel, H. A. (1962). Carcinoma of the gallbladder. *Am. J. Surg.*, **103**, 366–369
18. Keill, R. H. and DeWeese, M. S. (1973). Primary carcinoma of the gallbladder. *Am. J. Surg.*, **125**, 726–729
19. Klein, J. B. and Finck, F. M. (1972). Primary carcinoma of the gallbladder. *Arch. Surg.*, **104**, 769–772
20. Litwin, M. S. (1967). Primary carcinoma of the gallbladder. *Arch. Surg.*, **95**, 236–240
21. Andrews, E. C., Bennett, D. E. and Arhelger, R. B. (1969). Carcinoma of the gallbladder. *Southern Med. J.*, **62**, 573–578
22. Moossa, A. R., Anagnosr, M., Hall, A. W., Moraldi, A. and Skinner, D. B. (1975). The continuing challenge of gallbladder cancer. *Am. J. Surg.*, **130**, 57–62
23. Solan, M. J. and Jackson, B. T. (1971). Carcinoma of the gallbladder – a clinical appraisal and review of 57 cases. *Br. J. Surg.*, **58**, 593–597
24. Shieh, C. J., Dunn, E. and Standard, J. E. (1981). Primary carcinoma of the gallbladder: a review of a 16-year experience with the Waterbury Hospital Health Center. *Cancer*, **47**, 996–1004
25. Perpetuo, M., Valdivieso, M., Heilbrun, L. K., Nelson, R. S., Cohnor, T. and Budery, G. P. (1978). National history study of gallbladder cancer. *Cancer*, **42**, 330–335
26. Thorbjarnarson, B. and Glenn, F. (1959). Carcinoma of the gallbladder. *Cancer*, **12**, 1009–1015
27. Black, W. C., Key, C. R., Carmany, T. B. and Herman, D. (1977). Carcinoma of the gallbladder in a population of Southwestern American Indians. *Cancer*, **39**, 1267–1279
28. Burdette, W. J. (1957). Carcinoma of the gallbladder. *Ann. Surg.*, **145**, 832–843
29. Hart, J., Shani, M. and Modan, B. (1972). Epidemiological aspects of gallbladder and biliary tract neoplasms. *Am. J. Public Health*, **62**, 36–39
30. Steiner, P. E. (1954). *Cancer: Race and Geography*. pp. 186–199. (Baltimore: Williams & Wilkins)
31. Bornstein, F. P. (1970). Gallbladder carcinoma in the Mexican population of the Southwestern United States. *Pathol. Microbiol.*, **35**, 189–191
32. Retchenbach, D. D. (1967). Autopsy incidence of diseases among Southwestern American Indians. *Arch. Pathol.*, **84**, 81–86
33. Rudolph, R., Coher, J. J. and Gascoigne, R. H. (1970). Biliary cancer among Southwestern American Indians. *Arizona Med.*, **27**, 1–4
34. Isselbacher, K. J., Adams, R. D., Braunwald, E., Petersdorf, R. G. and Wilson, J. D. (eds.) (1980). *Harrison's Principles of Internal Medicine*, 9th Edn. (New York: McGraw Hill)
35. Aoki, K. and Ogawa, H. (1978). Cancer of the pancreas. International mortality trends. *World Health Statistical Report*, 1978, **31**, 2–27
36. Berg, J. W. and Connely, R. R. (1979). Updating the epidemiologic data on pancreatic cancer. *Semin. Oncol.*, **6**, 275–283
37. Morgan, R. G. (1977). Progress report – cancer of the pancreas. *Gut*, **18**, 580–596
38. Anderson, A., Bergdahl, L. and van der Linden, W. (1977). Malignant tumors of the extrahepatic bile ducts. *Surgery*, **81**, 198–202
39. Chandler, J. J. and Fletcher, W. S. (1963). A clinical study of primary carcinoma of the gallbladder. *Surg. Gynecol. Obstet.*, **117**, 297–300
40. Strom, B. L., Hibberd, P. L., Soper, K. A., Stolley, P. D. and Nelson, W. L. (1984). Epidemiology of cancers of the extrahepatic biliary tract: international variations. (Submitted for publication)
41. Graham, E. A. (1931). The prevention of carcinoma of the gallbladder. *Ann. Surg.*, **93**, 317–322
42. Kazmierski, R. H. (1951). Primary adenocarcinoma of the gallbladder with intramural calcification. *Am. J. Surg.*, 248–250
43. Fortner, J. G. and Randall, H. T. (1961). On the carcinogenicity of human gallstones. *Surg. Forum*, **12**, 155–156

44. Leitch, A. (1924). Gallstones and cancer of the gallbladder: an experimental study. *Br. Med. J.*, **2**, 451–454
45. Warren, R. and Balch, F. G. (1940). Carcinoma of the gallbladder – the etiological role of gallstones. *Surgery*, **7**, 657–665
46. Polk, H. C. (1966). Carcinoma and the calcified gallbladder. *Gastroenterology*, **50**, 582–585
47. Shepard, V. D., Walters, W. and Dockerty, M. B. (1942). Benign neoplasms of the gallbladder. *Arch. Surg.*, **45**, 1–18
48. Mancuso, T. F. and Brennan, M. J. (1970). Epidemiological considerations of cancer of the gallbladder, bile ducts and salivary glands in the rubber industry. *J. Occup. Med.*, **12**, 333–341
49. Wellington, D. G., MacDonald, E. J. and Wolf, P. F. (1979). *Cancer Mortality: Environmental and Ethnic Factors*. pp. 215–219. (New York: Academic Press)
50. Krain, L. S. (1972). Gallbladder and extrahepatic bile duct carcinoma. Analysis of 1808 cases. *Geriatrics*, **27**, 111–117
51. Horowitz, A. and Rosensweig, J. (1960). Carcinoma of the gallbladder – a real hazard. *J. Am. Med. Assoc.*, **173**, 234–236
52. Diehl, A. K. (1983). Gallstone size and the risk of gallbladder cancer. *J. Am. Med. Assoc.*, **250**, 2323–2326
53. Deyman, H., Gerbarg, D. S., Kelly, J. H., Parker, S. and Singer, J. (1961). Are gallstones and gallbladder carcinoma related? *J. Am. Med. Assoc.*, **176**, 450–451
54. Parkash, O. (1975). On the relationship of cholelithiasis to carcinoma of the gallbladder and on the sex dependency of the carcinoma of the bile ducts. *Digestion*, **12**, 129–133
55. Petrov, N. N. and Krotkina, N. A. (1947). Experimental carcinoma of the gallbladder. *Ann. Surg.*, **125**, 241–248
56. Fortner, J. G. (1955). The experimental induction of primary carcinoma of the gallbladder. *Cancer*, **8**, 689–700
57. Kowalewski, K. and Todd, E. F. (1971). Carcinoma of the gallbladder induced in hamsters by insertion of cholesterol pellets and feeding dimethynitrosamine. *Proc. Soc. Exp. Biol. Med.*, **136**, 482–486
58. Bain, G. O., Allen, P. B. R., Silbermann, O. and Kowalewski, K. (1959). Induction in hamsters of biliary carcinoma by intracholecystic methylcholantrene pellets. *Cancer Res.*, **19**, 93–96
59. Fortner, J. G. and Leffall, L. D. (1961). Carcinoma of the gallbladder in dogs. *Cancer*, **14**, 1127–1130
60. Nelson, A. A. and Woodard, G. (1953). Tumors of the urinary bladder, gallbladder, and liver in dogs fed *o*-aminoazotoluene or p-Dimethylaminoazobenzene. *J. Natl. Cancer Inst.*, **13**, 1497–1501
61. Sternberg, S. S., Popper, H., Oser, B. and Oser, M. (1960). Gallbladder and bile duct adenocarcinomas in dogs after long term feeding of aramite. *Cancer*, **13**, 780–789
62. Burrows, H. (1932). An experimental inquiry into the association between gallstones and primary cancer of the gallbladder. *Br. J. Surg.*, **20**, 607–629
63. Zeppa, R. and Womack, N. A. Carcinoma of the gallbladder: attempt of experimental induction. *Southern Med. J.*, **50**, 1267–1271
64. Friedman, G. D., Kannel, W. B. and Dawber, T. R. (1966). The epidemiology of gallbladder disease: observations in the Framingham Study. *J. Chron. Dis.*, **19**, 273–292
65. Bernstein, R. A., Giefer, E. E. and Vieira, J. J., *et al.* (1977). Gallbladder disease. II. Utilization of the life-table method in obtaining clinically useful information. *J. Chron. Dis.*, **30**, 529–541
66. Nilsson, S. (1966). Gallbladder disease and sex hormones: a statistical study. *Acta Chir. Scand.*, **132**, 275–279
67. Devor, E. J. and Buechley, R. W. (1980). Gallbladder cancer in Hispanic New Mexicans. I. General population 1957–1977. *Cancer*, **45**, 1705–1712
68. Sampliner, R. E., Bennett, P. H., Comess, L. J., Rose, F. A. and Burch, T. A. (1970). Gallbladder disease in Pima Indians. Demonstration of high prevalence and early onset by cholecystography. *N. Engl. J. Med.*, **283**, 1358–1364
69. Small, D. M. and Rapo, S. (1970). Source of abnormal bile in patients with cholesterol gallstones. *N. Engl. J. Med.*, **283**, 53–57
70. Thistle, J. L. and Schoenfield, L. J. (1971). Lithogenic bile among young Indian women.

Lithogenic potential decreased with chenodeoxycholic acid. *N. Engl. J. Med.*, **284**, 177–181
71. Bismuth, H. and Malt, R. A. (1979). Current concepts in cancer. Carcinoma of the biliary tract. *N. Engl. J. Med.*, **301**, 704–706
72. Bennion, L. J. and Grundy, S. M. (1978). Risk factors for the development of cholelithiasis in man. *N. Engl. J. Med.*, **299**, 1221–1227
73. Williams, C. N. and Johnston, J. L. (1980). Prevalence of gallstones and risk factors in caucasian women in a rural Canadian community. *Can. Med. Assoc. J.*, **120**, 664–668
74. Sarles, H., Hauton, J., Planche, N. E., Lafont, H. and Gerolami, A. (1970). Diet, cholesterol gallstones and composition of bile. *Am. J. Dig. Dis.*, **15**, 251–260
75. Pomare, E. W., Heaton, K. W., Low-Beer, T. S. and Espiner, H. J. (1976). The effect of wheat bran upon bile salt metabolism and upon the lipid composition of bile in gallstone patients. *Am. J. Dig. Dis.*, **21**, 521–526
76. Venick, L. J., Kuller, L. H., Lohsoonthorn, P., Rycheck, R. R. and Redmond, C. K. (1980). Relationship between cholecystectomy and ascending colon cancer. *Cancer*, **45**, 392–395
77. Boston Collaborative Drug Surveillance Program (1973). Oral contraceptives and venous thromboembolic disease, surgically confirmed gallbladder disease, and breast tumors. *Lancet*, **1**, 1399–1404
78. Boston Collaborative Drug Surveillance Program (1974). Surgically confirmed gallbladder disease, venous thromboembolism and breast tumors in relation to postmenopausal estrogen therapy. *N. Engl. J. Med.*, **290**, 15–19
79. Coronary Drug Project Research Group (1977). Gallbladder disease as a side effect of drugs influencing lipid metabolism. *N. Engl. J. Med.*, **296**, 1185–1190
80. Stolley, P. D., Tonascia, J. A., Tockman, M. S., Sartwell, P. E., Rutledge, A. H. and Jacobs, M. P. (1975). Thrombosis with low-estrogen oral contraceptives. *Am. J. Epidemiol.*, **102**, 197–208
81. Hikasa, Y., Nagase, M., Soloway, R. D., Tanimura, H., Setoyama, M., Kato, H., Kobayashi, N., Mukhaihara, S., Kamata, T., Muruyama, K. and Miki, K. (1981). Gallstones in Western Japan: Epidemiologic factors affecting the type and location of gallstones. *Arch. Jpn. Chir.*, **59**, 272–288
82. Bateson, M. C., MacLean, D., Ross, P. E. and Bonchier, I. A. D. (1978). Clofibrate therapy and gallstone induction. *Am. J. Dig. Dis.*, **23**, 623–628
83. Heaton, K. W. and Read, A. E. (1969). Gallstones in patients with disorders of the terminal ileum and disturbed bile salt metabolism. *Br. Med. J.*, **3**, 494–496
84. Weber, A. M., Ray, C. C., Morin, C. L. and Lasalle, R. (1973). Malabsorption of bile acids in children with cystic fibrosis. *N. Engl. J. Med.*, **289**, 1001–1005
85. Sapala, M. A., Sapala, J. A., Soto, A. D. R. and Bouwman, D. L. (1979). Cholelithiasis following subtotal gastric resection with truncal vagotomy. *Surg. Gynecol. Obstet.*, **148**, 36–38
86. Diaz-Buxo, J. A., Hermans, P. E. and Elveback, L. R. (1975). Prevalence of cholelithiasis in idiopathic late-onset immunoglobulin deficiency. *Ann. Intern. Med.*, **82**, 213–214
87. Van der Linden, W. and Lindeloj, G. (1965). The familial occurrence of gallstone disease. *Acta Genet. Basel.*, **15**, 159–164
88. Danzinger, R. G., Gordon, H., Schoenfield, L. J. and Thistle, J. L. (1972). Lithogenic bile in siblings of young women with cholelithiasis. *Mayo Clin. Proc.*, **47**, 762–766
89. Rios-Dalenz, J., Takabayashi, A., Henson, D. E., Strom, B. L. and Soloway, R. D. (1984). Cancer of the gallbladder in Bolivia: suggestions concerning etiology. (Submitted for publication)
90. Soloway, R. D. and Schoenfield, L. J. (1975). Effects of meals and interruption of the enterohepatic circulation on flow, lipid composition and cholesterol saturation of bile in man after cholecystectomy. *Am. J. Dig. Dis.*, **20**, 99–109
91. Wagner, C. I., Trotman, B. W. and Soloway, R. D. (1976). Kinetic analysis of biliary lipid excretion in man and dog. *J. Clin. Invest.*, **57**, 473–477
92. Carey, M. C., Wu, S-F. J. and Watkins, J. B. (1979). Solubility properties of sulfated monohydroxy bile salts. Relative insolubility of the disodium salt of glycolithocholate sulfate. *Biochem. Biophys. Acta*, **575**, 16–26
93. Takabayashi, A., Watkins, J. B., Soloway, R. D. and Trotman, B. W. (1980). The distribution of bile acids in cholesterol gallstones reflects co-precipitation or binding affinity as well as solubility. *Gastroenterology*, **79**, 1058–1059

94. Takabayashi, A., Watkins, J. B., Soloway, R. D., Rios-Dalenz, J. and Henson, D. E. (1980). Glycolithocholic acid is greatly increased in stones from patients with carcinoma of the gallbladder. *Gastroenterology*, **79**, 1059
95. Strom, B. L., Carson, J. L., Morse, M. L. and Soper, K. A. (1984). A novel approach to a long term post-marketing surveillance study, using Medicaid billing data. *Clin. Pharmacol. Ther.*, **35**, 278
96. Takabayashi, A., Balistreri, W. F., Watkins, J. B., Soloway, R. D., Rios-Dalenz, J. and Henson, D. W. (1981). Sulfation of lithocholic acid is incomplete in Bolivian patients with cholelithiasis and cancer of the gallbladder. *Gastroenterology*, **80**, 1352
97. Gorbach, S. L., Banwell, J. G., Jacobs, B., Chatterjee, B. D., Mitra, R., Sen, N. N. and Guha Mazumder, D. N. (1970). Tropical sprue and malnutrition in West Bengal. I. Intestinal microflora and absorption. *Am. J. Clin. Nutr.*, **23**, 1545
98. Hofmann, A. F. (1976). The enterohepatic circulation of bile in man. In Stollerman, G. H. (ed.) *Advances in Internal Medicine*. Vol. 21, pp. 501–534. (Chicago: Yearbook Medical Publishers)
99. Cowen, A. E., Korman, M. G., Hofmann, A. F. and Cass, O. W. (1975). Metabolism of lithocholate in healthy man. *Gastroenterology*, **69**, 59–66
100. Goodheart, G. L., Levison, M. E., Trotman, B. W. and Soloway, R. D. (1978). Pigment vs cholesterol cholelithiasis: bacteriology of gallbladder stones, bile and tissue correlated with biliary lipid analysis. *Am. J. Dig. Dis.*, **23**, 777–882
101. Mathan, V. I. (1973). Tropical sprue. In Sleisenger, M. H. and Fordtran, J. S. (eds.) *Gastrointestinal Disease. Pathophysiology, Diagnosis and Management*. pp. 978–988. (Philadelphia: W. B. Saunders)

12

Relationships between serum lipids and cholelithiasis: observations in the GREPCO study

M. ANGELICO and the GREPCO Group*

The association between coronary heart disease (CHD) and gallstone disease (GD) has been a matter of much controversy over recent decades[1,2]. Due to the high prevalence of both diseases in the free-living population, the coexistence of CHD and GD is relatively easily observed. However, demonstration of a real association based on epidemiological data is lacking[3], as it requires screening of population samples too large to be examined with objective diagnostic procedures.

One indirect way to predict the association between CHD and GD could be to find at least some common risk factors. Several conditions are suspected to be risk factors in the development of GD, but very few so far have been substantiated by prospective epidemiological studies. On the other hand, the risk factors for CHD are fairly well known and, among these, there is no question that serum lipids play a central role[4].

A number of clinical and experimental studies have supported the existence of a connection between the metabolism of plasma lipoprotein lipids and the development of cholesterol gallstones[5–8]. The exact nature of this connection, however, is not yet understood. We therefore reasoned that measuring serum lipid levels during an epidemiological survey primarily aimed at detecting GD in a free-living female population would probably have enabled us to confirm or refute the existence of a metabolic basis for a positive association between CHD and GD.

The results shown here indicate not only that one of the major risk factors for CHD, such as serum cholesterol, is not elevated among GD women, but also that serum cholesterol levels are inversely related to gallstones in a multiple logistic regression analysis.

* For the composition of the Group see p. xi

METHODS

The data reported in this paper are part of an extensive study on the epidemiology of GD and its related factors carried out in 1081 women, aged 20–64 years, employed in a public administration agency in Rome, Italy. Each woman was asked to take part in a generalized programme of preventive medicine not specifically limited to the evaluation of gallbladder status. The general aims, methodological details and prevalence data of this study are given in other chapters of this book and have been reported elsewhere[9]. In summary, screening operations consisted of a physical examination, echography of the liver and biliary tract, and cholecystography when necessary. Blood sampling and a questionnaire on family and personal history were also carried out. Blood samples were collected after a 12 h fast and analysed for total cholesterol, high-density lipoprotein (HDL) cholesterol, triglycerides, glucose and other parameters not relevant here. Cholesterol and triglycerides were analysed by automated enzymatic techniques[10]. HDL cholesterol was determined after heparine/$MnCl_2$ precipitation[11]. Our laboratory is engaged in the quality control programme for cholesterol and triglycerides of the WHO Regional Lipid Centre, Prague.

Data were statistically evaluated by Student's unpaired *t*-test, Fisher's exact Z-test[12], and multiple logistic function analysis[13]. Age standardization was performed by the direct method, using the whole sample as reference population.

RESULTS

Serum lipids in women with gallstones and with history of cholecystectomy

The following results refer to a population of 66 women with evidence of gallstones at echography and/or cholecystography, 36 with a positive history of cholecystectomy, and 979 women with no evidence of GD.

The mean, age-standardized levels of total serum cholesterol were not significantly different between the three groups of women. Mean HDL cholesterol was significantly lower ($p<0.05$) in women with gallstones than in those without gallstones. Mean serum triglyceride concentrations were significantly higher in women with gallstones ($p<0.01$) and in those with a history of cholecystectomy ($p<0.05$) than in women without GD.

The percentage of women with gallstones or history of cholecystectomy according to quartiles of serum lipid concentrations is shown in Table 1. The percentage of women with both gallstones and cholecystectomy increased with increasing triglyceride levels. A similar, although weaker, trend was present with respect to total serum cholesterol. The percentage of women with GD decreased with increasing values of HDL cholesterol, but this finding was the result of dishomogeneous data in women with gallstones and with history of cholecystectomy.

The association of serum lipid concentration with GD was studied by multivariate analysis, which was run separately for women with gallstones and women who had been cholecystectomized. The initial multiple logistic function model used comprised 19 variables, including, in addition to the

Table 1 Percentage of women with gallstones, history of cholecystectomy and gallstone disease according to quartiles of serum lipid concentrations

Serum lipid	*Quartiles** 1	2	3	4
Total cholesterol (mg/dl)	(<177)	(177–200)	(201–231)	(232)
Gallstones (%)	4.6	5.2	7.8	6.8
Cholecystectomy (%)	1.8	2.6	2.6	6.0
Gallstone disease (%)	6.4	7.8	10.4	12.8
HDL Cholesterol (mg/dl)	(<50)	(50–55)	(56–63)	(64)
Gallstones (%)	8.8	7.1	2.5	6.1
Cholecystectomy (%)	2.2	4.4	4.3	1.9
Gallstone disease (%)	11.0	11.5	6.8	8.0
Triglycerides (mg/dl)	(<61)	(61–78)	(79–105)	(106)
Gallstones (%)	4.4	4.7	7.4	7.9
Cholecystectomy (%)	0.7	2.5	3.7	6.0
Gallstone disease (%)	5.1	7.2	11.1	13.9

* Each quartile comprised approximately 270 women

concentration of serum lipids, age, body mass index, blood glucose, menopause, number of pregnancies, contraceptive use, family history of GD, history of weight reduction, smoking habits, alcohol consumption, use of hypolipidaemic drugs and dietary intake of butter, olive oil and polyunsaturated oils. Through a stepwise procedure we therefore selected the variables which contributed significantly ($p < 0.1$) to the fit of the observations. Five variables were found to be significantly related to the presence of gallstones, i.e. age, body mass index, serum triglycerides and number of pregnancies positively and serum cholesterol negatively. No association was found with the other lipid variables. Second-order terms were also tested to detect non-linearities or interactions between the above variables. A significant ($p < 0.05$) second-degree coefficient was found for serum cholesterol, indicating that its negative association with gallstones is not linear. A significant negative interaction was found between age and number of pregnancies (which is discussed elsewhere in this volume). The last equation of the stepwise procedure relative to women with gallstones is reported in Table 2, which shows only the variables and their second degree terms associated with gallstones with a p-value lower than 0.05.

The same initial multiple logistic function model was used to detect the association of serum lipids with a history of cholecystectomy. Table 2 also shows the final results emerging from the multiple stepwise procedure, after testing also for the second-degree terms of the significantly associated variables. A history of cholecystectomy was positively associated with age, serum triglycerides ($p < 0.05$) and blood glucose.

Prevalence of gallstone disease in hyperlipidaemias

Women with total serum cholesterol and/or triglycerides above the 95th percentile in the whole studied female population (i.e. total serum cholesterol

Table 2 Variables significantly associated with presence of gallstones at ultrasonography and with history of cholecystectomy in women: multiple logistic regression analysis

Presence of gallstones		*History of cholecystectomy*	
Variable	*T value*	*Variable*	*T value*
Age	4.14***	Age	2.66**
Triglycerides	2.74**	Triglycerides	2.51*
Body mass index	2.39*	Blood glucose	2.30*
Pregnancies	2.70**		
Pregnancies × age	−2.54*		
(Cholesterol)^2	−2.51*		

*=$p<0.05$; **=$p<0.01$; ***=$p<0.001$

higher than 280.6 mg/dl and/or serum triglycerides higher than 162.8 mg/dl) were arbitrarily defined as having hyperlipoproteinaemia (HLP). According to these criteria 34 women (3.1 % of the entire population) were classified as hypercholesterolaemic (H-CHO), 34 (3.1 %) as hypertriglyceridaemic (H-TG) and 20 (1.9 %) as mixed HLP (H-CHO-TG). In no cases was an alcohol-induced HLP present. Some of the clinical and biochemical data of HLP women and of the remaining 993 women with normal serum lipids are shown in Table 3. The prevalence of GD was significantly higher in H-TG women (26.5 %, $p<0.01$) and in women with H-CHO-TG (14.8 %, n.s.) vs. women with normal serum lipids (8.9 %). Conversely, none of the 34 women with H-CHO had evidence of gallstones, or had been cholecystectomized. To rule out the possible influence on these data due to differences in age and body mass index (which in fact were significantly higher in all the three groups of women with HLP), we calculated (Table 4) the expected number of cases of gallstones and cholecystectomies using the coefficients of risk derived from a multiple logistic function analysis including age and body mass index as independent variables. The results confirmed a prevalence of GD higher than expected in women with H-TG (26,5 % vs. 16.8 %, n.s.) and lower than expected in women with H-CHO (0 % vs. 15.0 %, $p<0.05$).

DISCUSSION

Two major observations may be referred to the previous epidemiological studies on GD in which serum lipids were measured:

(1) the diagnosis of gallstones was rarely based on objective diagnostic procedures, such as echography or cholecystography, prevalence data being generally derived from clinically diagnosed cases[1,8,14], and therefore not necessarily representative of unknown or asymptomatic cases;
(2) most of the subjects with GD so far screened for serum lipids were already cholecystectomized at the time of lipid measurement[1,15].

Our cross-sectional study provides for the first time data on serum lipid concentrations in a female adult population in whom the diagnosis of gallstones was basically assessed by ultrasound examination of the gall-

Table 3 Some clinical and biochemical data of normolipaemic women and women with hyperlipoproteinaemia (mean values ±SD)

	Normal serum lipids ($n=993$)	*Hypercholesterolaemia* ($n=34$)	*Hypertriglyceridaemia* ($n=34$)	*Mixed HLP*† ($n=20$)
Age (years)	39.7± 9.5	49.5± 7.0***	50.7± 9.1***	45.1±10.9**
Relative body weight (kg/height (cm)−100×100)	102.8±16.4	111.1±17.1**	117.5±15.2***	116.8±20.0*
Serum cholesterol (mg/dl)	197.4±34.8	301.9±19.3	205.1±34.8	321.2±34.8
Serum triglycerides (mg/dl)	79.6±26.6	115.0±26.6	203.5±35.4	238.9±79.6

*=$p<0.05$; **=$p<0.01$; ***=$p<0.001$ (significantly different from women with normal serum lipids)
† Mixed hyperlipoproteinaemia (i.e. serum cholesterol ≥280.6 mg/dl and serum triglycerides ≥162.8 mg/dl)

Table 4 Expected* and observed prevalence rates of gallstones, cholecystectomy and total gallbladder disease in women with hyperlipoproteinaemias (number of cases in parentheses)

	Expected prevalence rate (%)			*Observed prevalence rate* (%)		
	Gallstones	*Cholecystectomy*	*Total*	*Gallstones*	*Cholecystectomy*	*Total*
Hypercholesterolaemia (>280.6 mg/dl) (34 women)	9.4 (3.2)	5.6 (1.9)	15.0† (5.1)	— (0)	— (0)	— (0)
Hypertriglyceridaemia (>162.8 mg/dl) (34 women)	10.9 (3.7)	5.6 (2.0)	16.5 (5.7)	17.6 (6)	8.8 (3)	26.4 (9)
Mixed hyperlipoproteinaemia (20 women)	11.5 (2.3)	7.0 (1.4)	18.5 (3.7)	10.0 (2)	10.0 (2)	20.0 (4)

* The expected number of cases has been calculated by application to each hyperlipidaemic woman of the coefficient of risk relative to age and body mass index obtained in a multivariate analysis
† Significantly different ($p<0.05$) from the corresponding observed values (Z-test)

bladder, thus providing information also on asymptomatic cases. In addition our study considered cholecystectomized women separately from those with gallstones.

The most important fact emerging from this study is the demonstration of a negative independent association between the presence of gallstones and the total serum cholesterol concentration in a multivariate analysis. A similar negative correlation between the prevalence of known GD and serum cholesterol was observed in men before entry into the Coronary Drug Project[14]. This finding would not appear to support the existence of a basis for a positive association between CHD and GD, and furthermore suggests that low total cholesterol concentrations should be suspected as a possible risk factor in the development of gallstones.

Multivariate analysis did not show any association between total serum cholesterol levels and history of cholecystectomy. This suggests that cholecystectomy *per se* could modify serum cholesterol levels, either directly or as a consequence of behavioural or dietary changes after surgery. Apart from different statistical approaches, these data could also explain why the epidemiological studies in which only clinically diagnosed cases of GD were taken into consideration (i.e. essentially cholecystectomized cases), failed to demonstrate any relationship between serum cholesterol levels and the occurrence of GD[1,8].

As far as the possibility that low cholesterol concentrations represent a risk factor in the development of gallstones is concerned, this hypothesis is supported by the following observations. Firstly, it is well established that the prevalence of gallstones is higher among the females than the males[1]. This sex prevalence has been reported to decrease after menopause[16]. Serum cholesterol levels are higher in males than in females, but this difference disappears after menopause[17]. Thus, if high serum cholesterol levels are not only a positive risk factor for CHD, but also a negative risk factor for GD, it may explain, at least partially, why the occurrence of CHD is prevalent among males and that of GD among females. The disappearance of this difference after menopause would also, in this light, be possible.

Secondly, a very high prevalence of gallstone disease has been demonstrated in a population characterized by low serum cholesterol levels, such as Pima Indians[18].

Thirdly, clofibrate therapy in HLP has been shown to produce, as a side-effect, a rise in bile cholesterol saturation[19,20], thus enhancing the risk for cholesterol gallstone formation. An increased incidence of symptomatic GD was found in fact among clofibrate users in the Coronary Drug Project[14]. The occurrence of gallstones at autopsy has also been reported to be significantly higher in men ingesting a cholesterol-lowering diet for several years[21], although this result was not confirmed by another similar study[22]. Therefore it appears that use of drugs (and perhaps also of dietary measures) known to produce a hypocholesterolaemic effect results in an increase in bile lithogenicity, suggesting the existence of a causative inverse relationship between serum cholesterol levels and bile cholesterol saturation. The latter hypothesis is indeed supported by the results of the National Cooperative Gallstone Study[23], which demonstrated that chronic administration of chenodeoxycholic acid, a known gallstone-dissolving agent, significantly reduced bile cholesterol saturation, while it enhanced serum concentration of low-density lipoprotein cholesterol. Finally, a possible 'protective' role of abnormally high serum cholesterol levels against the occurrence of GD is supported by the finding that none of the women with H-CHO in the present study showed evidence of GD, while the expected prevalence rate was 15%.

Other major results from our study were: (a) the lack of independent associations between serum HDL cholesterol concentrations and presence of gallstones or history of cholecystectomy; (b) the demonstration of a positive independent association between GD and serum triglycerides. Furthermore the prevalence of GD in women with H-TG was found to be higher than the expected prevalence rate.

The absence of any significant relationship between HDL cholesterol concentration and GD is in contrast to a recent epidemiological report[8] in which an association between low levels of HDL cholesterol and history of GD was found in female twins. The reason for this contradiction is not obvious, but may well depend on the different approaches used for the diagnosis of GD. Conversely, the positive association of GD with serum triglyceride levels is in agreement with other biochemical[7,24], clinical[25] and epidemiological[8,15] studies, therefore underlining the fact that H-TG should be suspected as an independent risk factor in the development of gallstones.

References

1. Friedman, G. D. (1968). The relationship between coronary heart disease and gallbladder disease: a critical review. *Ann. Intern. Med.*, **68**, 222–235
2. Kaye, M. O. and Kern, F. (1971). Clinical relationship of gallstones. *Lancet*, **1**, 1228
3. Bennion, L. J. and Grundy, S. M. (1978). Risk factors for the development of cholelithiasis in man. *N. Engl. J. Med.*, **299**, 1221–1227
4. Glueck, C. J. (1983). Relationship of lipid disorders to coronary heart disease. *Am. J. Med.*, **74** (5A), Suppl. 10
5. Schwartz, C. C., Halloran, L. G., Vlahcevic, Z. R., Gregory, D. H. and Swell, L. (1978). Preferential utilization of free cholesterol from high density lipoprotein for biliary cholesterol secretion in man. *Science*, **200**, 62
6. Thornton, J. R., Heaton, K. W. and McFarlane, D. G. (1981). A relation between high density lipoprotein cholesterol and bile cholesterol saturation. *Br. Med. J.*, **283**, 1352–1354
7. Ahlberg, J., Angelin, B., Einarsson, K., Hellström, K. and Leijd, B. (1980). Biliary lipid composition in normo- and hyperlipoproteinemia. *Gastroenterology*, **79**, 90–94
8. Petitti, D. B., Friedman, G. D. and Klatsky, A. L. (1981). Association of a history of gallbladder disease with a reduced concentration of high density lipoprotein cholesterol. *N. Engl. J. Med.*, **304**, 1396–1398
9. GREPCO (Gruppo Romano per l'Epidemiologia e la Prevenzione della Colelitiasi). Prevalence of gallstone disease in an Italian adult female population. *Am. J. Epidemiol.* (In press)
10. Morisi, G., Macchia, T., Angelico, F., Pacioni, F. and Zucca, A. (1979). Determinazione automatica di trigliceridi, colesterolo, glucosio e acido urico. Prospettive di impiego in screenings di medicina preventiva. *Ann. Ist. Sup. Sanità*, **15**, 122
11. *Manual of Laboratory Operations, Lipid Research Clinic Program* (1974). DHEW Publ. N. (NHI) 75–328, Vol. 1, page 56
12. Remington, R. D. and Schork, M. A. (1970). In *Statistics with Applications to the Biological and Health Sciences* (Englewood Cliffs, NJ: Prentice-Hall)

13. *BMDP Statistical Software* (1981). Department of Biomathematics, University of California, Los Angeles. (University of California Press)
14. The Coronary Drug Project Research Group (1977). Gallbladder disease as a side effect of drugs influencing lipid metabolism. Experience in the Coronary Drug Project. *N. Engl. J. Med.*, **296**, 1185
15. Ahlberg, J., Angelin, B., Einarsson, K., Hellström, K. and Leijd, B. (1979). Prevalence of gallbladder disease in hyperlipoproteinemia. *Dig. Dis. Sci.*, **24**, 459
16. Horn, G. (1956). Observations on the aethiology of cholelithiasis. *Br. Med. J.*, **2**, 732
17. The Lipid Research Clinics (1980). *Population Studies Data Book*, vol. 1. The prevalence study. US Department of Health and Human Services. NIH publication, **80**, 1527
18. Sampliner, R. E., Bennett, P. H., Comess, L. J., Rose, F. A. and Burch, T. A. (1970). Gallbladder disease in Pima Indians. *N. Engl. J. Med.*, **283**, 1358–1364
19. Pertsemlidis, D., Panveliwalla, D. and Ahrens, E. H. Jr. (1974). Effects of clofibrate and of an estrogen-progestin combination on fasting biliary lipids and cholic acid kinetics in man. *Gastroenterology*, **66**, 565–573
20. Bateson, M. C., Maclean, D., Ross, P. E. and Bouchier, I. A. D. (1978). Clofibrate therapy and gallstone induction. *Dig. Dis.*, **23**, 623
21. Sturdevant, R. A. L., Pearce, M. L. and Dayton, S. (1973). Increased prevalence of cholelithiasis in men ingesting a serum cholesterol-lowering-diet. *N. Engl. J. Med.*, **288**, 24–27
22. Miettinen, M., Turpeinen, D., Karvonen, M. J. *et al.* (1976). Prevalence of cholelithiasis in men and women ingesting a serum cholesterol lowering diet. *Ann. Clin. Res.*, **8**, 111–116
23. Albers, J. J., Grundy, S. H., Cleary, P. A., Small, D. H., Lachin, J. M., Schoenfield, L. J. and The National Cooperative Gallstone Study Group (1982). The effect of chenodeoxycholic acid on lipoproteins and apolipoproteins. *Gastroenterology*, **82**, 638
24. Angelin, B., Einarsson, K., Hellström, K. and Kallner, M. (1976). Elimination of cholesterol in hyperlipoproteinemia. *Clin. Sci. Mol. Med.*, **51**, 393
25. Kadziolka, R., Nilsson, S. and Schersten, T. (1977). Prevalence of hyperlipoproteinemia in men with gallstone disease. *Scand. J. Gastroenterol.*, **12**, 353

13
Diabetes mellitus, obesity and cholelithiasis

W. C. KNOWLER, M. J. CARRAHER and D. J. PETTITT

In the United States and Europe most gallstone disease is due to cholesterol stones, for which the reported risk factors include family history of gallstones, obesity, severe bile acid malabsorption, clofibrate and oestrogen therapy, femaleness, and possibly pregnancy and diabetes[1]. In this report we review some previous publications concerning the two factors obesity and diabetes, and present additional data from the study of the Pima Indian population in Arizona, USA.

THE FRAMINGHAM STUDY

Details on the prevalence of clinically diagnosed gallstones in Framingham, Massachusetts were published in 1966[2]. The prevalence of gallstones was positively associated with obesity, estimated by relative weight, and with the number of pregnancies, and inversely associated with height. No relationship was found with diabetes, blood pressure, or serum cholesterol, although the number of diabetics in this study was small.

Table 1 shows three categories of subjects in the Framingham study. Some

Table 1 Relationship of relative weight to diagnosed gallbladder disease in Framingham (from Ref. 2)

		*Mean relative weight**		
Sex	*Age (years)*	*Disease at entry*	*Diagnosed within 10 years*	*No diagnosis*
Male	30–62	105	105	102
Female	30–39	107	99	97
	40–49	108†	112†	102
	50–62	115†	112	109

* Relative weight = subject's weight × 100/median weight for all Framingham individuals of same sex and height

† Significantly greater than the group with no diagnosis ($p < 0.05$)

had gallbladder disease at entry, when the study began; some had their first diagnosis within the first 10 years of the study; and some remained free of clinical disease throughout the study. For each of these groups the mean relative weight is shown for men aged 30–62 years and for women in three age groups. In the older women, relative weights were significantly higher in those with gallstone disease at the beginning of the study and in those who developed it during the study than in those who remained free of clinical disease. There were no significant differences in relative weight in the men, however.

EFFECT OF OBESITY IN THE OXFORD FAMILY PLANNING STUDY

The Oxford/Family Planning Association Contraceptive Study reported the incidence of cholelithiasis or cholecystitis treated by cholecystectomy[3]. The incidence of surgically confirmed gallbladder disease was strongly related to obesity (estimated by the body mass index, or Quetelet's index) at entry, as shown in Table 2. The incidence in those with body mass indices at least 30 kg/m^2 was over six times as high as in those with body mass indices under 20 kg/m^2. The relationship was affected little by adjustment for other risk factors.

Table 2 Incidence of surgically confirmed gallbladder disease by body mass index in women, aged 25–39 years: Oxford Family Planning Study (from Ref. 3)

	Crude		*Standardized‡*	
*Body mass index (kg/m^2)**	*Incidence†*	*Relative rate*	*Incidence§*	*Relative rate*
<20.0	0.96	1.00	1.04	1.00
20.0–22.4	1.05	1.09	1.09	1.05
22.5–24.9	1.46	1.52	1.42	1.36
25.0–27.4	2.00	2.08	1.81	1.74
27.5–29.9	3.94	4.09	3.39	3.26
≥30.0	6.26	6.49	5.76	5.54

* Body mass index = weight/height^2 in kg/m^2
† Incidence rate = new cases/1000 woman-years at risk
‡ Standardized rates are adjusted for all other measured risk factors
§ Test for linear trend in incidence rates: $p < 0.0001$

CHOLELITHIASIS, OBESITY AND DIABETES IN CANADIAN STUDIES

Adult women in two Canadian populations, one American Indian and one Caucasian, were studied by oral cholecystography[4,5]. In each group, cholelithiasis was positively associated with obesity, estimated by the body mass index or triceps skinfold thickness. Diabetes was not studied in these populations.

The association of symptomatic cholelithiasis and clinically diagnosed diabetes mellitus was assessed in a case–control study in Newfoundland[6]. The prevalence of known diabetes was compared in subjects undergoing cholecystectomy for cholesterol cholelithiasis and in subjects undergoing other surgical procedures. There was an inverse relationship, not statistically significant, between diabetes and cholelithiasis.

THE PIMA INDIAN CHOLECYSTOGRAPHY SURVEY

In the late 1960s a gallstone survey was conducted among the Pima Indians[7], as already discussed in Chapter 4. In this study gallstone disease, detected clinically or by oral cholecystography, was unrelated to relative body weight in either men or women. The total prevalence of gallbladder disease was also unrelated to diabetes, although in an earlier report of clinically diagnosed disease only, diabetes was more frequent in men with gallstone disease than in men without[8].

CLINICALLY DIAGNOSED GALLBLADDER DISEASE IN PIMA INDIANS

A longitudinal study of chronic diseases in this population was initiated in 1965[9]. Approximately every 2 years each community resident who was at least 5 years old was asked to participate in a biennial examination which included the systematic review of medical records for diagnosed gallstones based on X-ray or surgical evidence. Further cholecystographic surveys have not been performed. Each biennial examination included a modified glucose tolerance test during which the venous plasma glucose concentration was determined 2 h after a 75 g carbohydrate load. In some instances the fasting plasma glucose was also measured. Glucose tolerance was classified according to World Health Organization[10] criteria by the fasting (when available) and 2 h post-load plasma glucose concentrations. Table 3 shows the three categories defined by these criteria: normal glucose tolerance, impaired glucose tolerance, and diabetes. In the following paragraphs data on obesity, glucose tolerance, and clinically diagnosed gallbladder disease are used from the most recent biennial examination of each subject.

Table 4 shows age-adjusted prevalence rates of diagnosed gallstones according to the body mass index, or weight divided by the square of height, an estimate of obesity. In women only, the prevalence of gallbladder disease increased slightly with increasing obesity. Controlling for age with multiple logistic regressing analyses, the relationship between body mass index and disease was statistically significant ($p < 0.05$) in women but not in men.

Table 5 shows age–sex-specific prevalence of clinically diagnosed gallstones

Table 3 Diagnostic values for the oral glucose tolerance test, using a 75 g carbohydrate load: World Health Organization criteria (from Ref. 10)

	*Glucose concentration in venous plasma (mg/dl)**		
Category	*Fasting*		*Two-hour*
Normal	<140	and	<140
Impaired glucose tolerance	<140	and	140–199
Diabetes mellitus	≥140	or	≥200

* 140 mg/dl = 7.78 mmol/l; 200 mg/dl = 11.1 mmol/l

Table 4 Age-adjusted prevalence of diagnosed gallbladder disease by obesity in Pima Indians, aged ≥25 years

Sex	*Body mass index** (*kg/m²*)	*Age-adjusted prevalence*	*95 % confidence interval†*
Male	<25	7.3	4.5–10.0
	25–35	9.2	7.0–11.5
	≥35	7.2	3.3–11.1
Female	<25	35.8	29.1–42.6
	25–35	36.4	33.0–39.8
	≥35	39.9	34.3–45.5

* Body mass index = weight/height^2 in kg/m^2
† The methods of age adjustment and computation of confidence intervals for age-adjusted rates are described in Ref. 9

according to glucose tolerance. Adjusting for age and sex by the method of Mantel and Haenszel[11], the rates in those with impaired glucose tolerance or diabetes were significantly higher than in those with normal glucose tolerance ($p < 0.05$), but the impaired tolerant and diabetic groups did not differ significantly from each other.

In Table 6 the prevalence rates of diagnosed gallstone disease are age-adjusted to the 1970 US white census. In the women, gallstone disease was much more common in those with impaired glucose tolerance or diabetes than with normal glucose tolerance. A multiple logistic regression analysis revealed that the association with abnormal glucose tolerance could not be explained by associations with obesity. Thus the Pima Indian study provides evidence for a relationship of diagnosed gallstone disease not only with diabetes, but also with lesser degrees of impaired glucose tolerance.

METHODOLOGICAL ISSUES

Although this study provides evidence for associations of gallstone disease with impaired glucose tolerance and diabetes, not all studies have reached similar conclusions. Even the earlier Pima cholecystography study did not demonstrate an association with diabetes. Several methodological issues may account for some of the differences between findings. The formation of gallstones and the development of symptomatic, clinically diagnosed gallbladder disease may not share all the same determinants. Thus it is important to distinguish between reports of the total prevalence of gallstones and of clinically diagnosed disease only.

Classification of gallstone disease in different studies has been based on questions asked directly of the subject or on review of medical records. Diagnostic data have included surgical and autopsy findings and examination of previously undiagnosed subjects by cholecystography or ultrasound. Little epidemiological work has been done with ultrasound until recently, but it will probably be the method of choice in the future because it can be done safely and inexpensively on large numbers of subjects. Several other papers in this volume describe the use of ultrasound in large population surveys now under

Table 5 Prevalence of clinically diagnosed gallbladder disease by diabetes in Pima Indians

		Normal glucose tolerance		*Impaired glucose tolerance*		*Diabetes*	
Sex	*Age (years)*	*No. subjects*	*Prevalence (%)*	*No. subjects*	*Prevalence (%)*	*No. subjects*	*Prevalence (%)*
Male	5–14	643	0	35	0	2	0
	15–24	650	0.5	48	0	28	0
	25–34	217	1	49	0	86	2
	35–44	107	7	26	8	119	8
	45–54	64	14	23	0	99	10
	55–64	57	14	11	18	76	14
	65–74	39	5	15	33	67	31
	≥75	38	11	16	50	42	21
Female	5–14	537	0.2	29	0	6	0
	15–24	666	4	62	5	38	5
	25–34	287	18	68	21	102	18
	35–44	106	35	40	55	128	39
	45–54	55	45	22	41	169	52
	55–64	19	26	20	40	133	53
	65–74	24	54	20	60	103	57
	≥75	20	35	3	67	41	44

Table 6 Age-adjusted prevalence of diagnosed gallbladder disease by glucose tolerance in Pima Indians, aged ≥25 years

Sex	*Glucose tolerance*	*Age-adjusted prevalence (%)*	*95 % confidence interval**
Male	Normal	6.6	4.5– 8.8
	Impaired	9.2	5.0–13.3
	Diabetes	9.0	6.9–11.0
Female	Normal	26.8	22.6–31.1
	Impaired	33.9	27.5–40.3
	Diabetes	33.0	27.9–36.2

* The method of age adjustment and computation of confidence intervals for the age-adjusted rates are described in Ref. 9

way. Ultrasound is also being used in the current National Health and Examination Survey in the United States. These studies will allow the examination of large enough numbers of subjects to allow for better examination of associations with obesity and diabetes than have been possible in some of the earlier studies with sample sizes too small (especially of diabetics) for the detection of modest associations.

Diagnostic criteria for diabetes have differed widely between studies, and some reports were based only on known diabetes. Thus many people with lesser degrees of glucose intolerance, now classified as impaired glucose tolerance[10], would have been classified as non-diabetics if only symptomatic, diagnosed disease was ascertained. If the Pima Indian findings apply elsewhere, and subjects with impaired glucose tolerance have the highest prevalence of gallbladder disease (Table 6), then a relationship could easily be missed when only known diabetes is considered.

It must also be remembered that there may be true differences between populations in risk factors for gallstone disease. For example if American Indians have other, yet unidentified, risk factors, the role of obesity may be much less important than in Caucasians or other populations.

Acknowledgments

We thank the members of the Gila River Indian Community for their participation in these studies, the staff of the National Institute of Arthritis, Diabetes and Digestive and Kidney Diseases in Arizona for conducting the Pima Indian studies, and E. Begay for secretarial assistance.

References

1. Bennion, L. J. and Grundy, S. M. (1978). Risk factors for the development of cholelithiasis in man. *N. Engl. J. Med.*, **299**, 1161–1167, 1221–1227
2. Friedman, G. D., Kannel, W. B. and Dawber, T. R. (1966). The epidemiology of gallbladder disease: observations in the Framingham study. *J. Chron. Dis.*, **19**, 273–292
3. Layde, P. M., Vessey, M. P. and Yeates, D. (1982). Risk factors for gall-bladder disease: a cohort study of young women attending family planning clinics. *J. Epidemiol. Community Med.*, **36**, 274–278

4. Williams, C. N., Johnston, J. L. and Weldon, K. L. M. (1977). Prevalence of gallstones and gallbladder disease in Canadian Micmac Indian women. *Can. Med. Assoc. J.*, **117**, 758–760
5. Williams, C. N. and Johnston, J. L. (1980). Prevalence of gallstones and risk factors in Caucasian women in a rural Canadian community. *Can. Med. Assoc. J.*, **120**, 664–668
6. Honoré, L. H. (1980). The lack of a positive association between symptomatic cholesterol cholelithiasis and clinical diabetes mellitus: a retrospective study. *J. Chron. Dis.*, **33**, 465–469
7. Sampliner, R. E., Bennett, P. H., Comess, L. J., Rose, F. A. and Burch, T. A. (1970). Gallbladder disease in Pima Indians: demonstration of high prevalence and early onset by cholecystography. *N. Engl. J. Med.*, **283**, 1358–1364
8. Comess, L. J., Bennett, P. H. and Burch, T. A. (1967). Clinical gallbladder disease in Pima Indians: its high prevalence in contrast to Framingham, Massachusetts. *N. Engl. J. Med.*, **277**, 894–898
9. Knowler, W. C., Bennett, P. H., Hamman, R. F. and Miller, M. (1978). Diabetes incidence and prevalence in Pima Indians: a 19-fold greater incidence than in Rochester, Minnesota. *Am. J. Epidemiol.*, **108**, 497–505
10. WHO Expert Committee on Diabetes Mellitus (1980). Second Report, pp. 8–12. (Geneva: World Health Organization Technical Report Series 646)
11. Mantel, N. and Haenszel, W. (1959). Statistical aspects of the analysis of data from retrospective studies of disease. *J. Natl. Cancer Inst.*, **22**, 719–748

14
High-density lipoprotein–cholesterol and the risk of gallbladder disease

D. B. PETITTI

REVIEW OF PREVIOUS WORK

In 1979 we reported that women with a history of gallbladder disease were at higher risk of subsequently being hospitalized with an acute myocardial infarction[1]. Autopsy studies[2–3] have also found an increased prevalence of gallstones in patients dying with coronary heart disease, although this association has not been observed universally[4]. In addition, methodological problems are inherent in such investigations[5].

On the other hand, an association of gallbladder disease with acute myocardial infarction is plausible if both diseases have at least one common underlying pathophysiological mechanism. In our 1979 paper[1], we suggested that an association of lipid metabolism to both the risk of gallbladder disease and the risk of acute myocardial infarction would explain an association of gallbladder disease with an increased risk of acute myocardial infarction. The main constituent of gallstones in Americans is cholesterol. Thus, an association of gallbladder disease with cholesterol metabolism remained a plausible explanation despite the fact that epidemiological studies have not shown an association of total serum cholesterol with the risk of gallbladder disease[6]. The strong inverse association of the risk of acute myocardial infarction with the serum concentration of high-density lipoprotein–cholesterol HDL-C)[7] suggested that further study of it might be fruitful.

Table 1 shows the results of our analysis examining the prevalence of gallbladder disease with serum concentrations of total cholesterol, HDL-C, low-density lipoprotein–cholesterol (LDL-C), very low-density lipoprotein–cholesterol (VLDL-C), and triglyceride in 868 female twins participating in a special study of twins[8]. It should be noticed that the correlation of VLDL-C with tryglyceride concentration is 0.99. Thus, substitution of triglyceride for VLDL-C in any analysis yields results identical to those shown for VLDL-C. The importance of this observation will become

Table 1 Percentage of women reporting a history of gallbladder disease by quartile of serum lipid concentration (from Ref. 8)

	Quartile			
	I	*II*	*III*	*IV*
HDL–cholesterol	14.4	6.5	5.2	4.4
LDL–cholesterol	3.7	4.6	9.6	11.5
VLDL–cholesterol	1.6	4.3	7.8	16.9
Total cholesterol	2.8	5.3	9.5	12.6
Triglyceride	1.8	3.8	7.9	16.8

clear later. Table 1 shows that gallbladder disease is directly related to serum concentrations of total cholesterol, LDL-C, VLDL-C, and triglyceride and inversely related to the concentration of HDL-C in these women.

Table 2 shows the results of three multivariate analyses of these data in which a history of gallbladder was the dependent variable, and age was entered as a covariate along with the value of total cholesterol, HDL-C, LDL-C, or VLDL-C concentration. After control for age, the concentration of HDL-C remains highly significantly ($p = 0.005$) associated with the risk of gallbladder disease. There is no significant association with total cholesterol or LDL-C concentration after control for age, whereas the association with VLDL-C is significant ($p = 0.03$) at a lower level.

Table 3 shows the results of multivariate analyses in which age and Quetelet's body mass index were included as covariates along with either HDL-C, LDL-C, VLD-C, or total cholesterol. As in the previous analyses controlling only for age, neither total cholesterol concentration nor LDL-C concentration is significantly associated with the risk of gallbladder disease. After controlling for both Quetelet's index and age, the association of VLDL-C is also not significant. This suggests that the association of VLDL-C with the risk of gallbladder disease in these women shown in Tables 1 and 2 acts largely through the effects of age and body mass on the concentration of VLDL-C. In contrast, the association of risk of gallbladder disease with HDL-C concentration is independent of age and body mass.

Table 4 shows that the association of HDL-C with gallbladder disease is also

Table 2 Association of total cholesterol and cholesterol fractions with a history of gallbladder disease controlling for age (four separate analyses)

Lipid included in model	*Estimated relative risk**	*95 % confidence limits for relative risk*	*p value**
HDL–cholesterol	0.7†	0.6, 0.9	<0.001
LDL–cholesterol	1.0‡	1.0, 1.1	0.46
VLDL–cholesterol	1.1§	1.0, 1.3	0.03
Total cholesterol	1.0‡	1.0, 1.1	0.53

* Probability or relative risk for the lipid, controlling for age
† Decrease in relative risk per 10.0 mg of HDL–cholesterol per decilitre
‡ Increase in relative risk per 10.0 mg of cholesterol per decilitre
§ Increase in relative risk per 1.0 mg of VLDL–cholesterol per decilitre

Table 3 Association of total cholesterol and cholesterol fractions with a history of gallbladder disease controlling for age and Quetelet's index (four separate analyses)

Lipid included in model	*Estimated relative risk**	*95 % confidence limits for relative risk*	*p value**
HDL-cholesterol	0.8†	0.6, 0.9	<0.01
LDL-cholesterol	1.0‡	0.9, 1.1	0.88
VLDL-cholesterol	1.0§	0.9, 1.1	0.18
Total cholesterol	1.0‡	0.9, 1.1	0.86

* Probability or relative risk for the lipid, controlling for age and Quetelet's index
† Decrease in relative risk per 10.0 mg increase in HDL-cholesterol per decilitre
‡ Increase in relative risk per 10.0 mg increase in cholesterol per decilitre
§ Increase in relative risk per 10.0 mg increase in VLDL-cholesterol per decilitre

Table 4 Association of cholesterol fractions and other factors with a history of gallbladder disease (one analysis) (from Ref. 8)

Factor	*Estimated relative risk**	*95 % confidence limits for relative risk*	*p value**
Age	1.7†	1.3, 2.2	<0.01
Quetelet's index	1.7‡	1.2, 2.4	<0.01
HDL-cholesterol	0.8§	0.6, 1.0	0.02
Cigarette smoking	1.8	1.0, 3.3	0.05
Oestrogen use	2.0	1.1, 3.6	0.02
LDL-cholesterol	1.0	0.9, 1.1	0.92
VLDL-cholesterol	1.0	0.9, 1.1	0.81
Alcohol use	0.9	0.5, 1.6	0.79
Oral contraceptive use	0.7	0.4, 1.2	0.16

* Probability or relative risk for a single variable, controlling for all other variables in the table
† Increment in relative risk per decade of age
‡ Increment in relative risk per unit increase in Quetelet's index
§ Decrease in relative risk per 10 mg of HDL-cholesterol per decilitre

independent of a large number of other factors, including the concentrations of the other lipids. Thus, after simultaneous control in a multivariate analysis for age, Quetelet's index, cigarette smoking, oestrogen use, alcohol use, oral contraceptive use, and the concentrations of LDL-C and VLDL-C, HDL-C concentration remains significantly ($p<0.05$) associated with the risk of gallbladder disease. The association of HDL-C with the risk of gallbladder disease is inverse, a higher concentration of HDL-C being associated with a lower risk of gallbladder disease.

Thornton *et al.*[9] also found that serum HDL-C concentration was negatively correlated with bile saturation index (Table 5). The finding of a direct link between serum HDL-C concentration and the lithogenicity of bile firmly establishes a physiological basis for the epidemiological observation of the relation of HDL-C concentration to the risk of gallbladder disease.

Table 5 Correlation of bile cholesterol saturation and serum concentrations of total cholesterol, high-density lipoprotein cholesterol, and triglyceride (from Ref. 9)

Lipid	*Correlation with bile cholesterol saturation index (r)*	*p value*
Total cholesterol	0.319	ns*
HDL–cholesterol	−0.509	<0.01
Triglyceride	0.471	<0.02

* Not significant

FUNCTION OF HIGH-DENSITY LIPOPROTEIN

The function of HDL is not known with complete certainty[10]. It is postulated that it plays a role in the transport of cholesterol from the tissues to the liver[11] or that it acts as a scavenger of lipid and protein during normal plasma lipolysis[12]. High-density lipoproteins are derived directly from lecithin and free cholesterol and then secreted both from the liver and the intestine in a discoid form. The enzyme lecithin–cholesterol acyl transferase acts to transform the discoid particle to a spherical particle, which cholesterol ester enters. Catabolism and plasma clearance of high-density lipoprotein particles involves multiple mechanisms whose relative importance in man is unknown. However, the ultimate fate of cholesterol taken up by high-density lipoproteins is excretion in bile.

As pointed out by Thornton *et al.*[9], if cholesterol taken up by HDL were secreted into bile predominantly as cholesterol, then a higher concentration of HDL-C would be expected to increase the risk of cholelithiasis. On the other hand, if cholesterol taken up by HDL were secreted predominantly as bile acids, then the concentration of HDL-C would be expected to decrease the risk of gallbladder disease by decreasing bile saturation. This is, of course, what was observed in our epidemiological study and in the study of Thornton *et al.*[9]. There is also some direct evidence that free cholesterol from HDL-C is a primary precursor of bile acid synthesis in man[13]. The findings that the risk of acute myocardial infarction is increased in women with gallbladder disease; that gallbladder disease is inversely related to serum HDL-C concentration; and that HDL-C concentration is negatively correlated with bile saturation can all be understood based on knowledge of the function of high-density lipoprotein and the observation that the primary precursor of bile acid is free cholesterol derived from HDL-C.

CONTRADICTIONS

It is clear, however, that the serum concentration of HDL-C is not the sole determinant of the risk of cholelithiasis. If it were, one would expect that factors that raise HDL-C would lower the risk of gallbladder disease and vice-versa. Table 6 shows the association of a number of factors with gallbladder disease and with the serum concentration of HDL-C. White race (as compared with black), use of alcohol, cigarette smoking and obesity are 'consistent' risk factors. That is, each of these factors is associated with the risk of gallbladder

Table 6 Association of various factors with the risk of gallbladder disease and with HDL–cholesterol and triglyceride concentrations

Factor	*Association with gallbladder disease risk*	*Association with HDL–cholesterol concentration*	*Association with VLDL–cholesterol (triglyceride) concentration*	*Association with LDL–cholesterol concentration*
White race*	↑	↓	0	↓
Use of alcohol	↓	↑	↑	0
Cigarette smoking	↑	↓	0	0
Obesity	↑	↓	↑	↑
Female sex	↑	↑†	↓	↓
Exogenous oestrogen use	↑	↑†	↑	↑
Ageing	↑	↑†	↑	↑
Pima Indian race‡	↑	↑†	↑	↑
Type I diabetes	↑	↑†	↑	↑

* Compared with black race
† 'Inconsistent' risk factor (see text for explanation)
‡ Compared with white race

disease in a direction opposite the direction of its association with HDL-C concentration. In contrast, female sex, exogenous oestrogen use, ageing, Pima Indian race (as compared with white), and Type I diabetes are 'inconsistent' risk factors. Each is associated both with a higher risk of gallbladder disease and with a higher serum concentration of HDL-C.

Table 6 also shows the relation of each of these factors to the serum concentrations of VLDL-C (triglyceride) and LDL-C. The table shows that three of the four 'consistent' risk factors are either not associated with a difference in VLDL-C and LDL-C concentration, or are associated with a difference in VLDL-C and LDL-C concentration in a direction that is the same as the direction of their association with HDL-C. In contrast, four of the five 'inconsistent' risk factors are associated with a higher concentration of VLDL-C and LDL-C. These observations, together with the data shown in Tables 2 and 3, the studies of Thornton *et al.*[9], and those of van der Linden and Bergman[14] suggest the possibility that very low-density lipoproteins or triglyceride, as well as high-density lipoprotein, play an important role in the pathogenesis of cholelithiasis. Specifically, the observations suggest that a high concentration of VLDL-C (or triglyceride) may modify the effect of a given concentration of HDL-C on the lithogenicity of bile and the risk of cholelithiasis.

Alternatively, these inconsistences might be related to the different effects of these factors on the subfractions of HDL – HDL_2 and HDL_3; to the apolipoprotein constituents; or to gallbladder motility. Any of these subjects would be fruitful areas for further research on the pathogenesis of cholelithiasis.

References

1. Petitti, D. B., Wingerd, J., Pellegrin, F. and Ramcharan, S. (1979). Risk of vascular disease in

women: smoking, oral contraceptives, noncontraceptive estrogens, and other factors. *J. Am. Med. Assoc.*, **242**, 1150–1154
2. Tennant, R. and Zimmerman, H. M. (1931). Association between disease in the gall-bladder and in the heart, as evidenced at autopsy. *Yale J. Biol. Med.*, **3**, 495–503
3. Breyfogle, H. S. (1940). The frequency of coexisting gallbladder and coronary heart disease: a statistical analysis and biometric evaluation of 1,493 necropsies. *J. Am. Med. Assoc.*, **114**, 1434–1437
4. Barker, D. J., Gardner, M. J., Power, C. and Hutt, M. S. (1979). Prevalence of gallstones at autopsy in nine British towns: a collaborative study. *Br. Med. J.*, **2**, 1389–1392
5. Friedman, G. D., Kannel, W. B. and Dawber, T. R. (1966). The epidemiology of gall-bladder disease: observations in the Framingham Study. *J. Chron. Dis.*, **19**, 273–292
6. Friedman, G. D. (1968). The relationship between coronary heart disease and gallbladder disease: a critical review. *Ann. Intern. Med.*, **68**, 222–235
7. Rhoads, G. G., Gulbrandsen, C. L. and Kagan, A. (1976). Serum lipoproteins and coronary heart disease in a population of Hawaii Japanese men. *N. Engl. J. Med.*, **294**, 293–298
8. Petitti, D. B., Friedman, G. D. and Klatsky, A. L. (1981). Association of a history of gallbladder disease with a reduced concentration of high-density-lipoprotein cholesterol. *N. Engl. J. Med.*, **304**, 1396–1398
9. Thornton, J. R., Heaton, K. W. and MacFarlane, D. G. (1981). A relation between high-density-lipoprotein cholesterol and bile cholesterol saturation. *Br. Med. J.*, **283**, 1352–1354
10. Krauss, R. M. (1982). Regulation of high-density lipoprotein levels. *Med. Clin. North Am.*, **66**, 403–430
11. Glomset, J. A. (1968). The plasma lecithin:cholesterol acyltransferase reaction. *J. Lipid Res.*, **9**, 155–167
12. Levy, R. I. and Rifkind, B. M. (1980). The structure, function and metabolism of high-density lipoproteins: a status report. *Circulation*, **62** (Suppl IV), IV4–IV8
13. Halloran, L. G., Schwartz, C. C., Vlahcevic, Z. R., Nisman, R. M. and Swell, L. (1978). Evidence for high-density lipoprotein-free cholesterol as the primary precursor for bile-acid synthesis in man. *Surgery*, **84**, 1–6
14. van der Linden, W. V. and Bergman, F. (1977). An analysis of data on human hepatic bile. Relationship between main bile components, serum cholesterol and serum triglycerides. *Scand. J. Clin. Invest.*, **37**, 741–747

15
Intestinal metabolism of bile acids and cholelithiasis*

N. CARULLI, P. LORIA and D. MENOZZI

INTRODUCTION

In 1969 Cleave[1] proposed the term 'the saccharine disease' to include diverse conditions associated with overconsumption, such as obesity, diabetes and coronary heart disease, or attributed to colonic stasis such as constipation, haemorrhoids and diverticulosis. In the author's view such diseases share a common aetiological factor represented by the consumption of refined carbohydrates which has two effects: it increases the caloric intake/weight of ingested food ratio, and alters the colonic function due to the diminished ingestion of roughage, lost during the refining procedures.

From the epidemiological point of view the prevalence of these diseases in the western world has increased steadily during the past half-century and this can confidently be attributed to the changes of dietary habits that have taken place in this period. The same trend of prevalence characterizes gallstone disease, so that its inclusion in the 'saccharine' group has been proposed[2]. Indeed data obtained by some dietary surveys have revealed a higher caloric intake in subjects with gallstones than in normal persons[3–5]; the problem, however, is still controversial[6,7]. Recently it has been reported that subjects on diet rich in refined carbohydrate show an increase of bile cholesterol saturation[8,9].

Similarly lack of dietary vegetable fibre has been suggested as a possible cause of gallstones, based on epidemiological data showing a low prevalence of gallstones in African populations eating diets with higher fibre content than the western diet[2]. It must be stressed, however, that the pathophysiological link between dietary habits and gallstones is evolving and becoming more apparent as our knowledge of the natural history of the disease improves and its determinants are recognized. In this respect obesity is an emblematic condition since it is due to overconsumption and is associated with higher

* Abbreviations used in this paper: CA, cholic acid; CDCA, chenodeoxycholic acid; DCA, deoxycholic acid; LCA, lithocholic acid; UDCA, ursodeoxycholic acid

incidence of gallstones as confirmed by numerous epidemiological investigations[10-14].

The metabolic basis of cholesterol gallstones is the production by the liver of a bile supersaturated with cholesterol. This situation is caused by an increase of biliary cholesterol secretion, either absolute or relative to the secretion of bile acids. Indeed obese subjects show a bile saturation higher than that observed in non-obese controls matched for age, sex and race[15]. An absolute increase of biliary cholesterol secretion has been reported to be the underlying mechanism[15-17]. In other conditions the mechanism responsible for the occurrence of supersaturated bile, and hence the risk for gallstone formation, is not as clearly defined, mainly because the determinants of biliary cholesterol secretion are still poorly understood.

Low-Beer *et al.*[18] have proposed that the abundance of DCA into the bile acid pool might play a causative role in determining bile cholesterol supersaturation, thus predisposing to gallstone formation. As DCA is an intestinal metabolite of CA, this suggestion implies that colonic function has to be considered in the multifactorial aetiology of gallstones. This paper will briefly review the available evidence for the association between DCA and gallstones and the metabolic basis of this association.

INTESTINAL BILE ACID DEGRADATION

Cholic and chenodeoxycholic acids (CA and CDCA), synthesized by the liver, undergo bacterial degradation in the gut, mainly into the colon. Degradative reactions, by different bacterial enzymes, can occur at different sites of the ring system or at the side-chain of the molecule, giving rise to several compounds, some of which are not as yet defined[19].

In man the most important changes are the breakage of the amido bond of taurine and glycine conjugates of bile acids operated by bacterial hydrolases and the dehydroxylation of the unconjugated bile acid at the 7-position of the steroid ring. This latter reaction converts cholic acid (3α, 7α, 12α-trihydroxy-5β-cholanoic acid) to deoxycholic (3α, 12α-dihydroxy-5β-cholanoic acid) and chenodeoxycholic (3α, 7α-dihydroxy-5β-cholanoic) to lithocholic acid (3α-monohydroxy-5β-cholanoic).

The fate of the two secondary bile acids differs. One-third to one-half of formed DCA is absorbed, conjugated in the liver, excreted into the bile, and then reabsorbed as efficiently as the primary bile acids. In man its contribution to the pool is from 20 to 30 %. On the contrary lithocholic acid is poorly absorbed; in the liver it is conjugated with glycyne and taurine and it is partly sulphated at the 3-position and then excreted into the bile. This bile acid accounts for about 2 % of the biliary bile acids.

Factors influencing the formation of secondary bile acids and their contribution to the pool are not well defined. Theoretically an increased exposure of the bile acid pool to the intestinal flora would increase the degradation of bile acids; this could happen either because of an increased frequency of the enterohepatic cycling or because of a reduction of the elective absorptive site, i.e. the terminal ileum.

The first situation is best exemplified by cholecystectomy which abolishes somewhat the possibility of storing the bile acid pool during interprandial fasting, thus leading to an increased cycling. Indeed cholecystectomized patients have been shown to have an increased input and hence proportion of DCA into the pool[20–22]. The second instance could be represented by ileal resection or ileal diseases, both conditions associated with reduced bile acid absorption[23]. In this situation the extent of alteration of bile acid metabolism depends on the length of the resected or diseased ileum. In fact if ileal absorption of bile acids is greatly impaired, the colon is flooded with bile acids, cholegenic diarrhoea develops, bacterial attack decreases and intestinal metabolites are absorbed less. The net result will be that of a reduction of the bile acid pool, especially at expense of secondary bile acids. However in less dramatic situations an increased degradation of bile acid takes place, as demonstrated by a rise of deoxycholate into the pool in patients with ileal resection without diarrhoea[24]. Beside these pathological conditions, physiological factors such as age and diet, also seem to influence intestinal degradation and absorption of the secondary bile acids. Thus Van der Werf *et al.*[25] have studied bile acid metabolism in two age groups of subjects, reporting that elderly subjects show an increased intestinal 7α-dehydroxylation of bile acid as judged by the higher input of DCA into the pool. As for the responsible mechanism, the authors proposed the possibility of a decreased ileal absorption of CA together with a more effective absorption of the formed DCA.

The effect of the different constituents of the diet on bile acid degradation has not yet been studied extensively and the available information rests on a small number of epidemiological studies. Wynder and Reddy[26] have reported that the faecal excretion of bile acids, especially deoxycholic and lithocholic, is decreased in American vegetarians as compared with their compatriots eating a western mixed diet. Another study on vegetarians has shown that these subjects tend to have less deoxycholate and more cholate in their bile[27]. In addition the half-life of radioactive primary bile acids in the enterohepatic circulation of vegetarians was longer than in normal controls.

In contrast Huijbregts *et al.*[28] failed to reproduce these results in a small group of European vegetarians. In their study, in fact, it was found that the vegetarian diet was associated with a significantly increased 7α-dehydroxylation leading to a slightly higher input of deoxycholate into the pool.

Whether or not changes of bile acid metabolism associated with the vegetarian diet could be attributed to a higher intake of vegetable fibre is still a controversial issue. Studies carried out to investigate the effect of bran feeding on bile acid metabolism have reported a decreased[29–32], as well as an unchanged or even an increased, input of deoxycholate[33]. In another study on the effect of a high-fibre diet on morbidly obese patients, the most relevant finding was the shrinking of the total bile acid pool, due to an increased loss of bile acids[34].

Similarly inconclusive results have been reported on the effect of refined carbohydrates on deoxycholate formation. Substituting sugar for a normal diet was found to decrease biliary deoxycholate due to the better preservation of cholate into the enterohepatic circulations[35]. On the other hand subjects eating refined carbohydrate diets, as compared to those eating unrefined carbohydrate diets, were reported to show a trend towards an increased content of biliary deoxycholate[8].

Different diets may affect to a different extent the many variables, such as intestinal transit time, bacterial degradation and colonic absorption, contributing to the input of deoxycholate. Thus, unless controlled studies on large and homogeneous samples of populations on carefully standardized diets are performed, no clear-cut information can be obtained on any effect that dietary regimen might have on bile acid metabolism.

DEOXYCHOLIC ACID, BILE SATURATION AND GALLSTONES

Hoffman *et al.*[36], reporting on the baseline biliary data of 548 white American subjects with gallstones, participating in the National Cooperative Gallstone Study, attempted, by means of a multiple regression analysis, to quantitate the determinants of bile saturation. It was found that, at least for male patients, bile cholesterol was positively correlated with the proportion of DCA and negatively correlated with CDCA. These findings obtained in the largest group of gallstone patients give support to similar observations reported previously by several authors on smaller groups of subjects[20,37–40]. Whether the increased proportion of DCA precedes gallstone formation, or simply represents a secondary event that is the result of an increased cycling frequency of the bile acid pool due to the impaired storing capacity of the diseased gallbladder, cannot be decided from these observations. Certainly to find an increased percentage of DCA in the bile of subjects at high risk for developing gallstones would suggest that DCA may play a role in the events leading to the formation of gallstones.

In this respect Ahlberg *et al.*[41] have recently reported that in subjects with hyperlipidaemia types IV and IIb, both conditions carrying a high risk for gallstones, the proportion of DCA was significantly higher than in other hyperlipidaemic conditions and control subjects. Williams *et al.*[9] found the percentage of DCA to be correlated to biliary molar percentage of cholesterol, in a high-risk group of Canadian Indians.

To further assess the role of DCA in determining changes of bile saturation with cholesterol, two approaches have been used by several investigators: one consisting in the increase of the proportion of DCA, obtained by means of oral administration of the bile acid; the other, opposite to the first, in which DCA proportion was decreased by pharmacological or dietary means.

The reported results, as summarized in Table 1, are not concordant. In all subjects studied, DCA became the predominant bile acid in the pool; however in two studies only[18,42], the mean saturation index increased significantly, whereas in the others[43–45], no consistent changes of biliary lipid composition were observed. Duration of treatment, dosage and pretreatment value of bile saturation varied from study to study, although the discrepancy of the results cannot be entirely accounted for by these variables.

In healthy volunteers, DCA administered at low dosage for 2 weeks seemed to supersaturate the bile[18], whereas in other groups of healthy subjects treatment with higher doses, and for longer periods of time, did not produce

Table 1 Effect of DCA feeding on bile saturation

Subjects	No.	Dose (mg kg^{-1} day^{-1})	Duration (weeks)	DCA (%) Before	DCA (%) After	Saturation index	Authors
Healthy	16	100–150*	2	25	48	Increased	Low-Beer, 1975
Healthy	7	9.8	4–8	26	74	Unchanged	LaRusso, 1977
Healthy	8	10.7	3–4	26	87	Unchanged	Ahlberg, 1977
Gallstones	9	15.0	1–2	20	90	Unchanged	Carulli, 1980
Gallstones	8	15.0	3	20	78	Increased	Ponz de Leon, 1983

* mg/day

the same effect[43,44]. In two separate groups of gallstone patients the treatment with an equal dose resulted ineffective after 1–2 weeks[45], but it induced supersaturation of bile after 3 weeks[42].

More uniform results have been obtained with studies designed to investigate the effect of the reduction of DCA on biliary lipid composition. Table 2 summarizes such studies in which drugs or similar were used to change the bacterial flora activity without significantly altering the enterohepatic circulation of bile acids. The use of metronidazole[46] or ampicillin[47] has proved to be effective in reducing the proportion of bile biliary DCA, owing to the effect of these antibiotics on the bacterial flora. Similarly the administration of lactulose[48], or of *Streptococcus faecium*[49] led to a reduction of DCA, presumably through a mechanism somewhat different from that of antibiotics. In all these instances the reduction of DCA percentage was associated with a decrease in bile saturation. In two of these studies[46,49] bile saturation returned to the baseline value once the treatment was discontinued.

As discussed above, the effect of adding bran to the diet on the bile lipid composition is controversial; some studies showing a desaturating effect[30–32], others reporting no change[33]. It must be noticed, however, that in those studies in which bran administration produced a decrease of biliary deoxycholate it was associated with a reduced bile saturation, thus suggesting that the two effects are related.

Although the reduction of bile cholesterol saturation obtained with the above treatments is not of the same order of magnitude as that observed with

Table 2 Effect of drug-induced decrease of biliary DCA on bile saturation

Subjects	No.	Drug	Duration (weeks)	DCA (%) Before	DCA (%) After	Saturation index	Authors
Healthy	11	Metronidazole (2 g/day)	1.5	24	7	Decreased	Low-Beer, 1978
Gallstones	5	Ampicillin (2 g/day)	2–3	21	9	Decreased	Carulli, 1981
Healthy	10	Lactulose (40–60 g/day)	6	28	15	Decreased	Thornton, 1981
Healthy	8	*Streptococcus faecium* (750×10^6)	4	23	18	Decreased	Salvioli, 1982

the administration of CDCA, nevertheless it suggests that reduction of DCA may have some role in decreasing bile cholesterol.

MECHANISM OF DCA-INDUCED CHANGES OF BILE SATURATION

It is well established that CDCA administration is followed by a reduction of biliary cholesterol secretion and hence saturation, eventually leading to gallstone dissolution. This effect was thought to be specific of this bile acid so that its variations in the bile acid pool were considered determinant of the changes of saturation.

Low-Beer *et al.*[50] showed that feeding small doses of DCA to volunteers resulted in an increased DCA proportion at the expense of CDCA, while the proportion of CA remained unchanged. Subsequently the same authors extended this preliminary finding by investigating the kinetics of CDCA and CA in subjects taking DCA[51]. It was found that the expansion of the DCA pool was associated with a significant fall in both pool size and synthesis rate of CDCA, whereas CA was not affected. In addition, in a large number of subjects not taking any bile acid, the biliary proportion of DCA was inversely related to that of CDCA but not to that of CA. From this finding it was inferred that DCA administration may induce changes of bile saturation through a selective inhibition of CDCA synthesis.

This contention was not confirmed in other laboratories. La Russo *et al.*[43] demonstrated that DCA feeding in normal subjects depresses the synthesis and reduces the pool size of both primary bile acids. Ahlberg *et al.*[44] found an inverse relationship between the proportion of DCA and that of CDCA and CA, both in normal subjects fed DCA and in a large group of untreated hyperlipidaemic patients. Carulli *et al.*[45] reported that in patients with gallstones the administration of DCA is associated with a significant reduction of the pool size of both CDCA and CA. It must be added, however, that the dose of DCA used in the studies of Low-Beer and co-workers is far smaller than that used in the other studies. We do not know if this has any relevance to the discrepancy between the reported results.

An alternative mechanism by which DCA may influence bile saturation has been forwarded recently[47,52], and is based on the possibility that bile acids directly influence biliary lipid secretion by virtue of their detergent properties. In man, as in other animal species, biliary lipid secretion is closely linked to that of bile acids[53].

Molecules of the physiological bile acids have structural differences as to the number, the reciprocal position and orientation of the hydroxyl functions, which confer on them a different hydrophilic–hydrophobic balance. This aspect has been well quantified using high-pressure liquid chromatography and reverse-phase columns. With this system Armstrong and Carey[54] found that the order of elution of a mixture of bile acids is a function of their hydrophilicity. Hydrophilicity of the physiological bile acids, both free and conjugated, decreases in the order CA > CDCA > DCA > LCA, taurine conjugates being more hydrophilic than glycine conjugates. Such a characteristic is central to the lipid-solubilizing capacity of bile acids in that it has been shown that hydrophilicity correlates inversely with the micellar dissolution rate of cholesterol in model systems[54–56].

Whatever the intracellular site and the mechanism by which bile acids interact with cholesterol and phospholipid before their appearance in the bile, it may well be that the extent of this interaction, and hence the biliary output, is influenced by the detergent capacity of the bile acids. On this assumption we have conducted a study on T-tube patients, designed to assess the effect of individual bile acids on biliary lipid secretion. Bile acids investigated were DCA, CDCA, CA and UDCA. In the conditions of our study the replacement of the endogenous pool with individual bile acids was nearly complete. Biliary output of cholesterol and phospholipids was related linearly to that of bile acids, for the range of bile acid secretion observed.

The amount of cholesterol and phospholipid coupled to bile acids differed significantly depending on the bile acid secreted, being highest during DCA secretion followed, in decreasing order, by that observed during CDCA, CA and UDCA secretion[57].

Thus in our experimental conditions it seemed that biliary lipid output correlated to the hydrophilic–hydrophobic balance of the bile acids in the sense that the less hydrophilic (DCA) stimulated a secretion of cholesterol greater than more hydrophilic bile acids. These findings have been obtained in unphysiological conditions; nevertheless they provide a likely explanation for the changes of bile saturation observed during chronic bile acid feeding.

Taken as a mixture of bile acids the pool possesses a detergent capacity which can be considered the resultant of the lipid-solubilizing capacity of the bile acids present, in different proportions, in the pool. From the above considerations we may assume that a given bile acid pool will stimulate a secretion of cholesterol somewhat proportional to its detergent power. It follows that if the pool is enriched with a stronger detergent such as DCA the bile saturation should be increased, whereas it should be decreased by manipulations leading to a reduction of DCA.

As already discussed, a decrease of DCA proportion is associated with a fall of bile saturation whereas feeding of DCA does not always lead to the supersaturation, suggesting that a reduced detergency of the pool is more effective in desaturating bile than an increased detergency in supersaturating it. Undoubtedly bile acid pool composition is not the sole determinant of bile cholesterol saturation, and availability of cholesterol to be secreted into the bile would also be important.

References

1. Cleave, T. L., Campbell, G. D. and Painter, N. S. (1969). *Diabetes, Coronary Thrombosis and the Saccharine Disease.* 2nd edn. (Bristol: Wright)
2. Heaton, K. W. (1973). The epidemiology of gallstones and suggested aetiology. *Clin. Gastroenterol.*, **2**, 67–83
3. Sarles, H., Chalvet, H., Ambrosi, L., Gazeix, N. and D'Ortoli, A. (1957). Etude statistique des facteurs diététiques dans la pathologie de la lithiase biliaire humaine. *Sem. Hôp. Paris*, **33**, 3424–3438
4. Sarles, H., Chabert, C., Pommeau, Y., Save, E., Mouret, H. and Gerolami, A. (1969). Diet and

cholesterol gallstones. A study of 101 patients with cholelithiasis compared to 101 matched controls. *Am. J. Dig. Dis.*, **14**, 531–534
5. Sarles, H., Hauton, J., Planche, N. E., Lafont, H. and Gerolami, A. (1970). Diet, cholesterol gallstones and composition of the bile. *Am. J. Dig. Dis.*, **15**, 251–260
6. Sarles, H., Gerolami, A. and Bord, A. (1978). Diet and cholesterol gallstones. A further study. *Digestion*, **17**, 128–134
7. Reid, J. M., Fullmer, D. S., Pettigrew, K. D., Burch, T. A., Bennett, P. H., Miller, M. and Whedon, G. D. (1971). Nutrient intake of Pima Indian women: relationship to diabetes mellitus and gallbladder disease. *Am. J. Clin. Nutr.*, **24**, 1281–1289
8. Thornton, J. R., Emmett, P. M. and Heaton, K. W. (1983). Diet and gallstones: effects of refined and unrefined carbohydrate diets on bile cholesterol saturation and bile acid metabolism. *Gut*, **24**, 2–6
9. Williams, C. N., Johnston, J. L., McCarthy, S. and Field, C. A. (1981). Biliary lipid, bile acid composition and dietary correlations in Micmac Indian women. A population study. *Dig. Dis. Sci.*, **26**, 42–49
10. Gross, H. M. B. (1929). A statistical study of cholelithiasis. *J. Pathol. Bacteriol.*, **32**, 503–526
11. Marinović, I., Guerra, C. and Larach, G. (1972). Incidencia de litiasis biliar en material de autopsias y análisis de composición de los cálculos. *Rev. Med. Chil.*, **100**, 1320–1327
12. Van der Linden, W. (1961). Some biological traits in female gallstone disease patients: a study of body build, parity and serum cholesterol level with a discussion of some problems of selection in observational hospital data. *Acta Chir. Scand.* (Suppl.), **269**, 1–94
13. Friedman, G. D., Kannel, W. B. and Dawber, T. R. (1966). The epidemiology of gallbladder disease: observations in the Framingham study. *J. Chron. Dis.*, **19**, 273–292
14. Sturdevant, R. A. L., Pearce, M. L. and Dayton, S. (1973). Increased prevalence of cholelithiasis in men ingesting a serum-cholesterol-lowering diet. *N. Engl. J. Med.*, **288**, 24–27
15. Bennion, L. J. and Grundy, S. M. (1975). Effects of obesity and caloric intake on biliary lipid metabolism in man. *J. Clin. Invest.*, **56**, 996–1011
16. Shaffer, E. A. and Small, D. M. (1977). Biliary lipid secretion in cholesterol gallstone disease: the effect of cholecystectomy and obesity. *J. Clin. Invest.*, **59**, 828–840
17. Mabee, T. M., Meyer, P., DenBesten, L. and Mason, E. E. (1976). The mechanism of increased gallstone formation in obese human subjects. *Surgery*, **79**, 460–468
18. Low-Beer, T. S. and Pomare, E. W. (1975). Can colonic bacterial metabolites predispose to cholesterol gallstones? *Br. Med. J.*, **1**, 438–440
19. Macdonald, I. A., Bokkenheuser, V. D., Winter, J., McLernon, A. M. and Mosbach, E. H. (1983). Degradation of steroids in the human gut. *J. Lipid Res.*, **24**, 675–700
20. Hepner, G. W., Hofmann, A. F., Malagelada, J. R., Szczepanik, A. P. and Klein, P. D. (1974). Increased bacterial degradation of bile acids in cholecystectomized patients. *Gastroenterology*, **66**, 556–564
21. Pomare, E. W. and Heaton, K. W. (1973). The effect of cholecystectomy on bile salt metabolism. *Gut*, **14**, 753–762
22. Almond, H. R., Vlahcevic, Z. R., Bell, C. C., Gregory, D. H. and Swell, L. (1973). Bile acid pools, kinetics and biliary lipid composition before and after cholecystectomy. *N. Engl. J. Med.*, **289**, 1213–1216
23. Heaton, K. W. (1977). Disturbances of bile acid metabolism in intestinal disease. *Clin. Gastroenterol.*, **6**, 69–89
24. Abaurre, R., Gordon, S. G., Mann, J. G. and Kern, F. Jr. (1969). Fasting bile salt pool size and composition after ileal resection. *Gastroenterology*, **57**, 679–688
25. Van der Werf, S. D. J., Huijbregts, A. W. M., Lamers, H. L. M., Van Berge-Henegouwen, G. P. and Van Tongeren, J. H. M. (1981). Age dependent differences in human bile acid metabolism and 7α-dehydroxylation. *Eur. J. Clin. Invest.*, **11**, 425–431
26. Wynder, E. L. and Reddy, B. S. (1974). Metabolic epidemiology of colorectal cancer. *Cancer* (Suppl.), **34**, 801–806
27. Hepner, G. W. (1975). Altered bile acid metabolism in vegetarians. *Am. J. Dig. Dis.*, **20**, 935–940
28. Huijbregts, A. W. M., Van Schaik, A., Van Berge-Henegouwen, G. P. and Van der Werf, S. D. J. (1980). Serum lipids, biliary lipid composition, and bile acid metabolism in vegetarians as compared to normal controls. *Eur. J. Clin. Invest.*, **10**, 443–449

29. Pomare, E. W. and Heaton, K. W. (1973). Alteration of bile salt metabolism by dietary fibre (bran). *Br. Med. J.*, **4**, 262–264
30. Pomare, E. W., Heaton, K. W., Low-Beer, T. S. and Espiner, H. J. (1976). The effect of wheat bran upon bile salt metabolism and upon the lipid composition of bile in gallstone patients. *Am. J. Dig. Dis.*, **21**, 521–526
31. McDougall, R. M., Yakymyshyn, L., Walker, K. and Thurston, O. G. (1978). Effect of wheat bran on serum lipoproteins and biliary lipids. *Can. J. Surg.*, **21**, 433–435
32. Wicks, A. C. B., Yeates, J. and Heaton, K. W. (1978). Bran and bile: time-course of changes in normal young men given a standard dose. *Scand. J. Gastroenterol.*, **13**, 289–292
33. Huijbregts, A. W. M., Van Berge-Henegouwen, G. P., Hectors, M. P. C., Van Schaik, A. and Van der Werf, S. D. J. (1980). Effects of a standardized wheat bran preparation on biliary lipid composition and bile acid metabolism in young healthy males. *Eur. J. Clin. Invest.*, **10**, 451–458
34. Meyer, P. D., Den Besten, L. and Mason, E. E. (1979). The effects of a high-fiber diet on bile acid pool size, bile acid kinetics, and biliary lipid secretory rates in the morbidly obese. *Surgery*, **85**, 311–316
35. Hepner, G. W. (1975). Effect of decreased gallbladder stimulation on enterohepatic cycling and kinetics of bile acids. *Gastroenterology*, **68**, 1574–1581
36. Hofmann, A. F., Grundy, S. M., Lachin, J. M., Lan, S. P., Baum, R. A., Hanson, R. F., Hersh, T., Hightower, N. C. Jr., Marks, J. W., Mekhijan, H., Shaefer, R. A., Soloway, R. D., Thistle, J. L., Thomas, F. B., Tyor, M. P. and the National Cooperative Gallstone Study Group (1982). Pretreatment biliary lipid composition in white patients with radiolucent gallstones in the National Cooperative Gallstone Study. *Gastroenterology*, **83**, 738–752
37. Sjövall, J. (1960). Bile acids in man under normal and pathological conditions; bile acids and steroids. *Clin. Chim. Acta*, **5**, 33–41
38. Pomare, E. W. and Heaton, K. W. (1973). Bile salt metabolism in patients with gallstones in functioning gallbladder. *Gut*, **14**, 885–890
39. Van der Linden, W. and Bergman, F. (1977). An analysis of data on human hepatic bile. Relationship between main bile components, serum cholesterol and serum triglycerides. *Scand. J. Clin. Lab. Invest.*, **37**, 741–747
40. Bennion, L. J., Mott, D. M. and Howard, B. V. (1980). Oral contraceptives raise the cholesterol saturation of bile increasing biliary cholesterol secretion. *Metabolism*, **29**, 18–22
41. Ahlberg, J., Angelin, B. and Einarsson, K. (1980). Biliary lipid composition in normo- and hyperlipoproteinemia. *Gastroenterology*, **79**, 90–94
42. Ponz de Leon, M., Carulli, N., Iori, R., Loria, P. and Romani, M. (1983). Regulation of cholesterol absorption by bile acids: role of deoxycholic and cholic acid pool expansion on dietary cholesterol absorption. *Ital. J. Gastroenterol.*, **15**, 86–93
43. LaRusso, N. F., Szczepanic, P. A. and Hofmann, A. F. (1977). Effect of deoxycholic acid ingestion on bile acid metabolism and biliary lipid secretion in normal subjects. *Gastroenterology*, **72**, 132–140
44. Ahlberg, J., Angelin, B., Einarsson, K., Hellström, K. and Leijd, B. (1977). Influence of deoxycholic acid on biliary lipids in man. *Clin. Sci. Mol. Med.*, **53**, 249–256
45. Carulli, N., Ponz de Leon, M., Zironi, F., Iori, R. and Loria, P. (1980). Bile acid feeding and hepatic sterol metabolism: effect of deoxycholic acid. *Gastroenterology*, **79**, 637–641
46. Low-Beer, T. S. and Nutter, S. (1978). Colonic bacterial activity, biliary cholesterol saturation, and pathogenesis of gallstones. *Lancet*, **2**, 1063–1064
47. Carulli, N., Ponz de Leon, M., Loria, P., Iori, R., Rosi, A. and Romani, M. (1981). Effect of the selective expansion of cholic acid pool on bile lipid composition: possible mechanism of bile acid induced biliary cholesterol desaturation. *Gastroenterology*, **81**, 539–546
48. Thornton, J. R. and Heaton, K. W. (1981). Effects of lactulose on bile composition. In Paumgartner, G., Stiehl, A. and Gerok, W. (eds.) *Bile Acids and Lipids*, pp. 181–188. (Lancaster: MTP Press)
49. Salvioli, G., Salati, R., Bondi, M., Fratalocchi, A., Sala, B. M. and Gibertini, A. (1982). Bile acid transformation by the intestinal flora and cholesterol saturation in bile. Effects of Streptococcus faecium administration. *Digestion*, **23**, 80–88
50. Low-Beer, T. S., Pomare, E. W. and Morris, J. S. (1972). Control of bile salt synthesis. *Nature: New Biol.*, **238**, 215–216
51. Pomare, E. W. and Low-Beer, T. S. (1975). The selective inhibition of chenodeoxycholate

synthesis by cholate metabolites in man. *Clin. Sci. Mol. Med.*, **48**, 315–321

52. Carulli, N. and Ponz de Leon, M. (1982). How does bile acid pool composition regulate bile cholesterol saturation? *Ital. J. Gastroenterol.*, **14**, 179–183
53. Wagner, C. I., Trotman, B. V. and Soloway, R. D. (1976). Kinetic analysis of biliary lipid excretion in man and dog. *J. Clin. Invest.*, **57**, 473–477
54. Armstrong, M. J. and Carey, M. C. (1982). The hydrophobic-hydrophilic balance of bile salts. Inverse correlation between reverse-phase high performance liquid chromatographic mobilities and micellar cholesterol-solubilizing capacities. *J. Lipid Res.*, **23**, 70–80
55. Hegardt, F. G. and Dam, H. (1971). The solubility of cholesterol in aqueous solutions of bile salts and lecithin. *Z. Ernährungswiss.*, **10**, 223–233
56. Neiderhiser, D. H. and Roth, H. P. (1968). Cholesterol solubilization by solutions of bile salts and bile salts plus lecithin. *Proc. Soc. Exp. Biol. Med.*, **128**, 221–225
57. Carulli, N., Loria, P., Bertolotti, M., Ponz de Leon, M., Salvioli, G. F. and Iori, R. (1983). Physicalchemical characteristics (detergency) of bile acids (BA) as determinant of bile lipid secretion. *Gastroenterology*, **84**, 1367 (abstract)

Part 3
DATA FROM EPIDEMIOLOGY AND FROM TRIALS: LESSONS FOR CLINICAL PRACTICE

Chairmen: R. H. DOWLING and G. GIUNCHI

16
Gallbladder ultrasonography as a diagnostic tool in epidemiological screenings

L. LALLONI and the GREPCO Group*

Most *in vivo* studies on the epidemiology of gallstone disease have been performed by oral cholecystography. However, this technique has several disadvantages since it presents the hazards associated with X-ray exposure, is time-consuming, expensive and quite often does not offer a definite answer. All these limitations do not suggest the use of oral cholecystography as the technique of choice for epidemiological purposes.

The introduction of real-time ultrasonography for the detection of gallstones has markedly changed the epidemiological approach to the disease. Today it is possible to carry out screenings on a large scale on free-living population samples. Moreover, ultrasonography represents a rapid, easily repeatable procedure which has been shown to be as accurate as oral cholecystography[1–9].

This chapter reports ultrasonographic and cholecystographic results obtained within a survey on gallstone disease carried out by GREPCO on a sample of 1092 female civil servants in Rome. The general aims, screening procedures and prevalence data of the study are reported in Chapter 3 of this volume and have been described elsewhere[10,11].

Real-time ultrasonography of the liver and biliary tract was performed by the same physician of the echographic staff using linear array ALOKA equipment with a 3 MHz transducer. The women were examined, after an over-night fast, in the supine, left anterior oblique, and standing positions, with the consequent physiological relaxation of the gallbladder. Multiple scans of the right hypochondrium were obtained in the transverse, longitudinal and oblique planes. The woman's history was unknown to the physician of the echographic staff, except in the case of previous cholecystectomy. Ultrasound examination was considered conclusive in the presence of

* For the composition of the Group see p. xi

one of the following conditions: (1) non-shadowing echoes within a well-visualized gallbladder lumen; (2) shadowing echoes within a well-visualized gallbladder lumen; (3) non-visualization of the gallbladder lumen with high-level echoes and shadowing in the right hypochondrium. Figures 1–3 show three typical echograms.

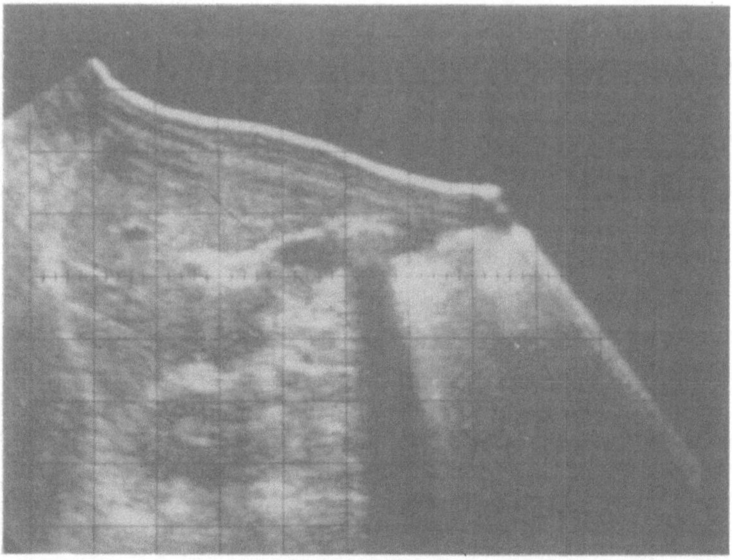

Figure 1 Shadowing echoes within a well-visualized gallbladder lumen

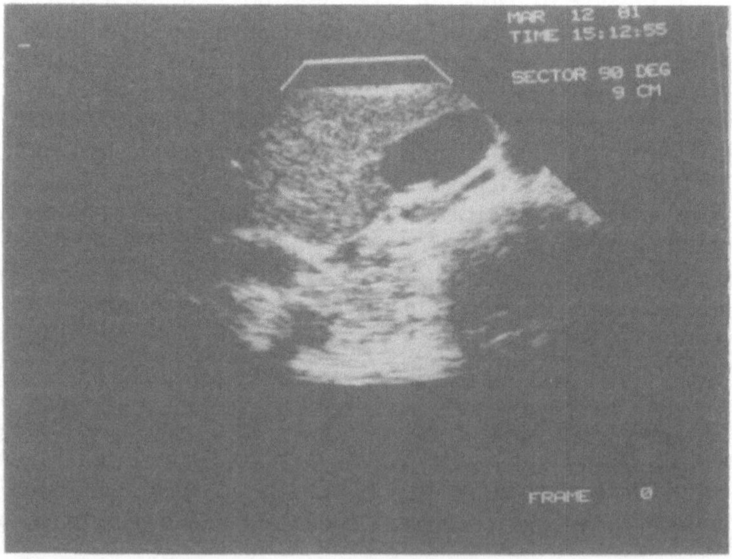

Figure 2 Non-shadowing echoes within a well-visualized gallbladder lumen

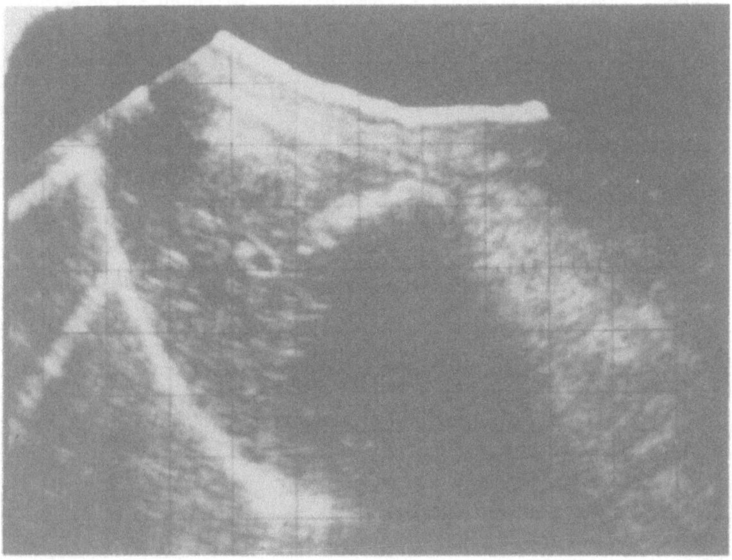

Figure 3 Non-visualization of the gallbladder lumen with high level echoes and shadowing in the right hypochondrium

In the case of non-visualization of the gallbladder the subject was re-examined on a subsequent day. If echography was still insufficient to draw definite conclusions because of body habitus, meteorism or presence of doubtful images, or if the presence of gallstones was suspected but not ascertained, the woman was referred to our outpatient service for a standard oral cholecystography. These women were defined as participants with doubtful or inconclusive ultrasound examination.

To validate the results of ultrasonography, all women with positive ultrasound examination of the gallbladder and a negative random sample were asked to have a standard oral cholecystography. Pregnant women, as well as those who had been submitted to oral cholecystography during the previous 12 months, were excluded. If, using the standard method, the gallbladder was unclearly or non-visualized, cholecystography was repeated after administration of a double dose of contrast medium. Cholecystograms were interpreted independently by two radiologists unaware of echographic findings. Concordant readings were obtained in all cases but one; agreement was finally reached on this cholecystogram also.

Ultrasound examination of the gallbladder was performed in 1092 women. Inconclusive or doubtful results were obtained in 31 women (2.8%) (Table 1); 22 were submitted to oral cholecystography which identified the presence of gallstones in four subjects. Nine women refused X-ray examination and were therefore excluded from prevalence data.

Thirty-eight women with positive ultrasound examination were submitted to oral cholecystography. The gallbladder was not visualized in 6 of them. Two women had positive echogram and negative cholecystogram, and it was

Table 1 Results of verification procedures for assessment of cholelithiasis

	No. of women	*Percentage*
Ultrasonography inconclusive, invited for cholecystography	31	100
Cholecystography not done	9*	29
Negative cholecystogram	18	58
Positive cholecystogram	4	13
Gallbladder not visualized on cholecystogram	0	0

*Excluded from calculation of prevalence data

Table 2 Results of verification procedures for assessment of cholelithiasis

	No. of women	*Percentage*
Ultrasonography positive, invited for cholecystography	64	100
Cholecystography not done, without record of positive cholecystogram	11	17.2
Cholecystography not done, with record of positive cholecystogram	15	23.4
Negative cholecystogram	2*	3.1
Positive cholecystogram	30	46.9
Gallbladder not visualized on cholecystogram	6	9.4

*Excluded from calculation of prevalence data

Table 3 Results of verification procedures for assessment of cholelithiasis

	No. of women	*Percentage*
Ultrasonography negative, random sample, invited for cholecystography	72	100
Cholecystography not done	14	19.4
Negative cholecystogram	58	80.6
Positive cholecystogram	0	0
Gallbladder not visualized on cholecystogram	0	0

impossible to reach a definite conclusion on their gallbladder status (Table 2).

Oral cholecystography was performed in 58 out of 72 women belonging to the negative random sample. A 100 % agreement between the two techniques was obtained (Table 3).

To estimate the prevalence of gallstone disease in the population under study, gallbladder status was defined as follows: (1) normal at echography and/or oral cholecystography; (2) presence of gallstones at echography and/or oral cholecystography; (3) presence of gallstones at echography and non-visualization of the gallbladder after a double dose of contrast medium at cholecystography; (4) presence of gallstones at oral cholecystography and inconclusive echography; (5) previous cholecystectomy. Conditions 2, 3, 4 and 5 defined gallstone disease.

In conclusion, in our experience ultrasonography proved to be a very accurate and reliable technique for the detection of gallstones. Its concordance with oral cholecystography (97.9 %), the low percentage of inconclusive examinations (2.8 %), the absence of risks and contraindications, quickness and easy repeatibility, as well as low costs, are all remarkable advantages which suggest ultrasonography as the technique of choice for epidemiological screenings.

References

1. Aron, S. and Rosenquist, C. J. (1976). Gray scale cholecystosonography: an evaluation of accuracy. *Am. J. Roentgenol.*, **127**, 817
2. Athey, P. A. and Martinez, E. J. (1979). Gray scale ultrasound of the gallbladder: a primary screening procedure for cholelithiasis. *Texas Med.*, **75**, 271
3. Nihan, P. (1978). Surgical and pathologic correlation of cholecystosonography and cholecystography. *Am. J. Roentgenol.*, **131**, 227
4. Cooperberg, P. L., Pon, M. S., Wong, P., Stoller, J. L. and Burhenne, H. J. (1979). Real-time high resolution ultrasound in the detection of biliary calculi. *Radiology*, **131**, 789
5. McCluskey, P., Prinz, R. A., Guico, R. and Greenlee, H. B. (1979). Use of ultrasound to demonstrate gallstones in symptomatic patients with normal oral cholecystograms. *Am. J. Surg.*, **138**, 655
6. Daly, R., Arnaud, J. P., Turbelin, J. M. and Adloff, M. (1980). Lithiase vésiculaire. Etude comparative de l'ultrasonographie vésiculaire et de la cholécystographie per os. *Nouv. Presse Méd.*, **25**, 9
7. Gonzalez, A. C. and Johnson, J. A. (1978). Ultrasonic examination of the gallbladder: a review. *Clin. Radiol.*, **29**, 171
8. Leopold, G. R., Amberg, Gosink, B. B. and Mittelstaedt, C. (1976). Gray scale ultrasonic cholecystography: a comparison with conventional radiographic techniques. *Radiology*, **121**, 445
9. McAvoy, J. M., Roth, J., Rees, W. V., Orr, F. and Dainko, E. A. (1978). Role of ultrasonography in the primary diagnosis of cholelithiasis. *Am. J. Surg.*, **136**, 309
10. Rome Group for Epidemiology and Prevention of Cholelithiasis (GREPCO) (1984). Prevalence of gallstone disease in an Italian adult female population. *Am. J. Epidemiol.*, **119**, 5
11. Rome Group for Epidemiology and Prevention of Cholelithiasis (GREPCO) (1982). Prevalenza della colelitiasi: osservazioni preliminari su un campione di popolazione lavorativa femminile. *Epatologia*, **28**, 79–88

17
Epidemiology and medical treatment of cholesterol gallstones: recurrence, post-dissolution management and the future

R. H. DOWLING

INTRODUCTION

The results of epidemiological studies, now based mainly on ultrasound screening, tell us that in developed societies the prevalence of gallstones is approximately 10%[1]. When combined with clinical assessment they also tell us that approximately two-thirds of gallstone carriers are unaware that they have stones[2,3]. In other words, the majority of gallstones diagnosed in this way are silent or asymptomatic. Indirect support for the concept that 'the innocent gallstone is not a myth'[4] comes from comparisons between prevalence rates for cholelithiasis and cholecystectomy rates in any given community. Even though the frequency with which cholecystectomy is carried out varies considerably from country to country[5], and despite the fact that surgical removal of the gallbladder is now the most common abdominal operation performed in Western society[6], it is clear that only a minority of gallstone carriers will ever come to surgery. By inference, therefore, the majority of patients with cholelithiasis are either unaware of their stones or have related symptoms which the patient, the doctor (or both) judge to be tolerable.

The increasing use of upper abdominal ultrasonography – (1) in patients with symptoms which suggest the possible presence of gallstones, (2) as part of routine physical examinations, or (3) in screening studies of segments of the population – will both unmask many previously undiagnosed stones and, at the same time, create an ethical and economical dilemma for those who make the diagnosis.

Should the patient be told that he or she has gallstones? Should the stones be treated actively, or should one simply adopt a watch-and-wait policy – treating symptoms if and when they arise? If one decides in favour of active treatment, should this be surgery or, in patients shown by subsequent cholecystectography to have radiolucent stones and a patent cystic duct, should it be medical dissolution therapy?

At present, there are no logical and scientifically based answers to these questions. Ideally, decisions about which of the therapeutic options is followed should be based on a knowledge of the risks and benefits of each approach. The risks and benefits of elective cholecystectomy are now well known and need not be re-stated here. Suffice to say that removal of the gallbladder is a safe and effective operation but, as with any abdominal surgery, cholecystectomy carries a small risk of morbidity and mortality.

The consequences of the conservative approach are less certain. The results of several classical studies on the natural history of untreated gallstone disease are available[7-9], but these were often based on studies in symptomatic patients, examined non-representative sections of the population[7] or, in some cases, were based on retrospective analyses which therefore suffer the defects of any retrospective study.

Based on experience gained over the last 12 years[10], the potential benefits and side-effects of medical treatment are now at least partly known. The purpose of this chapter, therefore, is to review briefly what is known about: (1) the efficacy of chenodeoxycholic acid (CDCA) and ursodeoxycholic acid (UDCA) in dissolving gallstones, (2) the factors influencing the response to treatment, (3) the reasons for patients 'dropping out', or being withdrawn from therapy, (4) the reliability of methods used to diagnose complete gallstone dissolution and to detect recurrence and (5) recurrence rates and post-dissolution management.

EFFICACY OF, AND FACTORS INFLUENCING THE RESPONSE TO, TREATMENT

When given in adequate doses (see below), CDCA and UDCA reduce biliary cholesterol secretion[11,12] and desaturate fasting duodenal bile[13,14], in most gallstone patients. However, the reported efficacy of these bile acid treatments in dissolving gallstones completely, varies considerably from centre to centre ranging from 13.5 % (by life-table analysis) after 2 years CDCA treatment in the so-called 'high-dose' group (750 mg/day which corresponds to 9.0 mg kg^{-1} day^{-1} in men and 10.6 in women) of the United States National Cooperative Gallstone Study (NCGS)[15] to approximately 80% with both bile acids in studies from Germany[16,17].

In the author's unit the final overall efficacy figure for CDCA in producing confirmed complete gallstone dissolution was just under 40 % of a largely unselected population of patients with radiolucent stones[18]. This figure rose to approximately 60 % in patients selected as being ideally suited for medical treatment – that is non-obese patients with small or medium-sized radiolucent gallstones measuring less than 15 mm in diameter[18]. If, in addition, we insisted on proof that the fasting duodenal bile had become desaturated in cholesterol during treatment, and demanded that the patients had completed not less than 12 months therapy, the cumulative efficacy rate rose to 80 %. It should be emphasized, however, that this latter figure represents the *maximum* possible dissolution rate which, short of exceptional luck, is unlikely to be achieved – because of unavoidable complications which lead to withdrawal or drop-out from therapy (see below).

Although intermediate results of many relatively short-term studies with UDCA (for example the results of partial and/or complete gallstone dissolution after 1 or 2 years treatment) are now available[19,20], final results, when treatment is stopped because of confirmed complete gallstone dissolution or therapeutic failure, are only now starting to appear[20,21,28].

All investigators agree that UDCA is a remarkably 'benign' bile acid treatment with virtually no side-effects. Unlike CDCA, which causes dose-related although often transient diarrhoea in 40–60 % of patients[10], modest hypertransaminasaemia in approximately 30 % of patients[10] and in the NCGS, at least, a slight but significant rise in fasting serum cholesterol levels[15], UDCA is virtually free from these problems. However, ursotherapy is associated with acquired gallstone opacification[22–24]. This also happens spontaneously[15] and is seen during chenotherapy[10,15,18,25,26], but there seems little doubt that it occurs more often during UDCA treatment. In the author's series[24], for example, it was seen in 19 of 119 patients with previously radiolucent stones treated with UDCA for 6 months or more. By life-table analysis this corresponds to an acquired gallstone opacification rate of 24.1 % at 3 years. Acquired calcification usually, but not invariably[15,24], halts subsequent gallstone dissolution. This may explain, at least in part, why, in the author's series, the efficacy of UDCA treatment in producing partial *plus* complete gallstone dissolution was relatively high and rapid, reaching a maximum of 77.4% at 3 years, while the rate for confirmed complete gallstone dissolution was as low as 20.3% at 3 years – again as judged by life-table analyses[24]. This contrasts with more optimistic results from Italy, Germany and the United States[17,27,28].

The factors governing efficacy are shown in Table 1. They include:

(1) the criteria used in the initial selection of patients for treatment;
(2) the dose and duration of therapy;
(3) the 'compliance' of patients in taking their prescribed bile acid doses;
(4) the accuracy of diagnostic methods used to detect partial and/or complete gallstone dissolution;
(5) the methods used to calculate the results – that is, which patients are included and which are excluded from the denominator when calculating percentage efficacy of treatment in producing partial and/or complete gallstone dissolution.

The best results are seen when, during the initial selection of patients for treatment, therapy is confined to non-obese patients who have a patent cystic duct – usually judged by opacification of the gallbladder during oral cholecystography – and radiolucent stones measuring less than 15 mm in diameter. Those with buoyant stones which 'float' or form a horizontal layer in the mixture of bile and contrast medium within the gallbladder when the patient is standing erect, do particularly well. Unfortunately such stones are rare, being seen in only 5 % of patients accepted for treatment in the author's unit[29]. However, in the series described by Fromm *et al.*[28], the percentage of patients with floating stones ranged from 42 % to 62 %.

Most clinicians treating gallstone patients now relate the amount of bile acid prescribed to the patient's body weight[10] and recommend doses of

Table 1 Factors governing the efficacy of CDCA and UDCA in dissolving gallstones

Initial patient selection
(a) Absolute
radiolucent gallstones
patent cystic duct
(b) Relative
non-obese patients
stones measuring <15 mm diameter
multiple stones
buoyant/floating stones
motivated (compliant) patients

Bile acid dose
(a) Proven
not less than 13–15 mg CDCA kg^{-1} day^{-1}
not less than 10 mg UDCA kg^{-1} day^{-1}
(b) Possible
daily bile acid dose taken at bedtime
accompanying low-cholesterol diet

Duration of treatment
Efficacy increases with time
Approx. 90% of patients with stones <15 mm diameter who are going to respond, will show radiological/ultrasonographic evidence of doing so within 12 months
Patients with stones >15 mm may require 2 years treatment before assessing ultimate outcome.

Methods used to calculate/express results
Life-table (actuarial) analysis is preferred method
Inclusion or exclusion from the denominator, of patients who:
(a) default from follow-up (drop-outs)
(b) withdraw from treatment because of:
complications of bile acid treatment
complications of gallstones
non-response
(c) are withdrawn from treatment by the physician

approximately 15 mg CDCA kg^{-1} day^{-1} and 10 mg UDCA kg^{-1} day^{-1}. There is little reliable information about short- and long-term compliance in patients taking these prescribed doses but, even in highly motivated patients supervised regularly by caring and enthusiastic physicians, the results of questionnaires completed by patients given other drugs suggest that compliance in taking bile acid treatment is likely to be far short of 100%.

The diagnostic accuracy of cholecystography in proving complete gallstone dissolution has recently been questioned[30,31]. Small residual stones or particles measuring <2 mm in diameter cannot be detected reliably by either cholecystography or ultrasonography. For this reason, since the introduction of bile acid dissolution therapy for gallstones, most investigators arbitrarily recommended 1–3 months further bile acid therapy after the initial on-treatment X-rays suggested completed gallstone dissolution. It would now seem sensible to supplement this with real-time ultrasonography (where available) of the gallbladder to minimize the chances of over-diagnosing complete gallstone dissolution when, in fact, residual gravel persists to act as a nidus for re-growth or recurrence of stones (see below).

Apart from the factors discussed above, another reason for the considerable discrepancies between reported efficacy rates of bile acid treatment in producing confirmed complete gallstone dissolution lies in the statistical methods used to calculate the results. Largely stimulated by the publication of the NCGS, many investigators now use actuarial life-table analyses to express their results[15]. This technique was 'borrowed' from oncology studies where cumulative survival rates were plotted as the percentage of patients remaining alive as a function of time and treatment. This method has advantages and disadvantages. It allows for the variable duration of follow-up in individual patients but provides a projected, rather than an actual, figure for percentage efficacy and it is sometimes difficult to extract 'raw data' from life-table results expressed in this way. Of greater importance is the need to agree uniform criteria for including or excluding from the analyses, results in patients who stopped treatment for whatever reason – before the final outcome of therapy has been established. Whether or not this is of major importance in any individual series will depend on the frequency of default or drop-out, the 'withdrawal' rate independent of how the decision to withdraw treatment is reached, and the complication rate – whether attributable to the gallstones or to the bile acid therapy. Such information is not always available in published reports and without it, valid comparisons of efficacy figures from different centres are difficult or impossible.

REASONS FOR 'DROP-OUT' AND WITHDRAWAL FROM THERAPY

By definition, if a patient defaults from treatment and follow-up, the reasons for his or her drop-out are likely to remain unknown. In some cases it may represent disenchantment with the often lengthy period of therapy and the need for follow-up, in some it may be because of side-effects of treatment (such as diarrhoea during CDCA therapy), whilst in others it may simply indicate poor motivation. Such withdrawals/drop-outs may, therefore, be considered as avoidable. Conversely, in other patients the reasons for withdrawal/drop-out may be inevitable and in these cases, the reasons can often be defined. These are summarized in Table 2.

Development of a non-functioning gallbladder

The natural history of untreated gallstone disease (Fig. 1) suggests that at an advanced stage in the evolution of the disease (Fig. 1 – Stage IV) the cystic duct becomes blocked and the gallbladder no longer opacifies during oral cholecystography*. There are only limited data available relating to the subsequent fate of these patients, but the frequency of surgical complications (such as cholecystitis, the development of hydrops of the gallbladder or

* There are many reasons other than a blocked cystic duct for non-visualization of the gallbladder during oral cholecystography: these have been reviewed elsewhere[32].

Table 2 Reasons for inevitable withdrawal/drop-out from bile acid treatment

Complications	*Estimated frequency*
(1) *Onset of 'surgical' complications* Severe and/or recurrent biliary colic Obstructive jaundice Cholecystitis Cholangitis Pancreatitis	Approx. 10%
(2) *Development of cystic duct obstruction* (=onset of an irreversible non-functioning gallbladder) often develops without symptoms	5–10%
(3) *Acquired gallstone calcification* (rim opacification) preventing subsequent gallstone dissolution	
during CDCA treatment	0–5%
during UDCA treatment	5–25%
(4) *Radiolucent non-cholesterol stones and/or non-dissolvable residue*	10–20%
(5) *Failure to respond to bile acid treatment* (persistence or recurrence of supersaturated bile despite adequate bile acid doses, good compliance and enrichment of biliary bile acids with prescribed agent). biological 'resistance' adaptive 'escape' from desaturating effect of treatment	Approx. 5%

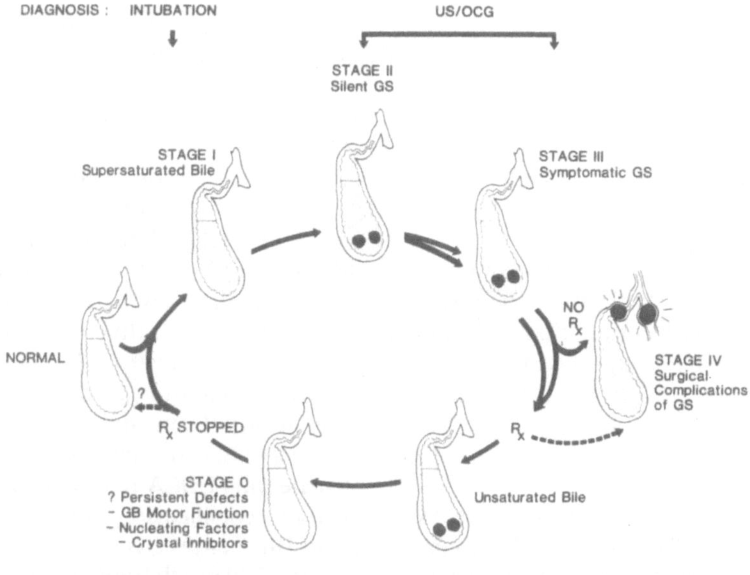

Figure 1 Schematic illustration of the gallstone formation, dissolution and recurrence cycle (based on earlier diagrams by Drs D. M. Small, A. F. Hofmann and C. Wolpers)

mucocoele formation and of empyaema of the gallbladder) in this subgroup of patients is likely to be higher than that seen in patients with a normally functioning gallbladder. This occurs in 5–10% of patients.

Onset of surgical complications

In addition to the complications of a blocked cystic duct described above, one must also consider complications of stone migration into the biliary tree such as severe and/or recurrent biliary colic, cholangitis, obstructive jaundice and pancreatitis.

In patients treated with CDCA in the author's unit, these 'surgical' complications of gallstones occurred in approximately 10% of the patients.

Whether or not these problems occurred more or less frequently than would have been seen in untreated patients, is unknown. However, the clinical impression that bile acid therapy 'protects' the patient from the onset of these complications (which usually require surgery), is partly supported by a supplementary retrospective analysis of the NCGS results by Jacobus *et al.*[33]. They showed that in patients with buoyant or 'floatable' stones, CDCA treatment significantly reduced the need for surgery, when compared with the placebo-treated group.

Acquired gallstone opacification (rim calcification)

This topic has already been discussed briefly above. The mechanism for the acquired calcification is not known but may be due directly to impaired calcium carbonate (probably vaterite) solubility in UDCA-rich bile[23] (E. Ros, personal communication). Alternatively, it may occur indirectly because bile acids which are markedly choleretic, such as UDCA, may affect biliary bicarbonate secretion[34] with secondary changes in bile pH and, as a result, in calcium carbonate solubility. A third hypothesis is that calcium may co-precipitate with glycoursodeoxycholic acid – which becomes a major biliary bile acid during UDCA treatment – to form calcium glycoursodeoxycholate[22]. If so, then in theory the calcification might be prevented by giving taurine supplements with the UDCA. (This is probably a cheaper and more effective way of enriching the biliary bile acids with tauroursodeoxycholate than by feeding the taurine conjugate of UDCA which, in any case, seems to be deconjugated in the gut and reconjugated in the liver with glycine, thereby defeating the object of the exercise)[35]. However, calcium glycoursodeoxycholate is, in fact, more soluble than calcium glycochenodeoxycholate (A. F. Hofmann, personal communication). If so and if, as is believed, gallstone calcification is more common during UDCA than during CDCA treatment, one might predict that the taurine plus UDCA regime would not prevent the problem of acquired gallstone calcification during UDCA treatment. This is amenable to proof and, in this context, the clinical results are infinitely more important than physicochemical predictions. The results of several such clinical studies are therefore awaited with interest.

Radiolucent non-cholesterol stones and/or residue

Although the majority of radiolucent stones are cholesterol-rich, some 10–20 % are not[36–38]. Therefore the selection of patients for medical treatment, based on the X-ray appearance of the stones, will inevitably mean that some patients, and in particular those with black pigment stones, will be inappropriately selected and treated. This is the main reason why the efficacy of bile acid therapy in producing complete gallstone dissolution can never reach 100 % and, indeed, is unlikely ever to exceed 80 %.

Biological resistance or non-response to CDCA and UDCA

This is defined as the persistance of supersaturated bile with unchanged gallstone size and number during prolonged (>1 year) treatment with 'adequate' (see above) bile acid doses and enrichment of the biliary bile acids to the expected degree, with the bile acid used in treatment. To date, this phenomenon has been described in approximately 5 % of patients treated with CDCA in one centre[39], but it may also occur with UDCA (Gleeson, Murphy and Dowling, unpublished observations).

The mechanism for this phenomenon is unknown but clinical observations suggest that in a small percentage of patients there may be an abnormal linkage between biliary cholesterol saturation (and perhaps also biliary cholesterol secretion) and the percentage of CDCA (or UDCA) in the biliary bile acids. In turn this may be due to abnormally high or unsuppressed rates of hepatic cholesterol synthesis – as judged by the activity of the rate-limiting enzyme for cholesterogenesis, HMGCoA reductase[39].

Fisher[40] has suggested that the summation of these inevitable complications will invariably reduce the maximum efficacy of bile acid treatment to approximately 33 % or less. However, this conclusion is based on the assumption that the list of inevitable complications (Table 2) will *necessarily* be cumulative. Fortunately, in our experience and in that of others, it is not – otherwise we could never have found a cumulative efficacy rate for confirmed complete gallstone dissolution with CDCA of 60 % in our prospective study[18].

THE RELIABILITY OF CHOLECYSTOGRAPHY AND ULTRASONOGRAPHY IN THE DIAGNOSIS OF GALLSTONE RECURRENCE

The reliability of cholecystographic and ultrasonographic techniques in the diagnosis of complete gallstone dissolution has already been discussed. It follows that if these investigations are normal when, in fact, gallstone particles or residue persist, not only will one over-diagnose complete gallstone dissolution but one will also over-estimate gallstone recurrence when, in reality, we are simply detecting small stones which have re-grown to a detectable size. Short of surgery (which would be difficult to justify in a patient whose stones had apparently been dissolved completely by medical treatment), there is no way of knowing which of the two techniques is most accurate in the narrow context of diagnosing complete gallstone dissolution during medical treatment.

The probability of false-negative or false-positive diagnoses would obviously be minimized if the findings obtained by both techniques (X-ray and ultrasound) were always in agreement but a recent report from the British Gallstone Study Group's post-dissolution trial suggests that there are appreciable discrepancies between the two diagnostic methods in detecting recurrent stones[41]. From a total of 71 cholecystograms performed, recurrent stones were diagnosed by oral cholecystography in 11 patients, and all 11 had an accompanying ultrasound which was positive in seven but which showed no stones in the remaining four. Conversely, of the 60 patients whose X-rays were normal, 56 had an accompanying ultrasound with concordant findings in 45 but discrepant findings in the remaining 11 where the diagnosis of stones was described as 'definite' in six and 'probable' in five.

There were also discrepant findings between separate ultrasound examinations. Of the 128 ultrasound studies, stones were diagnosed on 25 occasions, again some being described as definite and some as probable, and of these the ultrasound was repeated on 16 occasions which showed no stones in seven.

Considering that these patients were being followed with 6-monthly ultrasounds and yearly oral cholecystograms, it is not surprising that the recurrent stones were detected at an early stage when they were still small – usually measuring 2–3 mm in diameter. It follows that we are working at the lower limits of detection-sensitivity for both techniques. That being the case the discrepant results are not so surprising, but it is against this background that the reported rates of gallstone recurrence must be judged.

The results of three major post-dissolution studies are now available from London[42], Paris[43] and Rochester, Minnesota[44]. They suggest that when complete gallstone dissolution has been confirmed and treatment is stopped, stones recur in approximately 40–50 % of patients within 5 years. If stones are going to recur, most do so within the first 12–24 months of stopping treatment. How one can best prevent recurrence with post-dissolution treatment is at present unknown, but several national multi-centre trials are now in progress to answer this important question.

THE FUTURE

If, as a result of lessons learnt from epidemiological studies, ultrasonographic screening is to be carried out in large sectors of the community, we are likely to diagnose many thousands of patients with Stage II or Stage III gallstone disease (Fig. 1). It has been estimated that 30–60 % of these patients will be shown, by subsequent cholecystography and other studies, to have gallstones which are suitable for medical treatment. In the opinion of the author, if there is to be a significant role for gallstone dissolution therapy in the future, it must be as preventive medicine in the early stages of the disease – not so much to prevent the development of stones (since, by definition, these have already occurred) but to halt the progress of the disease and the subsequent development of surgical complications (Fig. 1).

We now know that, in selected patients, gallstone dissolution is possible; but if we are to consider medical therapy as a credible alternative to surgery or to an expectant approach in the future, we need to improve on considerably the present state-of-the-art (Table 3). We must achieve greater efficacy in producing complete gallstone dissolution and we need to be able to do this more rapidly than the 6–24 months required in successful cases at present[10].

Table 3 The future of gallstone dissolution therapy

Needed
More rapid gallstone dissolution
Greater efficacy in producing complete gallstone dissolution by:
(a) new bile acids
(b) other gallstone-dissolving agents
(c) adjuvant/potentiating therapy
More data on gallstone recurrence
Better post-dissolution management:
(a) with intermittent or continuous, low- or full-dose bile acid, other drug or dietary measures, to lower biliary cholesterol saturation
(b) identification and removal/inhibition of nucleating factors in bile
(c) identification and stimulation/administration of inhibitors of crystallization in bile
(d) stimulation of gallbladder contractile function?
Information about origin, chemical and physicochemical characteristics, physiological control and solubility/precipitation/dissolution characteristics of biliary calcium and bile pigments
Agents to dissolve calcium-containing and/or pigment-rich gallstones.

To this end we need to develop new gallstone-dissolving agents – whether bile acids and their derivatives or other substances – and we must consider the possibility of dual therapy with adjuvant or potentiating agents to speed up the dissolution process. Lessons from post-dissolution trials should teach us more about how gallstone recurrence may be prevented and, by extrapolation, how these findings may help to prevent primary gallstone formation in high-risk populations. At present, efforts have centred on methods of improving cholesterol solubility in bile, but over the past few years we have re-learned the lesson that supersaturated bile is not synonymous with inevitable gallstone formation. Other factors, such as the presence of nucleating agents or the absence of inhibitors of crystallization, may also be needed before gallstones occur. In preventing gallstone recurrence, therefore, and in the primary role of preventing gallstone formation, we need to learn much more about how the production of nucleating factors may be prevented and how the synthesis of crystal inhibitors may be promoted. Finally, we need to consolidate and extend our limited knowledge of biliary calcium metabolism with a view to understanding more about the formation of calcium-containing gallstones, and perhaps also about how they too may be dissolved by medical treatment.

Acknowledgements

Thanks are due to past and present colleagues in the author's Unit whose results form the basis for many of the opinions expressed in this chapter: in particular, the work of Drs D. Gleeson, P. Howard, P. N. Maton, G. M. Murphy and D. C. Ruppin, and the financial support of the Special Trustees of Guy's Hospital and of Gipharmex SpA Milan, are gratefully acknowledged. Miss Cathy Weeks kindly typed the script.

References

1. Ingelfinger, F. J. (1968). Digestive disease as a national problem. V. Gallstones. *Gastroenterology*, **55**, 102–104
2. Ricci, G. (1983). The Grepco Study: aims, methodology and prevalence data. In Abstracts of International Workshop on Epidemiology and Prevention of Gallstone Disease, Rome, December 1983
3. Barbara, L. (1983). Epidemiology of gallstone disease: the Sirmione Study. In Abstracts of International Workshop on Epidemiology and Prevention of Gallstone Disease, Rome, December 1983
4. Gracie, W. A. and Ransohoff, D. F. (1982). The natural history of silent gallstones: the innocent gallstone is not a myth. *N. Engl. J. Med.*, **307**, 798–800
5. Fisher, M. M. (1979). Perspectives in gallstones. In Fisher, M. M., Goresky, C. A., Shaffer, E. A. and Strasberg, S. M. (eds.) *Gallstones*, pp. 1–17. (New York: Plenum)
6. Holland, C. and Heaton, K. W. (1972). Increasing frequency of gallbladder operations in the Bristol clinical area. *Br. Med. J.*, **3**, 672–675
7. Lund, J. (1960). Surgical indications in cholelithiasis: prophylactic cholecystectomy elucidated on the basis of long-term follow-up on 526 nonoperated cases. *Ann. Surg.*, **151**, 153–162
8. Wenckert, A. and Robertson, B. (1966). The natural course of gallstone disease. Eleven-year review of 871 nonoperated cases. *Gastroenterology*, **50**, 376–381
9. Donaldson, R. M. Jr (1982). Advice for the patient with 'silent' gallstones. *N. Engl. J. Med.*, **307**, 815–817
10. Dowling, R. H. (1982). Cholelithiasis: medical treatment. *Clin. Gastroenterol.*, **12**, 125–178
11. Northfield, T. C., LaRusso, N. F., Hofmann, A. F. and Thistle, J. L. (1975). Biliary lipid output during three meals and an overnight fast. II. Effect of chenodeoxycholic acid treatment in gallstone subjects. *Gut*, **16**, 12–17
12. von Bergmann, K., Gutsfeld, M., Schulze-Hagen, K. and von Unruh, G. (1979). Effects of ursodeoxycholic acid on biliary lipid secretion in patients with radiolucent gallstones. In Paumgartner, G., Stiehl, A. and Gerok, W. (eds.) *Biological Effects of Bile Acids*. pp. 61–66. (Lancaster: MTP Press)
13. Thistle, J. L. and Schoenfield, L. J. (1971). Induced alterations in composition of bile of persons having cholelithiasis. *Gastroenterology*, **61**, 488–496
14. Maton, P. N., Murphy, G. M. and Dowling, R. H. (1977). Ursodeoxycholic acid treatment of gallstones. Dose–response study and possible mechanism of action. *Lancet*, **2**, 1297–1301
15. Schoenfield, L. J., Lachin, J. M., the NCGS Steering Committee and the NCGS Group (1981). National Cooperative Gallstone Study: A controlled trial of the efficacy and safety of chenodeoxycholic acid for dissolution of gallstones. *Ann. Intern. Med.*, **95**, 257–282
16. Leuschner, U. (1977). Dissolution of biliary cholesterol calculi using chenodeoxycholic acid. *Internist*, **18**, 114–115
17. Leuschner, U., Leuschner, M. and Stromm, W. D. (1982). Our 10 years' experience in gallstone dissolution. Comparison with the National Cooperative Gallstone (NCGS, USA) and the Tokyo Cooperative Gallstone Study (TCGS, Japan). *Gastroenterology*, **80**, 1113 (abstract)
18. Maton, P. N., Iser, J. H., Reuben, A., Saxton, H. M., Murphy, G. M. and Dowling, R. H. (1982). The final outcome of CDCA-treatment in 125 patients with radiolucent gallstones:

factors influencing efficacy withdrawal, symptoms and side effects and post-dissolution recurrence. *Medicine (Baltimore)*, **61**, 85–96
19. Dowling, R. H., Hofmann, A. F. and Barbara, L. (1978). *Workshop on Ursodeoxycholic Acid.* (Lancaster: MTP Press)
20. Bachrach, W. H. and Hofmann, A. F. (1982). Ursodeoxycholic acid in the treatment of cholesterol cholelithiasis: a review. *Dig. Dis. Sci.*, **27**, 737–761
21. Tokyo Cooperative Gallstone Study Group (1980). Efficacy and indications of ursodeoxycholic acid treatment for dissolving gallstones. *Gastroenterology*, **78**, 542–548
22. Bateson, M. C., Bouchier, I. A. D., Trash, D. B., Maudgal, D. P. and Northfield, T. C. (1981). Calcification of radiolucent gall stones during treatment with ursodeoxycholic acid. *Br. Med. J.*, **283**, 645–656
23. Raedsch, R., Stiehl, A. and Cyzgan, P. (1983). Ursodeoxycholic acid and gallstone calcification. *Lancet*, **2**, 1296 (Letter to editor)
24. Gleeson, D., Ruppin, D. C., Murphy, G. M. and Dowling, R. H. (1983). Second look at ursodeoxycholic acid (UDCA): high efficacy for partial but low efficacy for complete gallstone dissolution, and a high rate of acquired stone opacification. *Gut*, **24**, A999–A1000 (abstract)
25. Whiting, M., Jarvinen, V. and Watts, J. (1980). Chemical composition of gallstones resistant to dissolution therapy with chenodeoxycholic acid. *Gut*, **21**, 1077–1081
26. Sarva, R., Farivar, S., Fromm, H. and Poller, W. (1981). Study of the sensitivity and specificity of computerized tomography in the detection of calcified gallstones which appear radiolucent by conventional roentgenography. *Gastrointest. Radiol.*, **6**, 165–167
27. Roda, E., Bazzoli, F. and Labate, A. M. M. (1982). Ursodeoxycholic acid vs. chenodeoxycholic acid as cholesterol gallstone-dissolving agents: a comparative randomized study. *Hepatology*, **2**, 804–810
28. Fromm, H., Roat, J. W., Gonzalez, V., Sarva, R. P. and Farivar, S. (1983). Comparative efficacy and side effects of ursodeoxycholic and chenodeoxycholic acids in dissolving gallstones. *Gastroenterology*, **85**, 1257–1264
29. Ruppin, D. C., Maton, P. N., Williams, G. V., Merdith, T. J., Murphy, G. M., and Dowling, R. H. (1982). Ursotherapy for cholesterol gallstones? *Ital. J. Gastroenterol.*, **15**, (abstract; in press)
30. Somerville, K. W., Rose, D. H. and Bell, G. D. (1982). Gall-stone dissolution and recurrence: are we being misled? *Br. Med. J.*, **284**, 1295–1297
31. Shapero, T. F., Rosen, I. E., Milson, S. R. and Fisher, M. M. (1982). Discrepancy between ultrasound and oral cholecystography in the assessment of gallstone dissolution. *Hepatology*, **2**, 587–590.
32. Baddley, H., Nolan, D. J. and Slamon, P. R. (1978). *Radiological Atlas of Biliary and Pancreatic Disease.* (Aylesbury: HM&M)
33. Jacobus, D. P., Trout, J. R., Greenwell, B. E., Schoenfield, L. J. and Lachin, J. M. (1983). The natural history and the therapeutic response to chenodiol in patients with floatable stones in the National Co-operative Gallstone Study (NCGS). *Gastroenterology*, **84**, 1197 (abstract)
34. Dumont, M., Erlinger, S. and Uchman, S. (1980). Hypercholeresis induced by ursodeoxycholic acid and 7-ketolithocholic acid in the rat. Possible role of bicarbonate transport. *Gastroenterology*, **79**, 82–89
35. Batta, A. K., Salen, G., Shefer, S., Tint, G. S. and Dayal, B. (1982). The effect of tauroursodeoxycholic acid and taurine supplementation on biliary bile acid composition. *Hepatology*, **2**, 811–816
36. Bell, G. D., Dowling, R. H., Whitney, B. and Sutor, D. J. (1975). The value of radiology in predicting gallstone type when selecting patients for medical treatment. *Gut*, **16**, 359–364.
37. Trotman, B. W., Petrella, E. J., Soloway, R. D., Sanchez, H., Morris, T. A., III and Miller, W. T. (1975). Evaluation of radiographic lucency or opaqueness of gallstones as a means of identifying cholesterol or pigment stones. Correlation of lucency or opaqueness with calcium and mineral. *Gastroenterology*, **68**, 1563–1566
38. Bruusgaard, A., Sorensen, T. I. A., Justensen, T. and Krag, E. (1976). Bile acid metabolism after jejunoileal bypass operation for obesity. *Scand. J. Gastroenterol.*, **11**, 833–838
39. Maton, P. N., Murphy, G. M. and Dowling, R. H. (1980). Lack of response to chenodeoxycholic acid in obese and non-obese patients. *Gut*, **21**, 1082–1086
40. Fisher, M. M., Roberts, E. A., Rosen, I. E. and Wilson, S. R. (1982). The efficacy of

chenodeoxycholic acid in the dissolution of gallstones. In *Bile Acids and Cholesterol in Health and Disease*. I. Abstracts, 7th International Bile Acid Meeting, Basel, pp. 256–257
41. Gleeson, D., Ruppin, D. C. and Dowling, R. H. (1983). British Gallstone Study Group (BGSG) post-dissolution trial: interim report on overall recurrence rates and discrepancies between ultrasonography (US) and oral cholecystography (OCG). *Gut*, **24**, A1006 (abstract)
42. Ruppin, D. C. and Dowling, R. H. (1982). Is recurrence inevitable after gallstone dissolution by bile acid treatment? *Lancet*, **1**, 181–185
43. Toulet, J., Rousselet, J., Viteau, J.-M., Duchon, Y., Pagniez, R., Samain, B. and Vienne, J.-L. (1983). Récidives et prévention des récidives après dissolution de la lithiase vésiculaire par l'acide chénodésoxycholique chez 22 patients. *Gastroenterol. Clin. Biol.*, **7**, 605–609
44. Thistle, J. L. (1981). Medical treatment of gallstones. *Pract. Gastroenterol.*, **5**, 31–38

18
The role of diet in the aetiology of cholelithiasis

K. W. HEATON

TECHNIQUES FOR ELUCIDATING DIETARY FACTORS

Epidemiological and experimental techniques provide different but complementary information. With a disease which has a multi-factorial aetiology and an incompletely understood pathogenesis no single technique can be expected to reveal all the aetiological factors. Age, sex, race and other constitutional and hereditary factors interplay with, and modify, any environmental factors. Each technique has its own limitations and its own possibilities of bias, in both the collection and interpretation of data. The truth will only be revealed by an at-once broadminded and critical consideration of all the available data.

Inter-community comparisons

A good deal is known of the average person's dietary intake in different countries and, in Britain at least, in different parts of the same country. If we also knew the exact prevalence or, better still, incidence of gallstones in different countries and parts of a country, we could look for correlations between the two. Unfortunately, data for incidence are not available and data for prevalence are scanty and/or biased, being almost entirely based on autopsied patients at teaching hospitals.

In these circumstances the best that can be hoped for is some general impression about dietary patterns which encourage or discourage gallstone formation in a community.

Only a few authors have attempted a world-wide survey of gallstone prevalence[1-4] but it seems to be agreed that gallstones are rare in primitive, rural communities, are relatively uncommon in developing countries, and are common or very common in developed, westernized countries. This suggests only that something in the lifestyle, and possibly diet, of western countries favours the development of gallstones. There is no way of identifying the

Table 1 Ways in which modern western diets differ from primitive and traditional diets[5]

Increased	*Decreased*	*Unchanged*
*Total energy	Starch	Total protein
Total fats	*Dietary fibre (potassium)	
Animal fats		
Animal protein		
*Sugar		
*Cholesterol		
Salt (sodium)		
†Fruit and vegetables		
Chemical additives		
Alcohol		

* Factors which are suspected as favouring gallstones.
† In temperate climates

responsible factor or combination of factors, but it is perhaps worthwhile to list the ways in which modern western diets differ from primitive and traditional diets (Table 1).

Inter-community comparisons of gallstone prevalence within a country are rare. The only systematic one based on autopsy surveys is a study covering nine towns in England and Wales[6] and no data were given for dietary intakes.

Temporal changes

According to autopsy surveys, cholesterol-rich gallstones have become much commoner in Japan since the Second World War[7]. At the same time the diet has become westernized[8], with all the results listed in Table 1. Since the war there have been 2.5–6-fold increases in the frequency of gallbladder operations in England, France, Sweden, Canada, Greece and South Africa, which must be due in part to increases in the incidence of gallstones[4]. Eating habits have also changed since the war. It is difficult to make generalized statements about these changes, but there has certainly been increased processing of food, and populations have become generally fatter.

Case–control comparisons

These enable one to identify dietary risk-factors within a population provided there is a wide enough range of dietary intakes. If a food item has a threshold intake which is passed by the whole population then its effect may be missed. A genuine effect can also be missed if the numbers of cases and controls studied are too small, if some cases are wrongly diagnosed, if some of the controls have undiagnosed gallstones, if inappropriate controls are used (e.g. hospital patients with diet-induced diseases), if the technique used to determine dietary intakes is too crude and inaccurate, and if cases are interviewed after they have been diagnosed and have changed their diet. With so many pitfalls it is not surprising that, of the 11 case–control studies reported before 1984[9–19], not a single one is methodologically satisfactory and there is no uniformity in their results[20,21]. In particular they have all been too small. The desirable number of cases is at least 200[20] and the two largest series have included 101[11] and 160[19] patients.

However, there has now been published a case–control study from Adelaide[21] which has been designed to avoid all the known pitfalls. It includes 267 newly diagnosed cases of gallstones, 241 age- and sex-matched controls randomly selected from the same neighbourhood as the cases, and 359 hospital controls. Dietary intake was assessed by a food-frequency questionnaire, which is a validated technique, and was assessed 'blind' just before cholecystography in cases and hospital controls. The data were analysed in depth by multivariate analysis. The large numbers made it possible to compare cases and controls in different age groups as well as dividing them by sex.

The present discussion will refer only to the Adelaide study and to the next largest case–control study, which involved 160 cases and 160 hospital controls in Rome and Milan[19].

Associated diseases and metabolic disturbances

It has been postulated that two diseases which are each commoner in the presence of the other are likely to share a common cause[22]. There are, of course, other possible explanations, such as that one disease or its treatment may cause the other disease, but there is likely to be some truth in this hypothesis. Over the years many diseases have been linked with gallstones, but usually on inadequate statistical evidence[23]. At present the only diseases which can confidently be associated with gallstones are obesity, diabetes mellitus and, probably, hiatus hernia and diverticular disease of the colon[4,24–26] (I am excluding diseases which seem to cause gallstones by impairing the secretion of bile acids, namely chronic liver disease and ileal resection or disease). In addition, there is a strong association between gallstones and hypertriglyceridaemia.

The connections between gallstones, obesity, diabetes and hypertriglyceridaemia are remarkably close. If a person has any one of these four diseases he or she is at increased risk of having all the other three[1,27]. Moreover, gallbladder bile is more likely to be supersaturated with cholesterol in the presence of obesity[28], maturity onset diabetes[29] or hypertriglyceridaemia[30]. The apparent association with diabetes may in fact be due to the commonly associated obesity[29].

What do these associations teach us? What could be the common aetiological or pathogenetic factor? There are at least four possibilities:

(1) surplus energy intake or overnutrition; certainly calorie reduction cures most cases of maturity-onset diabetes and hypertriglyceridaemia as well as obesity;
(2) hyperinsulinaemia; this is a recognized feature of obesity, hypertriglyceridaemia and early diabetes, and the Adelaide case–control study has found gallstone patients to have raised fasting serum insulin[20];
(3) carbohydrate sensitivity and, specifically, sensitivity to rapidly

available carbohydrate; restriction of such carbohydrate is part of the standard treatment for obesity, diabetes and hypertriglyceridaemia;

(4) lack of dietary fibre is the best available theory for the causation of diverticular disease. As shown later, this can also be implicated in gallstone formation.

Animal experiments

There are several animal models for diet-induced cholesterol gallstone disease but their relevance to the human disease is not always clear. They involve highly artificial diets and very often the addition of pure cholesterol. Also, metabolism of cholesterol and bile acids varies considerably in different species. Animal studies will be considered further in later sections.

Human experiments

Because a change in the cholesterol saturation of gallbladder bile is likely to mean a change in the risk of forming gallstones some workers have investigated the effect of dietary change on the lipid composition of human bile. Bile has usually been obtained by intubating the duodenum and aspirating its contents after the gallbladder has been made to contract, for example by administering cholecystokinin. The lipid composition of this aspirate faithfully reflects that of gallbladder contents provided it is not too diluted by other secretions[31]. This approach is attractive and has been fruitful. However certain limitations must be remembered. Effects on bile seen in short-term studies may be transient. Conversely, a dietary change may take a long time to alter the bile, and long-term studies are lacking. Effects may be different in different groups of people, for example, in slim young men and in overweight, middle-aged women. Effects may vary according to the previous diet. In any case, supersaturation with cholesterol is not sufficient to explain cholesterol gallstone disease. Nucleating and anti-nucleating agents are also of critical importance[32,33].

CURRENT DIETARY THEORIES

The main theories are three: surplus energy (calories), high cholesterol intake, and the consumption of refined carbohydrates, better described as fibre-depleted foods. I will summarize the evidence and arguments for each in turn. They are not, of course, mutually exclusive.

High cholesterol intake

Epidemiologically, it may well be that western populations with a high prevalence of gallstones eat more cholesterol than people in developing countries but no statistical correlations have been demonstrated between cholesterol intake and gallstone prevalence. Case–control studies provide little support. In the Adelaide study[21] cholesterol intake was similar in male cases and their matched community controls. In female cases aged under 50 years intake was higher (284 ± 15 mg/day vs. 244 ± 11 in controls, $p < 0.05$), but in women over 50 intake was lower (235 ± 12 vs. 287 ± 18, $p < 0.05$). On multiple regression analysis, cholesterol was *negatively* associated with gallstones, but only in females and when included in a statistical model with fat or calories.

Human experiments have given conflicting results. Two American studies[34,35] found that adding cholesterol to the diet for 3 weeks raised the cholesterol content of bile. The first study[34] is hard to interpret because it involved adding egg yolks to a liquid formula diet and it is unsafe to extrapolate to a normal solid diet. Also, there was a significant rise in serum cholesterol during the experiment, whereas patients with gallstones do not have raised serum cholesterol levels – they may even be reduced[36] – and, other things being equal, there is no correlation between serum cholesterol and bile cholesterol saturation[37]. The second study[35] is also hard to interpret because as yet it has been published only as an abstract. However it purports to show that the saturation index of duodenal bile in seven healthy women rose from 0.89 ± 0.04 to 1.06 ± 0.04 ($p < 0.05$) when eggs were added to their diet to raise its cholesterol content from 500 to 1000 mg/day for 3 weeks. Also, in six women with radiolucent gallstones the saturation index rose from 1.28 ± 0.06 to 1.48 ± 0.05 ($p < 0.01$).

In opposition, Dam and his colleagues[38] fed five to ten eggs a day to young volunteers for 6 weeks and, despite a rise in the serum cholesterol, there was no tendency for the cholesterol content of bile to rise; in fact, in most subjects the bile acid/cholesterol ratio improved. Similarly, Andersén and Hellström[39] found no change in bile cholesterol saturation when five eggs a day were fed for 2 weeks.

Animal experiments certainly indicate that feeding cholesterol can induce supersaturated bile and cholesterol gallstones, at least in rodents like the mouse, prairie dog and gerbil, also the squirrel monkey[40]. However, it is very doubtful if these experiments are relevant to the human disease. Animals on these regimes become saturated with cholesterol, which is totally unlike the situation in gallstone patients. For example, in gerbils the serum cholesterol rose from 104 to 867 mg/dl. At the same time the liver became so stuffed with cholesterol it swelled to three times its normal size and most of the animals died[41]. In prairie dogs, serum cholesterol rose from 150 to over 1000 mg/dl[42,43], in mice from 108 to over 400 mg/dl[44] and in squirrel monkeys from 121 to 315 mg/dl[45]. Animal species vary greatly in how their bile responds to cholesterol feeding[46] and, in hamsters, bile saturation actually decreases[47]. In the author's view, animal models have not thrown any light on the dietary aetiology of human gallstones. They may even be misleading.

Surplus or high energy intake

The idea that excess of energy intake over expenditure predisposes to gallstones has to be attractive, if only because so many patients seen in clinical practice are clearly overweight. Furthermore, it is well documented that obese people synthesize excessive amounts of cholesterol and secrete excessive amounts of cholesterol in their bile so that their bile is almost always supersaturated with cholesterol[24,28]. However, the facts indicate that obesity is not a necessary cause for gallstones, since some gallstone patients are slim; nor is it a sufficient cause, since not all fat people have gallstones. All the same, it is undeniable that obesity is a risk factor for gallstones, at least in women. The Adelaide case–control study[21] found no difference in the Quetelet index (W/H^2) between male patients and their controls. Female patients were heavier than their hospital controls at all ages but only under the age of 50 were they heavier than their community controls. Other studies have pointed in the same direction – namely that obesity is a risk factor only at younger ages[20].

Surplus energy intake is not necessarily the same as high energy intake if by high is meant higher than average in the population. Dietary surveys indicate that fatter people do not eat more than thinner ones – they may even eat less because of their greater energy efficiency[48]. Nevertheless, the theory has gained some credence that high energy intake is a risk factor for gallstones. This theory arose from three case–control studies, carried out in Marseilles between 1956 and 1968[9–11], which all showed a higher energy intake in gallstone patients. However, these early examples of the case–control technique do not satisfy modern standards[20] and a difference in energy intake was not found in six other case–control studies[12–17], including a later one from Marseilles[12]. In the Adelaide study[21], a high energy intake increased the relative risk of gallstones in young and middle-aged women and in young men, but not in older subjects of both sexes (Fig. 1). These variations with age and sex help to explain the contradictory data obtained in smaller studies.

The idea that high energy intake is a causative factor was strengthened by a comparison of the published autopsy prevalence of gallstones in seven countries (France, Sweden, Portugal, South Africa, Uganda, India and Japan) and the estimated average intake of calories in these countries[49]. There appeared to be a good correlation, at any rate up to 3000 kcal (12.6 MJ)/day. However, no statistical testing was carried out and the prevalence rates were

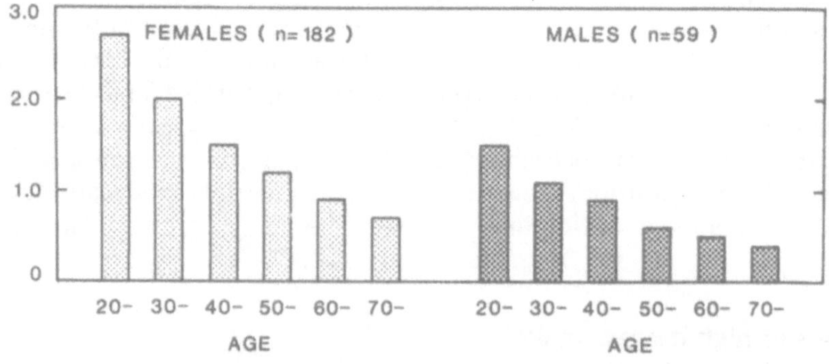

Figure 1 Relative risk of gallstones at different ages associated with an increase in calorie intake of 500 kcal/day: the Adelaide case–control study[21]

not age-standardized. Also correlations were present with animal fat and protein and no doubt they could be found with many other measures of affluence.

For an individual as opposed to a group of people a long-term increase in energy intake almost certainly increases the risk of gallstones if it results in increased body fat[28]. Studies on T-tube bile have suggested that, in the short term too, changes in energy intake may affect the cholesterol concentration of bile[50,51] but the situation was unphysiological and the changes in energy were drastic. In free-living middle-aged patients with radiolucent gallstones a 24 % change in energy intake (induced by changing sucrose intake) did not affect the cholesterol saturation of duodenal bile over a 6-week period[52].

If surplus (or high) energy intake is a risk factor, this implies that any dietary item or any eating habit which inflates energy intake will itself be a risk factor. The two dietary items which are most often blamed for inflating energy intake are refined carbohydrate, especially sugar, and fat. There is no evidence from epidemiology, case–control studies or human experiments to incriminate dietary fat in causing gallstones. There is, however, considerable evidence to incriminate refined carbohydrates.

Refined carbohydrates or fibre-depleted foods

The term refined carbohydrate was proposed by Cleave[53,54] to encompass all the carbohydrate-containing items in man's diet which have been artificially processed so as to remove a fibre-rich fraction. The main examples in western diets are sugars (white or brown) and syrups, which are fibre-free, and white flour which is, in effect, wholemeal flour from which the bran and germ have been removed. Trowell *et al.*[55] suggest that a better term is fibre-depleted foods, since white flour and other refined foods such as white rice are not by any means pure carbohydrate. Dietary fibre is defined[56] as the plant polysaccharides and lignin which escape digestion by the alimentary enzymes of man. It is composed chiefly of plant cell walls, which are complex, highly organized structures. Wheat bran contains about 40 % dietary fibre and is the richest source of fibre in the diet. About 50 % of bran fibre is fermented by anaerobic bacteria in the colon. Fibre from other sources is fermented more extensively and the resultant growth of bacteria is largely responsible for the greater bulk of the stools on a high-fibre diet[57]. The products of fermentation are the short-chain fatty acids – acetic, propionic and butyric – together with the gases hydrogen, CO_2 and in some people methane.

The consumption of fibre-depleted foods in place of natural, full-fibre foods is considered to have harmful effects in two main ways[53,54]. It provides insufficient fibre for the optimal function of the large intestine and it artificially inflates energy intake by making carbohydrate foods too easily ingested and digested.

The refined carbohydrate theory for gallstone formation can also be stated in two ways:

(1) refined or fibre-depleted foods lead to excessive energy intake and to

excessive insulin responses, either or both of which favour gallstone formation, probably by promoting cholesterol synthesis;

(2) lack of fibre in the diet leads to gallstones by altering bile acid metabolism, specifically by increasing the amount of deoxycholic acid which is formed in the colon from bacterial dehydroxylation of cholic acid.

It is difficult to test these hypotheses by traditional epidemiological techniques. Dietary fibre is hard to analyse and measure chemically, and data are not yet available for the fibre intakes of whole populations. However, the exchange of traditional, lightly processed diets for the modern western diet almost always involves a reduction in fibre intake and it always involves a greater intake of fibre-free sugars (Table 1). Hence, the fibre-depleted food theory could help to explain the marked geographical and historical variations in gallstone prevalence.

For more precise testing of this theory it is necessary to turn to case–control studies and experimental work.

Only one case–control study has looked specifically at the intake of refined sugars. Alessandrini and his colleagues in Rome and Milan[19] used a food-frequency questionnaire to compare the sugar and fibre intakes of 160 patients with radiolucent gallstones and 160 age- and sex-matched hospital controls, all with negative cholecystograms. The gallstone patients ate significantly more refined sugar, about 23 g/day vs. 19 g/day in the controls ($p<0.05$). Intakes were surprisingly low in both groups.

The Adelaide case–control study[21] looked at total sugar intake, which is composed mainly of refined sugar in most people, and also at sugar in drinks and sweets which is a large part of refined sugar intake. As shown in Table 2, total sugar intakes were considerably higher in both men and women with gallstones under the age of 50 but were not significantly different over the age of 50. Sugar in drinks and sweets was higher in all groups except the older men. These were the biggest and most consistent differences in any nutrient in this study. With the hospital controls there were trends in the same direction but these did not reach statistical significance.

Dietary fibre intakes were looked at by both Alessandrini *et al.*[19] and Scragg *et al.*[21]. The former found slight but significant ($p<0.05$) reductions in gallstone patients with total dietary fibre and fruit and vegetable fibre, but there was no difference in cereal fibre. As shown in Table 2, Scragg *et al.* found no difference in total dietary fibre intake in any age or sex group. However, on multivariate analysis fibre was negatively associated with gallstones in both sexes[21].

Hence case–control studies support the theory that refined carbohydrate in the form of sugars is an aetiological factor in gallstones. They give limited support to the idea that a low intake of dietary fibre is pathogenic.

Experimental studies in man

These consist of one study of the effects of refined carbohydrate in general and one of refined sugar in particular, together with several studies of the

Table 2 Daily intake of sugars and dietary fibre in patients with gallstones and matched community controls. The Adelaide case–control study[21]

	Females				*Males*			
	Age < 50		*Age* > 50		*Age* < 50		*Age* > 50	
	Cases	*Controls*	*Cases*	*Controls*	*Cases*	*Controls*	*Cases*	*Controls*
Sugars – total (g)	***147 ± 7	113 ± 4	128 ± 8	126 ± 7	*160 ± 15	121 ± 10	135 ± 12	153 ± 10
Sugars – drinks and sweets (g)	***53 ± 4	28 ± 3	**36 ± 4	23 ± 2	*58 ± 5	40 ± 7	46 ± 6	40 ± 5
Dietary fibre (g)	19.2 ± 0.8	17.7 ± 0.7	18.1 ± 0.9	21.9 ± 1.2	17.4 ± 2.1	18.3 ± 1.6	18.5 ± 2.2	22.6 ± 1.9

* $p < 0.05$, ** $p < 0.01$, *** $p < 0.001$

effect of wheat bran. All studies have involved analysing duodenal bile for its lipid composition and for the relative proportions of bile acids.

The effects of wheat bran on the cholesterol saturation of bile are shown in Fig. 2. In all four groups of subjects whose bile was initially supersaturated with cholesterol bile became less saturated, whereas in three groups with initially unsaturated bile there was no change[58-62]. Thus bran appears to have a consistent normalizing effect on bile. However, this effect is relatively weak and in only a minority of subjects did bran convert supersaturated into unsaturated bile.

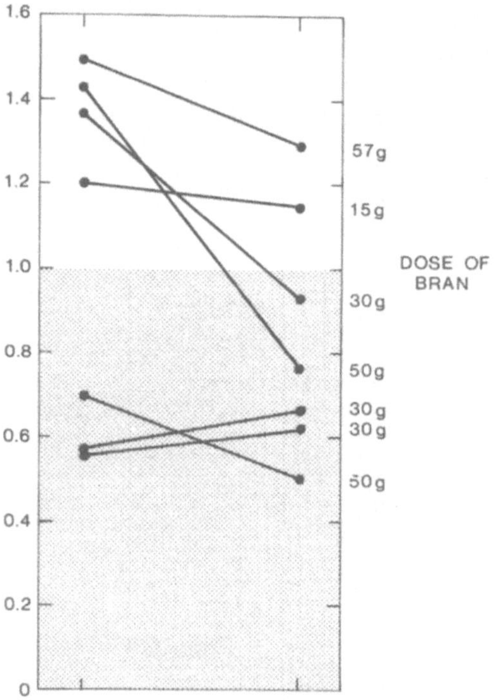

Figure 2 Cholesterol saturation index of duodenal bile in seven groups of subjects before and during treatment with wheat bran in the daily dose stated. Each point represents a mean value for a group[58-62]

The mode of action of bran has not been proved. However, in all groups of subjects in whom bile has become less saturated there has also been a fall in the proportion of deoxycholate in the bile acid pool. This is probably relevant because, besides bran, there are five other measures which lower the deoxycholate content of bile at the same time as making it less saturated with cholesterol. These are treatment with metronidazole[63], ampicillin[64] or lactulose[65], oral administration of *Streptococcus faecium*[66] and the reversal of hypothyroidism with thyroxine treatment[67].

Deoxycholic acid is a secondary bile acid; that is, a bacterial breakdown product of an original or primary bile acid, in this case the dehydroxylation product of cholic acid.

Measures which increase the deoxycholic acid content of bile tend to raise the cholesterol saturation of bile and people with gallstones tend to have an increased proportion of deoxycholic acid in their bile[68,69]. Why deoxycholic acid should favour more saturated bile is uncertain but there are two possible explanations[69]. First, being the most detergent of the major bile acids, deoxycholic acid may leach out excessive amounts of cholesterol from the liver cell as it is being secreted into the bile. Second, deoxycholic acid displaces chenodeoxycholic acid from the bile (either by competing with it for intestinal absorption or by suppressing its synthesis) and this removes an agent which is known to lower cholesterol secretion. Whatever the mode of action of deoxycholic acid, bran may act by reducing it.

Bran may reduce the amount of circulating deoxycholate in two ways. First, it provides solid matter in the colon to which deoxycholic acid would tend to adsorb[70]. Second, up to 50% of bran is metabolized by bacteria to short-chain fatty acids. These could lower the pH in the right colon below the point at which bacterial dehydroxylases are active – a mechanism which also accounts for the action of lactulose[65].

Thornton *et al.*[71] studied the effects on bile of replacing refined carbohydrate in the diet with full-fibre foods. Thirteen women with asymptomatic, radiolucent gallstones were studied after 6 weeks on a diet containing frequently consumed amounts of refined sugar and fibre-depleted starch and again after 6 weeks on a diet devoid of these products but with free access to all full-fibre foods. The cholesterol saturation index of bile averaged 1.50 on the fibre-depleted diet and 1.20 on the full-fibre diet. The index was lower on the full-fibre diet in all but one person, and she ate immoderately of nuts and, unlike the rest, gained weight. There was little change in the deoxycholate percentage in bile, so it was not thought that the beneficial effect of full-fibre foods was the same as the bran effect. It was speculated that benefit was due to the drastic reduction in the intake of refined sugars (from 106 to 6 g/day). However, a subsequent 6-week crossover study comparing two diets which were closely similar except for their sucrose contents (112 and 16 g/day respectively) showed no difference in bile saturation index[52]. Thus the beneficial effect of the full-fibre diet is still unexplained.

ANIMAL EXPERIMENTS

No animal experiments have been reported which were designed to test the hypothesis that refined carbohydrates favour gallstone formation. However, many lithogenic dietary regimes have been reported and, while the diets vary widely, they have one feature in common – they are all semi-synthetic or semi-purified[72]. In practice this means that their carbohydrate component is always in refined or fibre-depleted form, usually glucose or sucrose, but sometimes corn starch. The idea that lack of fibre explains the lithogenicity of these diets is supported by two observations. First, in the hamster the diet loses

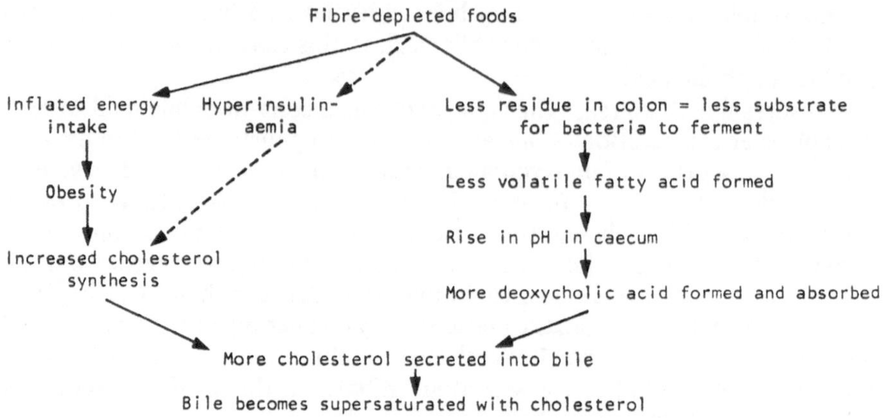

Figure 3

its lithogenic effect if it is supplemented with bulking agents such as agar and carboxymethyl cellulose, or even if the animal is allowed to eat the straw laid on the floor of its cage[73]. Second, in the rabbit, stones dissolve rapidly if ordinary chow is fed.

CONCLUSIONS

Eating refined carbohydrates rather than full-fibre foods inflates energy intake and depresses fibre intake. In the short term it makes bile more saturated with cholesterol, at least in susceptible people, though the mechanism is unknown and seems not to be loss of a 'bran effect'. In the long term, if obesity results from this or any eating habit the formation of gallstones will again be promoted. Patients with gallstones tend to eat more sugar than other people in a western community but their fibre intake is similar (and low). Populations prone to cholesterol gallstones tend to be on western-style diets which are low in fibre and high in refined or fibre-depleted carbohydrate foods. A high intake of cholesterol may be an additional factor.

A unifying hypothesis to show the postulated links between fibre-depleted foods and cholesterol gallstones is shown in Fig. 3.

References

1. Heaton, K. W. (1973). The epidemiology of gallstones and suggested aetiology. *Clin. Gastroenterol.*, **2**, 67–83
2. Burkitt, D. P. and Tunstall, M. (1975). Gallstones: geographical and chronological features. *J. Trop. Med. Hyg.*, **78**, 140–144
3. Brett, M. and Barker, D. J. P. (1976). The world distribution of gallstones. *Int. J. Epidemiol.*, **5**, 335–341
4. Heaton, K. (1981). Gallstones. In Trowell, H. C. and Burkitt, D. P. (eds.) *Western Diseases: their Emergence and Prevention*. pp. 47–59. (London: Arnold)

5. Trowell, H. (1981). Hypertension, obesity, diabetes mellitus and coronary heart disease. In Trowell, H. C. and Burkitt, D. P. (eds.) *Western Diseases: their Emergence and Prevention.* pp. 3–32. (London: Arnold)
6. Barker, D. J. P., Gardner, M. J., Power, C. and Hutt, M. S. R. (1979). Prevalence of gallstones at necropsy in nine British towns: a collaborative study. *Br. Med. J.*, **2**, 1389–1392
7. Kameda, H. (1967). Gallstones, compositions, structural characteristics and geographical distribution. In *Proceedings of 3rd World Congress of Gastroenterology, Tokyo 1966*, Vol. 4, pp. 117–124. (Basel: Karger)
8. Hikasa, Y., Nagase, M., Tanimura, H., Shioda, R., Setoyama, M., Kobayashi, M., Mukaihara, S., Kamata, T., Maruyama, K., Kato, H., Mori, K. and Soloway, R. D. (1980). Epidemiology and etiology of gallstones. *Arch. Jap. Chir.*, **49**, 555–571
9. Sarles, H., Chalvet, H., Ambrosi, L. and D'Ortoli, G. (1957). Etude statistique des facteurs diététiques dans la pathogénie de la lithiase biliaire humaine. *Sem. Hop. Paris*, **58**, 3424–3428
10. Hauton, J. (1967). Cholelithiasis. Third World Congress of Gastroenterology, Tokyo. *Recent Adv. Gastroenterol.*, **4**, 109–116
11. Sarles, H., Chabert, C., Pommeau, Y., Save, E., Mouret, H. and Gérolami, H. (1969). Diet and cholesterol gallstones. A study of 101 patients with cholelithiasis compared to 101 matched controls. *Am. J. Dig. Dis.*, **14**, 531–537
12. Sarles, H., Gérolami, A. and Bord, A. (1978). Diet and cholesterol gallstones. A further study. *Digestion*, **17**, 128–134
13. Coste, T., Karsenti, P., Berta, J. L., Cubeau, J. and Guilloud-Bataille, M. (1979). Facteurs diététiques de la lithiase biliare: comparaison de l'alimentation d'un groupe de lithiasiques à l'alimentation d'un groupe témoin. *Gastroenterol. Clin. Biol.*, **3**, 417–424
14. Wheeler, M., Hills, L. L. and Laby, B. (1970). Cholelithiasis: a clinical and dietary survey. *Gut*, **11**, 430–437
15. Burnett, W. (1971). The epidemiology of gallstones. *Tijdschrift voor Gastroenterologie*, **14**, 79–89
16. Reid, J. M., Fullmer, S. D., Pettigrew, K. D., Burch, T. A., Bennett, P. H., Miller, M. and Whedon, G. D. (1971). Nutrient intake of Pima Indian women: relationships to diabetes mellitus and gallbladder disease. *Am. J. Clin. Nutr.*, **24**, 1281–1289
17. Smith, D. A. and Gee, M. I. (1979). A dietary survey to determine the relationship between diet and cholelithiasis. *Am. J. Clin. Nutr.*, **32**, 1519–1526
18. Williams, C. N. and Johnson, J. L. (1980). Prevalence of gallstones and risk factors in Caucasian women in a rural Canadian community. *Canad. Med. Assoc. J.*, **120**, 664–668
19. Alessandrini, A., Fusco, M. A., Gatti, E. and Rossi, P. A. (1982). Dietary fibres and cholesterol gallstones: a case control study. *Ital. J. Gastroenterol.*, **14**, 156–158
20. Scragg, R. K. R. (1983). Diet, Obesity, Plasma Lipids and Insulin in Gallstone Disease. *Ph.D thesis*, University of Adelaide
21. Scragg, R. K. R., McMichael, A. J. and Baghurst, P. A. (1984). Diet, alcohol, and relative weight in gall stone disease: a case-control study. *Br. Med. J.*, **288**, 1113–1119
22. Burkitt, D. P. (1969). Related disease – related cause? *Lancet*, **2**, 1229–1231
23. Kaye, M. D. and Kern, F. (1971). Clinical relationships of gallstones. *Lancet*, **1**, 1228–1230
24. Bennion, L. J. and Grundy, S. M. (1978). Risk factors for the development of cholelithiasis in man. *N. Engl. J. Med.*, **299**, 1161–1167; 1221–1227
25. Capron, J-P., Payenneville, H., Dumont, M., Dupas, J-L. and Lorriaux, A. (1978). Evidence for an association between cholelithiasis and hiatus hernia. *Lancet*, **2**, 329–331
26. Capron, J-P., Piperaud, R., Dupas, J-L., Delamarre, J. and Lorriaux, A. (1981). Evidence for an association between cholelithiasis and diverticular disease of the colon: a case-controlled study. *Dig. Dis. Sci.*, **26**, 523–527
27. Heaton, K. W. (1979). Diet and gallstones. In Fisher, M. M., Goresky, C. A., Shaffer, E. A. and Strasberg, S. M. (eds.) *Hepatology – Research and Clinical issues*, Vol. 4. *Gallstones*, pp. 371–389. (New York: Plenum)
28. Bennion, L. J. and Grundy, S. M. (1975). Effects of obesity and caloric intake on biliary lipid metabolism in man. *J. Clin. Invest.*, **56**, 996–1011
29. Haber, G. B. and Heaton, K. W. (1979). Lipid composition of bile in diabetics and obesity-matched controls. *Gut*, **20**, 518–522

30. Ahlberg, J., Angelin, B., Einarsson, K., Hellström, K. and Leijd, B. (1980). Biliary lipid composition in normo- and hyperlipoproteinemia. *Gastroenterology*, **79**, 90–94
31. Vlahcevic, Z. R., Bell, C. C., Juttijudata, P. and Swell, L. (1971). Bile-rich duodenal fluid as an indicator of biliary lipid composition and its applicability to detection of lithogenic bile. *Am. J. Dig. Dis.*, **16**, 797–802
32. Burnstein, M. J., Ilson, R. G., Petrunka, C. N., Taylor, R. D. and Strasberg, S. M. (1983). Evidence for a potent nucleating factor in the gallbladder bile of patients with cholesterol gallstones. *Gastroenterology*, **85**, 801–807
33. Gollish, S. H., Burnstein, M. J., Ilson, R. G., Petrunka, C. N. and Strasberg, S. M. (1983). Nucleation of cholesterol monohydrate crystals from hepatic and gallbladder bile of patients with cholesterol gallstones. *Gut*, **24**, 836–844
34. DenBesten, L., Connor, W. E. and Bell, S. (1973). The effect of dietary cholesterol on the composition of human bile. *Surgery*, **73**, 266–273
35. Lee, D. W., Gilmore, C. J., Bonorris, G. G., Cohen, H., Marks, J. W., Meiselman, M. S. and Schoenfield, L. J. (1983). Effect of dietary cholesterol on biliary lipids in women with and without gallstones. In Paumgartner, G., Stiehl, A. and Gerok, W. (eds.) *Bile Acids and Cholesterol in Health and Disease* (Falk Symposium 33). pp. 237–238. (Lancaster: MTP Press)
36. Van der Linden, W. (1961). Some biological traits in female gallstone-disease patients. *Acta Chir. Scand. Suppl.* 269
37. Thornton, J. R., Heaton, K. W. and Macfarlane, D. G. (1981). A relation between high-density-lipoprotein cholesterol and bile cholesterol saturation. *Br. Med. J.*, **283**, 1352–1354
38. Dam, H., Prange, I., Jensen, M. K., Kallehauge, H. E. and Fenger, H. J. (1971). Studies on human bile. IV. Influence of ingestion of cholesterol in the form of eggs on the composition of bile in healthy subjects. *Z. Ernährungswiss.*, **10**, 178–187
39. Andersén, E. and Hellström, K. (1979). The effect of cholesterol feeding on bile acid kinetics and biliary lipids in normolipidemic and hypertriglyceridemic subjects. *J. Lipid Res.*, **20**, 1020–1027
40. Van der Linden, W. and Bergman, F. (1977). Formation and dissolution of gallstones in experimental animals. *Int. Rev. Exp. Pathol.*, **17**, 173–233
41. Bergman, F. and van der Linden, W. (1971). Reaction of the mongolian gerbil to a cholesterol-cholic acid-containing gallstone inducing diet. *Acta Pathol. Microbiol. Scand.*, **79**, 476–486
42. Brenneman, D. E., Connor, W. E., Forker, E. L. and DenBesten, L. (1972). The formation of abnormal bile and cholesterol gallstones from dietary cholesterol in the prairie dog. *J. Clin. Invest.*, **51**, 1495–1503
43. Chang, S-H., Ho, K-J. and Taylor, C. B. (1973). Cholesterol gallstone formation and its regression in prairie dogs. *Arch. Pathol.*, **96**, 417–426
44. Tepperman, J., Caldwell, F. T. and Tepperman, H. M. (1964). Induction of gallstones in mice by feeding a cholesterol-cholic acid containing diet. *Am. J. Physiol.*, **206**, 628–634
45. Osuga, T. and Portman, O. W. (1971). Experimental formation of gallstones in the squirrel monkey. *Proc. Soc. Exp. Biol. Med.*, **136**, 722–726
46. Ho, K-J. (1976). Comparative studies on the effect of cholesterol feeding on biliary composition. *Am. J. Clin. Nutr.*, **29**, 698–704
47. Dam, H., Prange, I. and Sondergaard, E. (1968). Alimentary production of gallstones in hamsters. 20. Influence of dietary cholesterol on gallstone formation. *Z. Ernährungswiss.*, **9**, 43–49
48. Keen, H., Thomas, B. J., Jarrett, R. J. and Fuller, J. H. (1979). Nutrient intake, adiposity, and diabetes. *Br. Med. J.*, **1**, 655–658
49. Sarles, H., Gerolami, A. and Cros, R. C. (1978). Diet and cholesterol gallstones. A multicenter study. *Digestion*, **17**, 121–127
50. Sarles, H., Hauton, J., Lafont, H., Teissier, N., Planche, N. E. and Gérolami, A. (1968). Rôle de l'alimentation sur la concentration du cholestérol biliaire chez l'homme lithiasique et non-lithiasique. *Clin. Chim. Acta*, **19**, 147–155
51. Sarles, H., Crotte, C., Gerolami, A., Mulé, A., Domingo, N. and Hauton, J. (1971). The influence of calorie intake and of dietary protein on the bile lipids. *Scand. J. Gastroenterol.*, **6**, 189–191

52. Werner, D., Emmett, P. M. and Heaton, K. W. (1984). The effects of dietary sucrose on factors influencing cholesterol gallstone formation. *Gut*, **25**, 269–274
53. Cleave, T. L. and Campbell, G. D. (1966). *Diabetes, Coronary Thrombosis and the Saccharine Disease*. (Bristol: Wright)
54. Cleave, T. L. (1974). *The Saccharine Disease*. (Bristol: Wright)
55. Trowell, H. C., Burkitt, D. P. and Heaton, K. W. (eds.) (1984). *Dietary Fibre, Fibre-depleted Foods and Disease*. (London: Academic Press)
56. Trowell, H. C., Southgate, D. A. T., Wolever, T. M. S., Leeds, A. R., Gassull, M. A. and Jenkins, D. J. A. (1976). Dietary fibre redefined. *Lancet*, **1**, 967
57. Stephen, A. M. and Cummings, J. H. (1980). Mechanism of action of dietary fibre in the human colon. *Nature*, **284**, 283–284
58. Pomare, E. W., Heaton, K. W., Low-Beer, T. S. and Espiner, H. J. (1976). The effect of wheat bran upon bile salt metabolism and upon the lipid composition of bile in gallstone patients. *Am. J. Dig. Dis.*, **21**, 521–526
59. Watts, J. McK., Jablonski, P. and Toouli, J. (1978). The effect of added bran to the diet on the saturation of bile in people without gallstones. *Am. J. Surg.*, **135**, 321–324
60. McDougall, R. M., Yakymyshyn, L., Walker, K. and Thurston, O. G. (1978). The effect of wheat bran on serum lipoproteins and biliary lipids. *Can. J. Surg.*, **21**, 433–435
61. Tarpila, S., Miettinen, T. A. and Metsäranta, L. (1978). Effects of bran on serum cholesterol, faecal mass, fat, bile acids and neutral sterols, and biliary lipids in patients with diverticular disease of the colon. *Gut*, **19**, 137–145
62. Huijbregts, A. W. M., van Berge-Henegouwen, G. P., Hectors, M. P. C., van Schaik, A. and van der Werf, S. D. J. (1980). Effects of a standardised wheat bran preparation on biliary lipid composition and bile acid metabolism in young healthy males. *Eur. J. Clin. Invest.*, **10**, 451–458
63. Low-Beer, T. S. and Nutter, S. (1978). Colonic bacterial activity, biliary cholesterol saturation, and pathogenesis of gallstones. *Lancet*, **2**, 1063–1065
64. Carulli, N., Ponz de Leon, M., Loria, P., Iori, R., Rosi, A. and Romani, M. (1981). Effect of the selective expansion of the cholic acid pool on bile lipid composition: possible mechanism of bile acid induced biliary cholesterol desaturation. *Gastroenterology*, **81**, 539–546
65. Thornton, J. R. and Heaton, K. W. (1981). Do colonic bacteria contribute to cholesterol gallstone formation? Effects of lactulose on bile. *Br. Med. J.*, **282**, 1018–1020
66. Salvioli, G., Salati, R., Bondi, M., Fratalocchi, A., Sala, B. M. and Gibertini, A. (1982). Bile acid transformation by the intestinal flora and cholesterol saturation in bile. Effects of Streptococcus faecium administration. *Digestion*, **23**, 80–88
67. Angelin, B., Einarsson, K. and Leijd, B. (1983). Bile acid metabolism in hypothyroid subjects: response to substitution therapy. *Eur. J. Clin. Invest.*, **13**, 99–106
68. Low-Beer, T. S. and Pomare, E. W. (1975). Can colonic bacterial metabolites predispose to cholesterol gallstones? *Br. Med. J.*, **1**, 438–440
69. Heaton, K. W. (1984). Bile salts. In Wright, R., Millward-Sadler, G. H., Alberti, K. G. M. M. and Karran, S. (eds.) *Liver and Biliary Disease*. 2nd Edn. (London: Saunders) In press.
70. Eastwood, M. A. and Hamilton, D. (1968). Studies on the adsorption of bile salts to non-absorbed components of diet. *Biochim. Biophys. Acta*, **152**, 165–173
71. Thornton, J. R., Emmett, P. M. and Heaton, K. W. (1983). Diet and gallstones: effects of refined and unrefined carbohydrate diets on bile cholesterol saturation and bile acid metabolism. *Gut*, **24**, 2–6
72. Heaton, K. W. (1975). Gallstones and cholecystitis. In Burkitt, D. P. and Trowell, H. C. (eds.) *Refined Carbohydrate Foods and Disease. Some Implications of Dietary Fibre*. pp. 173–194. (London: Academic Press)
73. Hikasa, Y., Matsuda, S., Nagase, M., Yoshinaga, M., Tobe, T., Maruyama, I., Shioda, R., Tanimura, H., Muraoka, R., Moroya, H. and Togo, M. (1969). Initiating factors of gallstones, especially cholesterol stones (III). *Arch. Jap. Chir.* **38**, 107–124

19
Pathogenic and clinical relationships between endemic salmonellosis and gallstone disease

F. NERVI, B. PAZ and F. MONTIEL

Typhoid fever is endemic in many areas of the world, including Egypt, Mexico, Central and South America[1]. An index of the epidemiological significance of this important disease in different countries is given by the mortality rate, as shown in Fig. 1. Well-known associations between *Salmonella typhi* and the gallbladder are the chronic carrier state, acute cholecystitis, as a complication that develops during the evolution of typhoid fever[2] and gallbladder cancer[3].

The population of endemic areas is continuously exposed to *Salmonella typhi* infection. It is common that adults from these areas will acquire substantial resistance to successive exposures to the bacteria; they may even develop bacteraemia without symptoms[4]. Under these conditions the biliary tract of these subjects may be frequently infected with *Salmonella typhi* and other *Salmonellae*, including *paratyphi* A and B. A chronic carrier state may result if a previous mucosal lesion exists in the gallbladder, as is commonly found in gallstone disease[2]. The majority of chronic carriers of *Salmonella typhi* are subjects with gallstones[5,6].

Because Chile has a high prevalence of cholesterol gallstones[7] and salmonellosis is endemic, we looked for potential changes of bile composition and bile acid metabolism in a series of patients with typhoid fever. We hypothesized that the common involvement of the enterohepatic organs, during the course of typhoid fever, might favour the production of lithogenic bile. Secondly, we studied prospectively the incidence of *Salmonella typhi* in bile cultures obtained in a series of patients operated on because of symptomatic gallbladder disease. The objective of this study was to answer the question whether *Salmonella* might be a frequent aetiological factor of acute cholecystitis in patients with gallstones, in the absence of clinical typhoid fever.

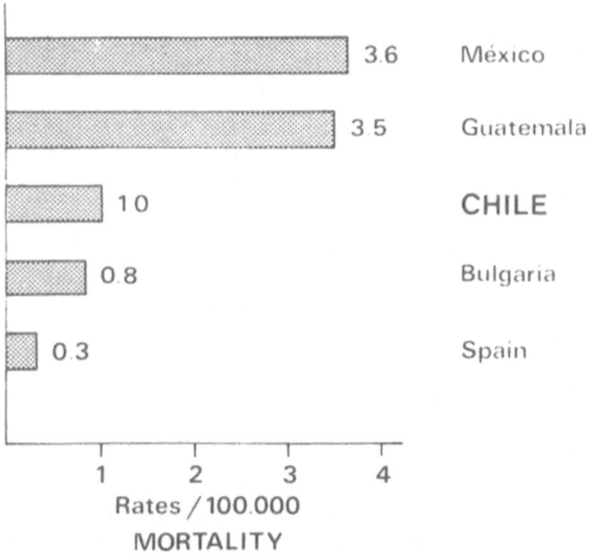

Figure 1 Mortality rates of typhoid fever in different countries (World Health Organization, 1977)

BILIARY LIPID COMPOSITION AND BILE ACID POOL SIZE DURING THE EVOLUTION OF TYPHOID FEVER

In addition to classical ileitis, *Salmonella typhi* induces a diffuse inflammation of the jejunum with important alterations of the epithelial lining of the villi and crypt glands. These histological changes are found very early in biopsy specimens obtained from volunteers challenged with an infecting dose of oral *Salmonella typhi*[8]. Electron microscopy of biopsy specimens from the small intestine in experimental infection in the guinea pig, has demonstrated marked degenerative changes in the microvilli of the enterocytes[9]. Similarly, during the septicaemic phase of the disease the gallbladder becomes constantly involved[2].

To disclose a potential lithogenic effect of typhoid fever in our population, mediated by modifications of bile composition, we studied a group of 11 patients with bacteriological confirmation of typhoid fever (either by positive blood or bile culture), that were in the second week of the clinical disease[10]. The parameters measured in this group were compared with those from a group of six control subjects of similar age and social background. None of the patients were receiving antibiotics at the time of the study, or had diarrhoea. Oral cholecystography was normal in all the subjects in this study.

Total biliary lipid concentration measured in duodenal bile was significantly lower by 50 % in typhoid patients, but cholesterol saturation remained in the normal range, as shown in Table 1. The presence of unconjugated bilirubin was not investigated in the duodenal bile samples, however Salmonellae extracts obtained by sonication lacked β-glucuronidase activity

Table 1 Effect of typhoid fever on biliary lipid concentration and cholesterol saturation in duodenal bile

Group	*Total biliary lipids* (*g* %)	*Cholesterol saturation* (%)
Control subjects (6)	3±1.2	105±29
Patients with typhoid fever (11)	1.5±0.6*	122±38

Duodenal bile was obtained by intubation after 12 h of fasting and a duodenal infusion of 30 ml of an 8 % amino acid solution to contract the gallbladder[31]. There were seven men and four women in the typhoid group (mean age 22±5), and three men and three women in the control group (mean age 26±5). Total biliary lipids represents the sum of bile salt, phospholipid and cholesterol concentration. Cholesterol saturation was calculated according to Holzbach[32]. Figures represent the mean ±SD

* Significantly different from controls; $p<0.02$, Student's t test

(unpublished observations from this laboratory). The lower concentration of biliary lipids found in typhoid patients may indicate a diseased gallbladder with functional impairement of mucosal concentration and/or muscular contraction. However, it may also be possible that cholecystokinin secretion from the duodenal mucosa is decreased in typhoid patients after the challenge with the amino acid solution to contract the gallbladder.

The size of the bile acid pool remains in the normal range in typhoid patients, although there are substantial changes in its composition (Fig. 2). Chenodeoxycholic pool size significantly increased in typhoid patients from 1.4±0.2 to 1.9±0.2 g per 70 kg of body weight. There is a reciprocal change in the size of the deoxycholic pool; it decreased 50% from 0.6±0.2 to 0.3±0.1 ($p<0.01$).

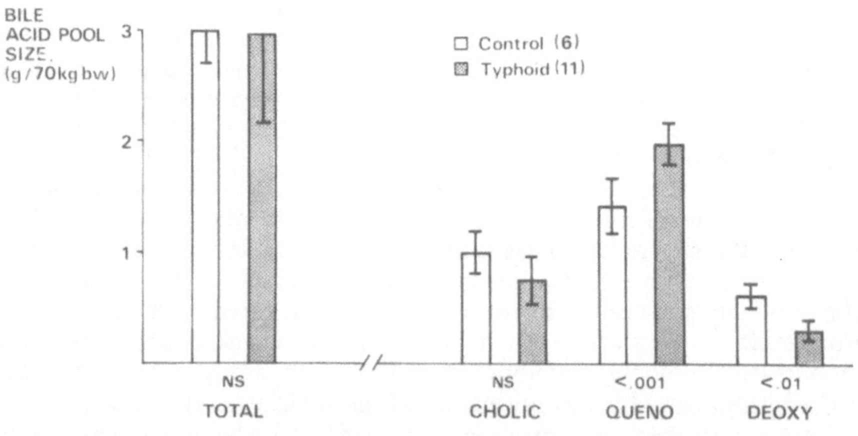

Figure 2 Effect of typhoid fever on bile acid pool size and composition. Bars represent the mean±1 SD. A fasting duodenal bile sample was obtained as described in Table 2. The bile acid pool was labelled with an oral dose of 5 μCi of [^{14}C]cholic acid. Patients with typhoid fever had a caloric intake of 1150±570 (SD) calories per day the week prior to the study, compared to a mean ingestion of 2563±570 calories per day in controls

These results indicate that neither the ileopathy of typhoid fever nor the invasive process of the proximal small intestine in the early phases of the disease, alter the mechanisms of bile acid reabsorption as is commonly found in Crohn's ileitis[11]. The important changes in bile acid composition observed in the patients that we studied are probably the consequence of a reduced cycling of the bile acid pool during typhoid fever[12]. Presumably this effect is secondary to the reduced ingestion of food observed in these patients, as shown in Fig. 2. A similar effect has been found in normal subjects with decreased gallbladder stimulation due to restriction of protein and fat intake[13].

The theory that bacterial infection might be an important aetiological factor of cholesterol gallstone disease was a widely held opinion in the past[14–16]. Our study does not support the hypothesis that *Salmonella typhi* infection may participate as a lithogenic factor through modifications of biliary lipid composition. The finding that biliary lipids concentration was lower in patients with typhoid fever might indicate the presence of a diseased gallbladder. If this interpretation proves to be correct, it may be possible that *Salmonella* infection of the gallbladder may favour other steps of gallstone formation, such as cholesterol crystallization or stone growth.

EFFECT OF *SALMONELLA TYPHI* ON THE CLINICAL PRESENTATION OF GALLSTONE DISEASE

In 1981 a prospective study was initiated to study the incidence of *Salmonella* infection of the biliary tract in patients with symptomatic gallstone disease. Because it is known that chronic carriers in endemic areas represent 2–5 % of the population[17,18], the majority of which are adults with gallstones, we arbitrarily chose to study approximately 300 patients subjected to cholecystectomy at the Hospital Clínico de la Universidad Católica. The study was finished during the course of 1983.

The patients were classified as cases of acute or chronic cholecystitis, before the results of the bile cultures were known. The diagnostic criteria considered both the clinical picture and the histopathology of the gallbladder[19]. A patient was classified as a case of acute cholecystitis when there were biliary colics with acute inflammation of the gallbladder and/or two or more of the following signs: (a) pain in the right upper quadrant; (b) axillar temperature over 37.5 °C; (c) palpable abdominal mass and (d) blood white cells $>10\,000/mm^3$. Chronic cholecystitis was diagnosed when patients were subjected to elective cholecystectomy because of previous biliary colics and presented with chronic inflammatory changes of the gallbladder. Bile cultures were performed according to standard bacteriological techniques for aerobic and anaerobic bacteria[20].

The general characteristics of the population studied are presented in Table 2. As expected, positive bile cultures were significantly more frequent in acute than in chronic cholecystitis, as is commonly found in Europe[21] and in the United States[22]. Less than 5 % of the patients presented cholecystitis without stones. Common duct stones were significantly more frequent in

Table 2 General characteristics of the population subjected to a cholecystectomy and whose biles were cultured

	Cholecystitis		
	Acute (*n*=131)	*Chronic* (*n*=205)	*p**
Age	58±17†	48±15†	<0.005
Female patients	63%	76%	<0.02
Choledocolithiasis	28%	18%	<0.05
Positive cultures	73%	31%‡	<0.005

* Significance was assessed by 'Z' test, except in the case of the age of the groups, in which a *t* test was performed

† Represent the mean ± 1 SD

‡ Five positive bile cultures to *Staphyloccocus epiderdimidis* were eliminated from the calculation, because they were considered contaminants

acute cases, 28 % compared to 18 % in chronic cholecystitis. This factor, and the significantly higher mean age of the acute patients, may explain the higher proportion of positive cultures in acute cholecystitis, since it is known that these two factors increase the frequency of positive cultures obtained from operated patients[23].

The overall incidence of *Salmonella* infection was 5 % of the operated patients: 1.5 % of the patients with chronic cholecystitis and 10.5 % of the patients with acute cholecystitis. All these cases had gallstones and more than 50 % of their weight was cholesterol in a series of six patients, including three cases with chronic cholecystitis.

The bacterial species found with higher frequencies are presented in Fig. 3. There were no differences in the distribution of the commoner species between the patients with acute or chronic cholecystitis. *Escherichia coli, Streptoccocus* D and No-D, *Klebsiella, Enterobacter* and anaerobes were the principal species found. This pattern is similar to that found in other countries[21,22,24]. However, as shown in Fig. 4, *Salmonella* was found in 4.7 % of the positive bile cultures of patients with chronic cholecystitis compared to 14.7 % of the acute cases ($p < 0.03$). The clinical history of these patients was carefully re-evaluated to discard those patients that could have developed acute cholecystitis during the course of clinical typhoid fever. Only two of 14 patients with acute cholecystitis *Salmonella*-positive were considered to have typhoid fever complicated by acute cholecystitis. If a 'Z' test is performed considering only the 12 patients without typhoid fever, then again the difference between acute and chronic cholecystitis with *Salmonella*-positive bile culture remains statistically significant at the $p < 0.05$ level. The mean age of the patients with acute cholecystitis *Salmonella*-positive was similar to the mean age of the total group of patients with chronic cholecystitis. In addition, the frequency of choledocholithiasis in the patients with acute cholecystitis *Salmonella*-positive was only 7.2 %. Therefore, it can be concluded that neither age nor common bile obstruction could have increased the frequency of *Salmonella* infection in the biliary tree of the patients with acute cholecystitis.

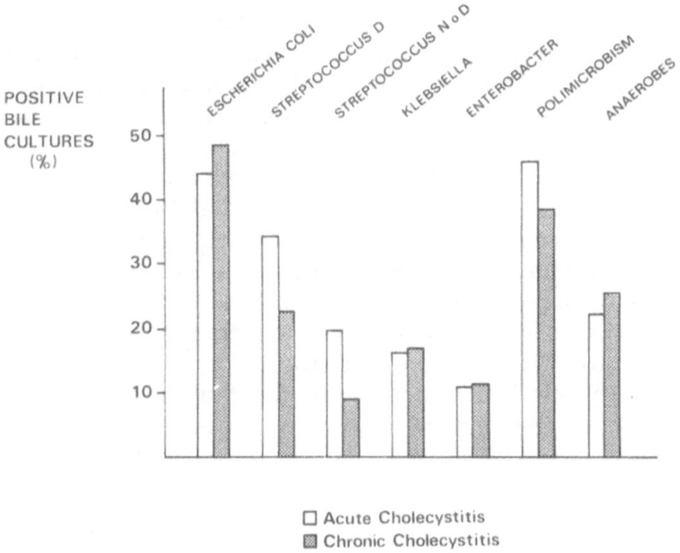

Figure 3 Incidence of different bacterial species in cases of acute and chronic cholecystitis with positive bile culture

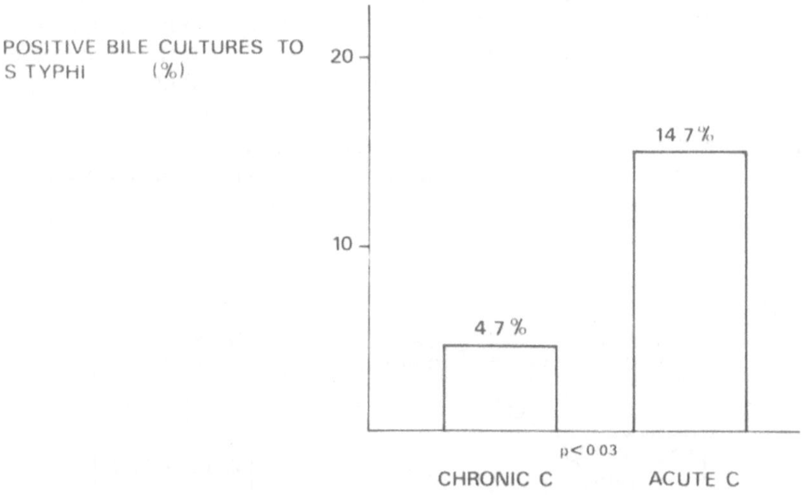

Figure 4 Incidence of *Salmonella* in cases of acute and chronic cholecystitis with positive bile cultures. One patient with chronic cholecystitis had a positive bile culture to *Salmonella paratyphi* B and three patients with acute cholecystitis had positive bile culture to *Salmonella paratyphi* (one A and two B)

The histopathology of gallbladder from patients who had undergone cholecystectomy and presented *Salmonella* in their bile cultures, was similar to that of the patients with negative or positive bile cultures to other bacteria.

It is now generally accepted that the primary aetiological factor of acute cholecystitis is the cystic duct obstruction by a gallstone, in the majority of the patients[25]. Biliary infection would have a minor role in the initiation of acute cholecystitis. Our results imply that *Salmonella typhi* may be an important initiating factor of acute cholecystitis in endemic areas, in the absence of a typhoid syndrome. A further implication is that the overall incidence of *Salmonella* infection obtained from bile cultures of patients operated on because of symptomatic gallbladder disease in endemic areas, cannot be extrapolated to the general population of subjects harbouring gallstones, as a measure of the true frequency of chronic carriers[26,27]. In addition, this study raises the question whether other bacteria can be common initiating factors of acute cholecystitis. This hypothesis implies that virulence factors may be present only in some strains of the bacteria commonly found in the biliary tract.

DISCUSSION

The apparent interrelationships between endemic salmonellosis and gallstone disease are presented in Fig. 5, and can be summarized in four points. First, the high prevalence of gallstones is one of the major determinants of the numbers of chronic carriers of *Salmonella typhi* in areas with high prevalence of typhoid fever, such as Chile. The high number of chronic carriers maintains the endemic cycle and interferes with effective control of typhoid fever.

Second, the association of the chronic carrier state with gallstones, two important risk factors of gallbladder cancer, may explain the high frequency of this cancer in Chile. The mortality rate of gallbladder cancer is approximately 7 per 100 000 in Chile[28], one of the highest in the world. Gallbladder cancer represents the second most frequent digestive cancer (gastric cancer has a mortality rate of 23 and colon cancer only of 3 per 100 000).

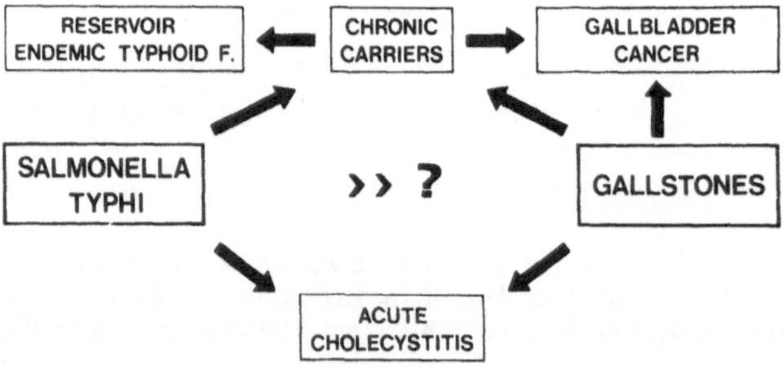

Figure 5 Apparent interrelationships between endemic salmonellosis and gallstone disease

Third, typhoid fever or *Salmonella* infection do not significantly affect biliary lipid composition to facilitate the production of a supersaturated bile. There is no evidence of a potential aetiological role of this infection in the pathogenesis of gallstone disease through this mechanism.

Fourth, besides the well-known capacity of *Salmonella typhi* and *S. paratyphi* to induce acute cholecystitis, as a complication during the evolution of typhoid fever, these bacteria may induce acute cholecystitis in the absence of a typhoid syndrome, as was previously shown at the end of the last century[29]. Our finding of an important incidence of *Salmonella* infection in the population of patients with acute cholecystitis may in part explain the high frequency of cholecystectomy in Chile because of acute gallbladder disease. Approximately 40 000 cholecystectomies are performed per year in that country; 35 % of this total represents emergency operations performed, presumably, because of acute cholecystitis[30].

We can conclude that the natural history of gallstone disease may be more aggressive in those areas in which *Salmonella typhi* is endemic, such as Mexico, Central and South America.

Acknowledgments

The authors wish to thank Irene Vicente, Cecilia Valdés, Carolina Céspedes and Pamela Nazal for collecting the bile cultures. Patricia Cavalla, Ana María Ramos, Angela Solari and Beatriz Ronco gave excellent technical assistance. We also wish to thank Miriem Aguad for typing this manuscript. This study was supported by Grants 10/80 and 94/82 from the Dirección de Investigación de la Pontificia Universidad Católica de Chile.

References

1. W.H.O. *World Health Statistics Annual* (1977). (Geneva: World Health Organization)
2. Scott, A. J. (1971). Bacteria and disease of the biliary tract. *Gut*, **12**, 487–492
3. Diehl, A. K. (1980). Epidemiology of gallbladder cancer: a synthesis of recent data. *J. Natl. Cancer Inst.*, **65**, 1209–1214
4. Hornick, R. B., Greisman, S. E., Woodward, T. E., Dupont, H. L., Dawkins, A. T. and Snyder, M. J. (1970). Typhoid fever: pathogenesis and inmunologic control. *N. Engl. J. Med.*, **283**, 686–691
5. Ames, W. R. and Robins, M. (1943). Age and sex as factors in the development of the typhoid carrier state, and a method for estimating carrier prevalence. *Am. J. Publ. Health*, **33**, 221–230
6. Vogelsang, T. M. and Boe, J. (1948). Temporary and chronic carriers of *Salmonella typhi* and *Salmonella paratyphi* B. *J. Hyg.*, **46**, 252–261
7. Marinović, I., Guerra, C. and Larach, G. (1972). Incidencia de litlasis biliar en material de autopsias y análisis de composición de los cálculos. *Rev. Med. Chile*, **100**, 1320–1327
8. Sprinz, H., Gangarosa, E. J., Williams, M., Hornick, R. B. and Woodward, T. E. (1966). Histopathology of the upper small intestines in typhoid fever. *Am. J. Dig. Dis.*, **11**, 615–624
9. Takeuchi, A. (1967) Electron microscope studies of experimental Salmonella infection. I. Penetration into the intestinal epithelium by Salmonella typhimurium. *Am. J. Pathol.*, **50**, 109–119
10. Nervi, F., Covarrubias, C., Valdivieso, V., Zunino, E., Salcedo, M., Solari, A. and Ronco, B. (1983). Evidencia de hipofunción vesicular y cambios del pool de ácidos biliares en fiebre tifoidea. *Rev. Med. Chile*, **111**, 796–801

11. Vantrappen, G., Ghoos, Y., Rutgeerts, P. and Janssens, S. (1977). Bile acid studies in uncomplicated Crohn's disease. *Gut*, **18**, 730–735
12. Covarrubias, C., Nervi, F., Valdivieso, V., Zunino, E., Salcedo, M., Solari, A. and Ronco, B. (1983). The effect of typhoid fever on bile acid pool size and composition. *J. Infect. Dis.*, **147**, 361
13. Hepner, G. H. (1975). Effect of decreased gallbladder stimulation on enterohepatic cycling and kinetics of bile acids. *Gastroenterology*, **68**, 1574–1581
14. Rosenow, E. C. (1916). The etiology of cholecystitis and gallstones and their production by the intravenous injection of bacteria. *J. Infect. Dis.*, **19**, 527–556
15. Brown, R. O. (1919). A study on the etiology of cholecystitis and its production by the injection of streptococci. *Arch. Intern. Med.*, **23**, 185–189
16. Rains, A. J. (1962). Research concerning the formation of gallstones. *Br. Med. J.*, **2**, 685–691
17. Stokes, A. and Clarke, C. (1916). A search for typhoid carriers among 800 convalescents. *Lancet*, **1**, 566–569
18. Armijo, R., Pizzi, A. and Lobos, H. (1967). Prevalencia de portadores tíficos después del tratamiento con cloranfenicol. *Bol. Of. Sanit. Panam.*, **62**, 295–302
19. Edlund, Y. and Zettergreen, L. (1958). Histopathology of the gallbladder in gallstone disease related to clinical data. With a proposal for uniform surgical and clinical terminology. *Acta Chir. Scand.*, **116**, 450–460
20. Lennette, E. H., Balows, A., Hausler, W. J. Jr. and Truant, J. P. (1980) *Manual of Clinical Microbiology*. 3rd Edn. (Washington: American Society for Microbiology)
21. Bergan, T., Doblong, I. and Liavag, I. (1979). Bacterial isolates in cholecystitis and cholelitiasis. *Scand. J. Gastroenterol.*, **14**, 625–631
22. Mason, G. R. (1968). Bacteriology and antibiotic selection in biliary tract surgery. *Arch. Surg.*, **97**, 533–537
23. Wilson, S. E., Finegold, S. M. and Williams, R. A. (1982). *Intraabdominal Infection*. pp. 113–125. (New York: McGraw-Hill)
24. Dije, M., MacDonald, A. and Smith, G. (1978). The bacterial flora of the biliary tract and liver in man. *Br. J. Surg.*, **65**, 285–287
25. Way, L. W. and Sleisenger, M. H. (1983). Acute cholecystitis. In Sleisenger, M. H. and Fordtran, J. S. (eds.) *Gastrointestinal Disease*. 3rd Edn. pp. 1374–1383. (Philadelphia: W. B. Saunders)
26. Levine, M. M., Black, R. E., Lanata, C. and the Chilean Typhoid Committee (1982). Precise estimation of the numbers of chronic carriers of Salmonella typhi in Santiago, Chile, an endemic area. *J. Infect. Dis.*, **146**, 724–726
27. Nervi, F., Raddatz, A. and Zamorano, N. (1984). Overestimation of the numbers of chronic carriers of Salmonella typhi in Santiago. *J. Infect. Dis.* (In press)
28. Medina, E. and Csendes, A. (1983). Características epidemiológicas del cáncer en Chile. *Rev. Med. Chile*, **111**, 69–75
29. Cushing, H. W. (1898) Typhoidal cholecystitis and cholelithiasis. *Bull. Johns Hopkins Hosp.*, **9**, 91–96
30. Fernández, M. (1979) Litiasis biliar en Chile. Encuesta nacional. *Rev. Chil. Cir.*, **31**, 47
31. Go, U. L., Hofmann, A. F. and Summerskill, W. H. (1970) Pancreozymin bioassay in man based on pancreatic enzyme secretion: potency of specific aminoacids and other digestive products. *J. Clin. Invest.*, **49**, 1558–1564
32. Holzbach, R. T., March, M., Olszewski, M. and Holan, K. (1973). Cholesterol solubility in bile. Evidence that supersaturated bile is frequent in healthy man. *J. Clin. Invest.*, **52**, 1467–1479

20
Clinical symptoms and gallstone disease: lessons from a population study

L. CAPOCACCIA and the GREPCO Group*

From a clinical point of view gallstone disease is one of the best-known diseases. Most treatises deal with the clinical aspects of biliary stones in a rather uniform way: i.e., biliary colics and related 'dyspeptic' symptoms are commonly associated with stones. Nonetheless, few clinical data[1] derived from epidemiological surveys are available. A particular aspect, which may be the most important for a clinician, is represented by asymptomatic gallstones. It is a problem which has drawn the attention of many authors from the very beginning of the study of gallstone disease. It is evident that only an epidemiological study can provide an answer to the problem, though recent papers have largely contributed to improving our knowledge[2,3].

Within the data collected from the GREPCO study, many have been purposely directed to the above aspects. This paper is thus aimed at defining the sensitivity, specificity and predictive value of the symptoms and signs commonly related to gallstones.

MATERIAL AND METHODS

Our data concern 1081 women of a population of 1439 working and free-living females, aged 20–64 years. Details are reported in other papers in this book and have been partly published[4].

The questionnaire was completed by the participants and subsequently checked with each woman by a member of the clinical staff. Part of the questionnaire concerned the occurrence of abdominal symptoms. Each woman was asked (a) whether during the last 5 years she had ever suffered from abdominal pain (b), if so, to indicate, on an appropriate figure, the main site of the pain, (c) whether the pain lasted more than $\frac{1}{2}$ h, (d) whether the pain was so severe that she had to lie down, and (e) whether she had taken

* For the composition of the Group, see p. xi

antispasmodics to relieve the pain. The women were also requested to define whether the pain had a time relationship to the taking of meals.

As to dyspeptic symptoms, the question asked was: 'During the last 5 years have you often suffered from . . .' for each of the following: 'belching', 'heartburn', 'nausea', 'vomiting', 'bloated feeling after meals', 'intolerance to fatty or fried foods', 'heavy feeling on the right side', 'headache' and 'daily bowel movements'.

The women aware of having gallstones were defined as those non-cholecystectomized who responded positively to the question: 'Have you ever had gallstones?'

Statistical analyses were performed using the 'Z' test[5]. The predictive value was calculated dividing the number of gallstone women with biliary colic (as defined from the obtained results, see 'Results and Discussion' section) divided by the total of women with the colic. Multivariate analysis was performed by the multiple logistic function[6] in order to identify the set of variables with the best predictive capacity. The variables included were 35 and concerned only anamnestic and physical findings.

RESULTS AND DISCUSSION

Dyspeptic symptoms

No difference was observed between women with or without gallstones. At variance, cholecystectomized women showed higher frequency of vomiting, heavy feeling on the right side and intolerance to fatty meals. Our data are very similar to those reported in men by Bainton *et al.*[1] and indicate that symptoms of dyspepsia often attributed to gallstones discriminate poorly between those with and those without stones. It is not easy to comment on the observed greater frequency of some of the dyspeptic symptoms (vomiting, intolerance to fatty meals and heavy feeling on the right hypochondrium) in the cholecystectomized population. It could in fact be inferred that the so-called post-cholecystectomy syndrome is a real entity in our population; unfortunately, our questionnaire did not include the question whether such symptoms had their onset after or before surgery (Table 1).

Biliary colic

At least one episode of abdominal pain in the last 5 years was present in 66.6 % of gallstone and in 59.4 % of non-gallstone women: this difference was not statistically significant. Significant differences were instead found between women with and those without gallstones (34.8 % vs. 20.7 %) when the abdominal pain was better defined in its localization (the right hypochondrium or epigastrium) and duration (more than $\frac{1}{2}$ h). The further characterization of the pain through questions (d) and (e) of the clinical questionnaire (see Material and Methods) has further improved the specificity but also unacceptably decreased the sensitivity of the pain: in fact, 20.4 % of gallstone women answered positively to the question (e) vs. 7.7 % of non-

Table 1 Prevalence (%) of dyspeptic symptoms

Symptoms	*(1) Women without gallstones (n=979)*	*(2) Women with gallstones (n=66)*	*(3) Cholecystectomized women (n=36)*
Headache	52.8	42.5	43.7
Itching	12.0	10.6	12.5
Belching	19.1	29.8	21.9
Heartburn	20.2	21.7	28.1
Nausea	17.6	8.5	12.5
Vomiting	7.9	2.1	18.7*†
Abdominal postprandial blowing	44.6	40.3	59.3
Intolerance to fatty meals	31.3	21.3	46.9†
Heavy feeling at the right hypochondrium	23.0	29.8	46.3*
Diarrhoea	1.9	1.5	2.8
Constipation	5.4	6.1	5.5

* Statistical difference vs. (1): $p<0.05$
†Statistical difference vs. (2): $p<0.05$

gallstone women, whereas 15.9% of the former had been obliged to take antispasmodics vs. 4.5 % of non-gallstone women (Table 2). Thus, we have defined as representative of a *biliary colic* a pain localized at the right hypochondrium or epigastrium lasting more than ½ h. *Women with symptomatic gallstones were thus defined as those women with evidence of gallstones who had experienced a biliary colic* as specified above. The overall results in our population indicate that 34.8 % of gallstones were symptomatic and 65.2 % asymptomatic. No time relationship was found between biliary colic and meals. Prevalence of biliary colic was not different between women aware or unaware of having gallstones. It is noteworthy that 58 % of cholecystectomized people responded positively to the question: '. . . have you pain at the right hypochondrium or epigastrium of more than half an hour after cholecystectomy?'

Table 2 Prevalence (%) of abdominal pain (biliary colic) in the last 5 years

Definition of the pain	*Women without gallstones (n=957)*	*Women with gallstones (n=66)*	*Statistical significance*
Abdominal pain	59.4	66.6	n.s.
Pain on the right hypochondrium or epigastrium lasting more than ½ h*	20.7	34.8	$p<0.01$
As above, restricting patient to bed rest	7.7	20.4	$p<0.001$
As above, obliging patient to take antispasmodics	4.5	15.9	$p<0.001$

* This pain was defined as biliary colic

Predictive value of biliary colic

Considering the value of biliary colic in diagnosing gallstones, some considerations deserve attention. As shown in Table 3, the sensitivity of biliary colic is rather low and unrelated to the age, reaching, as mentioned before, an overall mean value of 34.8 %, which means that almost two-thirds of gallstone women did not suffer from this symptom. The specificity of biliary colic has instead resulted as rather high and age-dependent, reaching an overall mean value of almost 80 %; nonetheless, this means that one-quarter of non-gallstone women (i.e. a very large number of women when this one-quarter is related to the entire population we studied) may have presented with what could be defined as a biliary colic. Thus, the value of biliary colic in predicting the presence of gallstones in women when measured with Bayes' equation has been only slightly higher than the true prevalence of gallstone disease. This fact may explain why the prevalence of women aware of having gallstones was not different between symptomatic and asymptomatic subjects. In other words, our data suggest that in the absence of more specific findings, such as jaundice or fever, the diagnosis of cholelithiasis is often fortuitous.

Table 3 Sensitivity, specificity and positive predictive value of biliary colic for the presence of gallstones, according to age

Age (years)	*Sensitivity* (%)	*Specificity* (%)	*Predictive value** (%)
20–29	33.3	76.6	2.7
30–39	35.3	78.1	6.6
40–49	44.4	80.2	12.1
50–59	26.3	82.0	15.6
60–64	33.3	86.2	41.2
Total	34.8	79.3	9.8

* Calculated according to Bayes' theorem

Prediction of cholelithiasis by multivariate analysis

In order to obtain diagnostic criteria of better predictive value than the mere presence of biliary colic, we have determined the coefficient of probability of having gallstones by means of the multilogistic function analysis, which included, as independent variables, a series of 35 first-level (anamnestic and physical) data. Among these independent variables, only the following five proved to be associated with the disease: age, number of pregnancies, body mass index, biliary colic and biliary colic restricting the patient to bed rest. A percentage of probability of having gallstones has then been attributed to each subject. The whole population has subsequently been divided into deciles, according to the above probability. The results are represented in Table 4.

It is evident that the use of the five selected variables is actually capable of identifying a subgroup of population with a very high probability of having stones. In our case it was possible to select a population with a more than 10 %

Table 4 Multivariate analysis including the following five variables which proved to be associated with the disease: age, parity, obesity, biliary colic and biliary colic restricting to bed

Decile	*Subjects*	*Expected rate*	*Observed rate*	*Expected proportion*	*Observed proportion*
1	98	0.4	1.0	0.7	1.7
2	98	0.9	0.0	1.5	0.0
3	97	1.7	3.1	2.8	5.0
4	97	2.7	4.1	4.5	6.7
5	98	3.4	1.0	5.7	1.7
6	97	4.6	4.1	7.5	6.7
7	98	6.0	7.1	9.8	11.7
8	97	7.5	4.1	12.2	6.7
9	97	10.5	12.4	17.0	20.6
10	97	23.8	24.8	38.5	40.0

The observed population has been divided into deciles according to the estimated probability of being a case. For each decile the following parameters have been computed: the expected rate of cases, the proportion of expected cases over the total of expected cases, and the proportion of observed cases over the total of observed cases

probability of having gallstones, which corresponds to more than 55 % of the total expected cases. In other words, had we been aware of this finding, the examination of only one-fifth of the population would have permitted the detection of three-fifths of the women with stones. There is little doubt that, apart from epidemiological considerations, this procedure could offer many advantages in terms of identification and early treatment of gallstones.

References

1. Bainton, D., Davies, G. T., Evans, K. T. and Gravelle, I. H. (1976). Gallbladder disease. Prevalence in a South Wales industrial town. *N. Engl. J. Med.*, **294**, 1147–1149
2. Gracie, W. A. and Ransohoff, D. F. (1982). The natural history of silent gallstones: the innocent gallstone is not a myth. *N. Engl. J. Med.*, **307**, 798–800
3. Ransohoff, D. R., Gracie, W. A., Wolfenson, L. B. and Neuhauser, D. (1983). Prophylactic cholecystectomy or expectant management for silent gallstones. *Ann. Intern. Med.*, **99**, 199–204
4. The Rome Group for Epidemiology and Prevention of Cholelithiasis (GREPCO) (1984). Prevalence of gallstone disease in an Italian adult female population. *Am. J. Epidemiol.* In press).
5. Remington, R. D. and Schark, M. A. (1970). *Statistics with Applications to the Biological and Health Sciences*. p. 81. (Englewood Cliffs, NJ: Prentice-Hall)
6. Walker, S. H. and Duncan, O. B. (1967). Estimation of probability of an event as a function of several independent variables. *Biometrika*, **54**, 167–179

21
Problems in determining the prognosis of asymptomatic gallstones

G. D. FRIEDMAN

ABSTRACT

Decisions as to whether to perform prophylactic cholecystectomy on patients with asymptomatic gallstones require better information on the rate of development of complications than presently exists. The published data are scanty, are probably applicable only to whites, frequently do not clearly define the symptom status of patients at entry to the study, and contain little information that identifies subgroups with differing prognoses. Efforts to overcome these deficiencies and problems encountered in the design of a new follow-up study are described. In the absence of cholecystograms performed routinely on asymptomatic persons it is difficult to assemble a cohort of patients with silent gallstones suitable for a follow-up study. Other methods of identifying such patients may require that follow-up for the study start later than the time when stones were first demonstrated. Characteristics that should be ascertained at entry include demographic and important clinical features, the number and type of stones and the patient's symptoms. Follow-up should include the various complications of cholelithiasis, and whether cholecystectomy was later performed. All dates on which these significant events occur should be noted.

The medical profession continues to debate what to do for the patient with asymptomatic gallstones. One point of view, often held by surgeons, is that cholecystectomy should be performed immediately. The rationale for this approach may be stated as follows: cholecystectomy is quite safe when the patient is asymptomatic and it will prevent later complications resulting from gallstones. If one waits for symptoms to develop, the patient will be sick and older and much less able to tolerate surgery. Further, if the stones are not removed the patient is at risk of developing cancer of the gallbladder, which is usually incurable by the time it is discovered.

The other policy, often advocated by internists, is that cholecystectomy should not be performed unless and until the patient develops clear-cut symptoms or complications of cholelithiasis. The rationale for this approach is as follows: although prophylactic cholecystectomy is relatively safe, some otherwise healthy patients will die due to the surgery or anaesthesia. In terms of years of life lost, this tragic and unnecessary early mortality more than makes up for the greater mortality, surgical and otherwise, if complications occur later; and in many persons with gallstones these complications never occur. Also, routine identification and removal of all gallbladders with stones would be a very costly policy and would overload our surgical resources. Further, the risk of gallbladder cancer in persons with gallstones is very low and there is recent evidence[1] that cholecystectomy increases the risk of colon cancer, a much more common malignancy.

Resolution of this dilemma rests to a large extent on determining the rate at which complications develop in persons with asymptomatic gallstones. There is surprisingly little information about this, and examination of the few published studies points up another critical question – what do we mean by 'asymptomatic gallstones' and how often are patients who are discovered to have gallstones truly asymptomatic?

LITERATURE REVIEW

The six studies that I know of, on the prognosis of asymptomatic gallstones, are summarized in Table 1. Note first that in three or four of them, the patients were not all strictly asymptomatic; in fact, it is rather difficult to be sure of the clinical status of many of the patients as judged by some of the reports. The reported rate of development of complications ranged from about 1.1 % per year in persons with silent or truly asymptomatic stones to about 6.3 % per year for persons some of whom were symptomatic and some of whom were asymptomatic. The number of subjects in most of these studies has been rather small; altogether they total 1198. There are little or no data on non-whites. Only the recent study by Gracie and Ransohoff[7] used a reasonably sophisticated actuarial analysis to determine the probability of complications.

I am aware of two detailed decision analyses of immediate operation for asymptomatic gallstones vs. watchful waiting, based on computer analysis. These have employed some of the above complication rates, plus other published data on operative mortality and complications, survival rates from population life-tables, and economic data. Fitzpatrick *et al.*[8] found little difference between the two approaches to treatment, in terms of average life expectancy. 'Good-risk' patients lost, on average, 2 weeks of life, using a wait-and-see approach. 'Poor-risk' patients gained up to 1 month of life by deciding against immediate surgery. These conclusions were based on the 6.3% annual complication rate from the study by Wenckert and Robertson[6], which is probably too high. Fitzpatrick *et al.* also calculated the costs of screening all US 50-year-olds and 60-year-olds with cholecystograms each year and of operating on all with stones detected. This totalled $1.1 billion per year in the US using the now-too-low cost estimates of $50 per cholecystogram, $2000 per operation, and income losses of $1000. Cancers of the gallbladder and

Table 1 Studies of the prognosis of asymptomatic gallstones

Authors	*Year*	*Subjects*	*Initial symptom status*	*Length of follow-up*	*Annual rate of development of complications**	*Conclusion as to immediate surgery*
Peterson[2]	1915	51 women with gallstones discovered during pelvic surgery and who replied later to the author's inquiry	Either asymptomatic or symptoms did not 'over-shadow the importance of the pelvic condition'	Not stated – probably over 5 years in many cases	Cannot tell from data presented (37.2 % had symptoms referable to gallbladder)	Remove gallstones during pelvic surgery if can be done without much additional risk to patient
Truesdell[3]	1944	36 women with gallstones discovered at laparotomy and who did not die or have cholecystectomy shortly thereafter	'Quiescent or symptomless'	'Up to 20 years or more'	Cannot tell from data presented (50 % had gallbladder removed or were not asymptomatic)	Operate
Comfort *et al.*[4]	1948	112 patients at Mayo Clinic with asymptomatic gallstones discovered, 1925–34, at laparotomy for another condition. Average age 48 years, sex and race distribution not stated	Asymptomatic	14–23 years	About 1.1 %/year (19 % in average of 18–19 years)	Elective, let patient decide

Lund[5]	1960	25 men, 70 women admitted to a surgical service, Copenhagen, Denmark	Asymptomatic or slight symptoms	5–20 years	Probably about 3 %/year in men, 6 %/year in women (total 32 % of men, 52 % of women)	Operate
Wenckert and Robertson[6]	1966	781 patients with abnormal cholecystograms in Malmö, Sweden, 1951 and 1952, and not operated on for 1 year	Apparently mixed asymptomatic and symptomatic	11 years	Conflicting statements: 3.8 %/year (35 % in 11 years) or 6.3 % (51 % in 11 years)	Operate
Gracie and Ransohoff[7]	1982	123 (110 men, 13 women) healthy white faculty members, University of Michigan	Asymptomatic or non-specific symptoms	Up to 21 years	About 1.3 %/year (18 % in 15 years)	Do not operate

* Annual rate of complications $= 1 - (1 - \text{percentage with complications})^{\frac{1}{\text{no. of years}}}$

colon were not entered into the equation. For the individual patient, the authors concluded that considerations other than mortality, such as risk of morbidity and patient's peace of mind, should be the main determinants of whether to operate immediately or not.

In the other decision analysis, published recently by Ransohoff *et al.*[9], life expectancy was slightly better for patients who do not receive immediate cholecystectomy; the average difference was 4 days of life for a 30-year-old man and 18 days of life for a 50-year-old man. For women of these ages the average loss of life would be 1 day and 12 days, respectively. The difference in monetary costs also favoured watchful waiting rather than immediate cholecystectomy. The complication rate used in this study was 2 % per year for the first 5 years, 1 % per year during the second 5 years, and 0.5 % per year thereafter, based on the study of Gracie and Ransohoff[7]. In both of the above decision analysis studies higher complication rates were also fed into the computer. Expectant management was still preferable in the second study if the annual rate of development of biliary pain was raised to 5.4 %, and of other complications, to 0.6 %. In the first study there were some shifts in preference between the two approaches when the assumptions about complication rates were altered, but the differences in average life expectancy continued to be minimal.

NEED FOR MORE INFORMATION ABOUT THE RATE OF DEVELOPMENT OF COMPLICATIONS: APPROACH TO A NEW STUDY

One of the weakest links in the chain of evidence needed to arrive at a decision about asymptomatic gallstones is the information available about the rate of development of complications. It has been based on a few studies covering relatively few subjects, and all or nearly all of these subjects probably have been of the white race. The symptom-status of the subjects has often been unclear or mixed in these reports. Little effort has been devoted to identifying subgroups of these patients with markedly differing prognosis, if there be such.

A major problem has involved the definition of asymptomatic gallstones and the applicability of this label to patients for whom a decision is required. No doubt there are patients with truly asymptomatic gallstones. These stones are discovered when a cholecystogram is performed as part of a thorough health evaluation of the sort that is sometimes given to executives. Or such stones may be discovered during an ultrasonographic or surgical exploration of the abdomen done because of other present or suspected conditions. Also, if calcified, stones may show up on an X-ray of the abdomen. However, most patients in whom gallstones are discovered have received a cholecystogram because of abdominal symptoms that raised the question of gallbladder disease in the physician's mind. These symptoms, such as vague epigastric pain, food intolerance, or dyspepsia, may or may not have anything to do with the gallbladder – it is very difficult to be sure. If gallstones are found, and no other cause is identified, one is tempted to blame the symptoms on the stones, but this may well be incorrect[10]. On the other hand we cannot be sure that the stones are not responsible. At present it seems important to differentiate, as best we can, gallstones that are totally silent and discovered quite by accident, and those that are discovered because the patient has come to the doctor because of abdominal symptoms that are not classical biliary pain.

The Kaiser-Permanente Medical Care Program in Northern California provides comprehensive outpatient and inpatient medical care on a prepaid basis to 1.8 million subscribers. The subscribers comprise all racial and socioeconomic groups. A prepaid medical programme has no economic incentive to perform unnecessary surgery; it is unlikely that cholecystectomy would be performed unless the need were clear. In this setting, follow-up data in routine medical records should be available on large numbers of people with gallstones. Therefore, we felt that we might be able to conduct an extensive and valuable study of the rate of development of complications in persons with gallstones. By describing our efforts to set up such a study, I hope to illustrate some general problems that hamper the investigation of this question. My recommendations regarding how to conduct the study will, no doubt, be modified after ours is completed.

COHORT IDENTIFICATION

The first major task in a follow-up study of persons with asymptomatic gallstones is to identify a cohort of such individuals. To avoid having to wait for many years to see the results, it is preferable to identify and define a study cohort in the past and conduct an historical cohort study rather than a prospective cohort study. The first place to look for gallstones would, of course, be in old files of X-ray reports, seeking both abnormal cholecystograms and calcified gallstones on abdominal X-rays. I learned, to my sorrow, that our X-ray departments throw away their old reports and old films after they are 5 years old. Thus, anyone whom we could identify with gallstones by this means would have been known to have the stones for only 0–5 years. Copies of the X-ray reports are, of course, kept much longer in the medical records of patients, but there is no easy way to know which patients' charts to look into. Ultrasonography records also were not the answer. This is a relatively new procedure and the numbers of unsuspected gallstones discovered incidentally several years ago were too few to yield a good-sized study group.

Our organization does provide health appraisals for its subscribers in the form of multiphasic health checkups (MHCs), but these have never included cholecystography. During the early phases of the MHC programme, in the mid-1960s, abdominal X-rays were performed on each patient, but they were discontinued when they did not appear to be a cost-effective screening tool. Again to my sorrow I learned that, unlike the other MHC data, the findings on these abdominal films were not stored in computer records.

There were, however, questionnaire items in the MHC that seemed promising. During the 8-year period, 1964–72, patients were asked whether (a) a doctor told them that they had gallbladder disease before 1 year ago, or (b) in the past year, and (c) whether they had gallbladder surgery before 1 year ago, or (d) any surgery (type not recorded) in the past year. Using these four questions we formed five preliminary groups for study as shown in Table 2.

We checked on the actual status of the examinees at the time of MHC by reviewing a sample of their medical charts. The results were as shown in Table 3.

Thus, using the MHC questionnaire data for screening purposes, we could identify two groups that contained substantial numbers of people whom we could follow up to determine the prognosis of asymptomatic or mildly symptomatic stones; these were groups 3 and 5, containing a total of 3266 persons. Our pilot study indicated that medical record review would reduce this number to about 700 confirmed cases. In the sample of records reviewed, the first X-ray evidence of stones was recorded anywhere from 10 years before to 7 years after the MHC. Follow-up time after the MHC ranged from 1 to 19 years.

Table 2

Presumed status	*Criteria*	*Number*
(1) Gallbladder removed	yes to c	4018
(2) Gallbladder possibly removed in previous year	yes to a or b, no/? to c, yes to d	312
(3) Gallstones present	yes to a or b, no to c and d	2454
(4) Gallbladder disease unlikely	no to a, b and c	160 528
(5) Gallstones present; removal uncertain	yes to a or b, no/? to c and d	812
(6) Everybody else	all others	38 765

Table 3

Presumed status	*No. reviewed*	*Results*
(1) Gallbladder removed	17	All confirmed
(2) Gallbladder possibly removed	14	Three (21 %) had had stones removed by cholecystectomy; the others had no stones or no relevant information
(3) Gallstones present	39	Eight (21 %) had documented stones
(4) Gallbladder disease unlikely	(Not evaluated further)	
(5) Gallstones present; removal uncertain	26	Six (23 %) had documented stones

One other source of computer-stored data was evaluated. Between 1967 and 1973 diagnoses made in one of our outpatient clinics were stored in a computer. There were approximately 1000 patients with a computer-recorded diagnosis of gallbladder disease in this dataset. Review of charts of a sample of 30 of these patients revealed seven who had documented asymptomatic or mildly symptomatic gallstones. In this group follow-up duration after X-ray evidence ranged from 8 to 13 years. This source of cases should therefore add about 200 to the 700 obtained by screening of MHC questionnaires.

Entry of each patient into actuarial analysis

In deriving cases by scanning questionnaires and clinic records in this way, we must think very carefully about when to enter each patient into our follow-up. Let us consider, for example, a patient who reported having gallstones on an MHC questionnaire in 1970, and whose medical record indicates that they were first documented by X-ray in 1960. That patient should be entered into follow-up in 1970, and in an actuarial analysis should be regarded as contributing only information starting in the tenth year after gallstones are demonstrated. We must resist the temptation to use the first 10 years of experience with documented gallstones, of this patient. If we used that first 10 years of experience we would bias our study toward finding a better prognosis, since we have discovered and selected this patient for study only because she survived with her gallstones unremoved until the time of the MHC. Someone who had gallstones discovered in 1960, and who had them removed in 1963 because they were bothering her, or who died of ascending cholangitis due to a common duct stone, would never have been included in our study group. We can only perform an unbiased follow-up if we start at the index MHC, which brought the patient into the study. Similarly, we must not include the discovery-till-surgery experience of those patients who at index MHC said that they had had their gallbladders removed, because we would again have lost the sicker patients, i.e. those who had been operated upon and who had died because of the surgery or other reasons.

DATA COLLECTION

The data to be collected must satisfy certain requirements. We must ascertain the clinical and demographic characteristics of the patients at entry to follow-up, so that we can describe the group we are studying and identify subgroups with different complication rates. We must record the evidence that documents the presence of gallstones and describes them, and do our best to ascertain the symptoms of the patient or absence thereof up to the time when gallstones were demonstrated. We must then record the important events and complications that occur during follow-up. The dates at which all of these events occurred – plus the date of entry to, and end of, follow-up – must be noted.

Characteristics at entry

The demographic characteristics needed are age, sex, and race or ethnic group. Occupation, educational level and/or other measures of socioeconomic status or lifestyle may also prove valuable. Some basic clinical characteristics such as the presence or absence of alcoholism, diabetes mellitus, and obesity (including actual height and weight) should be recorded. In ascertaining the patient's symptom status it should be determined whether the patient has ever experienced typical biliary pain or attacks of acute cholecystitis. If so, she would ordinarily be a candidate for immediate cholecystectomy and is not appropriate for inclusion in a study of asymptomatic or mildly symptomatic gallstones. However, if a goodly number of such patients who were not immediately operated upon can be identified, a separate follow-up of that group would be of interest, particularly to see how often such patients become persistently asymptomatic once they have recovered from their acute attack. Another important symptom that would usually indicate that the stones are causing problems and should be removed is, of course, obstructive jaundice. The mild or non-specific symptoms that can accompany gallstones are many. Examples are indigestion or dyspepsia, intolerance of fatty or other foods, and vague or mild abdominal pain. It is important to determine whether some other cause for these symptoms, such as peptic ulcer, was discovered.

The type of, and findings on, objective demonstration of gallstones need to be recorded. There may be calcified gallstones seen on a simple X-ray of the abdomen. Radio-opaque or radiolucent stones may appear in a cholecystogram, or the latter may show a non-functioning gallbladder with no stones visible. Other objective demonstrations of gallstones may come from ultrasonographic examinations of the abdomen, or by surgeons' palpation during laparotomy. The number, size and X-ray appearance (lucent vs. opaque) of the stones should be noted. As mentioned above, follow-up should ordinarily start when the stones were first objectively documented, unless a later event, such as completion of a health questionnaire, is really what calls the patient to the investigator's attention. The time interval between objective documentation and that later event should be noted.

Follow-up data

The complications to look for during follow-up include troublesome biliary pain, acute cholecystitis, and obstructive jaundice or ascending cholangitis due to ductal obstruction by stones. These ordinarily require surgical intervention, and the first time that one of these occurs should be regarded as the time that the patient has developed a complication and is no longer asymptomatic or mildly symptomatic. One may, of course, study complications individually and, for example, continue regarding a patient as being at risk of cholangitis after biliary pain occurs, if the gallbladder is not removed. Carcinoma of the gallbladder is another complication that represents a failure of expectant management of asymptomatic gallstones. Pancreatitis may also be such a complication and should be noted. If a patient remains asymptomatic but later undergoes an elective cholecystectomy, this should be recorded and follow-up of the patient (as a person with asymptomatic gallstones) should be ended at the time of this operation.

Complications of both early and late surgery for gallbladder disease are an important consideration in deciding how to manage the patient. The investigator may wish to record these in the selected study group or may choose instead to rely on the larger published series. If a large study group is to be followed up beyond the time of cholecystectomy, the occurrence of carcinoma of the colon should be noted. It would be of interest to determine whether the incidence of colon cancer is greater or less in persons after cholecystectomy than in persons with asymptomatic gallstones, and whether it is higher in either of these groups than in the general population.

DATA ANALYSIS

Methods of data analysis for a study of this sort have been discussed comprehensively by Lee[11]. Some basic needs to keep in mind are to determine complication rates for individual years (e.g. year 1, year 5, year 10) or for small groups of years (e.g. years 1–5, years 6–10) and to have each subject contribute all his or her experience from the time of entry into follow-up either until a complication develops or until follow-up is ended. It is important to compare complication rates in clinically and demographically different subgroups in order to identify characteristics of prognostic significance.

References

1. Vernick, L. J. and Kuller, L. H. (1982). A case–control study of cholecystectomy and right-side colon cancer: the influence of alternative data sources and differential interview participation proportions on odds ratio estimates. *Am. J. Epidemiol.*, **116**, 86–101
2. Peterson, R. (1915). Gall-stones during the course of 1,066 abdominal sections for pelvic disease. *Surg. Gynecol. Obstet.*, **20**, 284–291
3. Truesdell, E. D. (1944). The frequency and future of gallstones believed to be quiescent or symptomless. *Ann. Surg.*, **119**, 232–245
4. Comfort, M. W., Gray, H. K. and Wilson, J. M. (1948). The silent gallstone: a ten to twenty year follow-up study of 112 cases. *Ann. Surg.*, **128**, 931–937
5. Lund, J. (1960). Surgical indications in cholelithiasis: prophylactic cholecystectomy elucidated on the basis of long-term follow-up on 526 nonoperated cases. *Ann. Surg.*, **151**, 153–162
6. Wenckert, A. and Robertson, B. (1966). The natural course of gallstone disease: eleven-year review of 781 nonoperated cases. *Gastroenterology*, **50**, 376–381
7. Gracie, W. A. and Ransohoff, D. F. (1982). The natural history of silent gallstones: the innocent gallstone is not a myth. *N. Engl. J. Med.*, **307**, 798–800
8. Fitzpatrick, G., Neutra, R. and Gilbert, J. P. (1977). Cost-effectiveness of cholecystectomy for silent gallstones. In Bunker, J. P., Barnes, B. A. and Mosteller, F. (eds.) *Costs, Risks and Benefits of Surgery*. pp. 246–261. (New York: Oxford University Press)
9. Ransohoff, D. F., Gracie, W. A., Wolfenson, L. B. and Neuhauser, D. (1983). Prophylactic cholecystectomy or expectant management for silent gallstones: a decision analysis to assess survival. *Ann. Intern. Med.*, **99**, 199–204
10. Price, W. H. (1963). Gall-bladder dyspepsia. *Br. Med. J.*, **2**, 138–141
11. Lee, E. T. (1980). *Statistical Methods for Survival Data Analysis*. (Belmont, California: Lifetime Learning Publications)

22
Cholecystectomy and large bowel cancer

V. SPERANZA and S. LEARDI

A high risk of large bowel cancer is reported in patients who have undergone cholecystectomy (Table 1). Pathophysiologic changes, resulting from cholecystectomy, most probably play an important role in colorectal carcinogenesis.

PATHOPHYSIOLOGY

Removal of the gallbladder means that there is no longer a reservoir for the bile. This leads to a constant stream of bile from the liver to the intestinal lumen throughout the 24 h, even during fasting, with constant and continuous absorption of bile acids in the ileocaecal tract. The increased enterohepatic turnover results in a negative feedback which inhibits hepatic synthesis of primary bile acids. Consequently there is a progressive decrease in production, which falls to 45 % in the case of cholic acid and to 74 % for chenodeoxycholic[1].

The continuous presence in the ileocaecal tract of a bile acid pool, altered both in quantity and quality, affects the enzymatic activity of the colonic bacterial flora, particularly the anaerobic species (*Bacteroides* and *Clostridia*)[2]. This explains the increase in the processes of deconjugation and dehydroxylation, with a consequently greater conversion of primary bile acids into secondary (deoxycholic) in cholecystectomized patients, than in normal[3]. In its turn, this intestinal absorption of deoxycholic acid negatively influences hepatic synthesis of primary bile acids.

Table 1 Relative risk of the colorectal cancer after cholecystectomy

Authors	*Relative risk*
Turnbull *et al.*, 1981	2.7
Linos *et al.*, 1981	1.7
Vernick and Kuller, 1981	1.7
Turunen *et al.*, 1981	1.5

In cholecystectomized patients, therefore, the pool of both primary acids seems to be reduced, but there is a notable increase of secondary (deoxycholic) acid[1]. The latter may possibly be converted by the anaerobic colonic flora into a carcinogenic substance such as methylcholanthene and/or its metabolites[4].

Experimental studies on animals, for example rats, who have no gallbladder, indicate that the presence of deoxycholic acid in the lumen of the colon may trigger off a carcinogenic process, or at least might hasten those already determined by other stimuli[5,6].

Furthermore increased faecal excretion of deoxycholic acid is significantly more noticeable in patients with colonic neoplasms than in normal subjects, or in those with non-neoplastic gastrointestinal diseases[7,8]. On the basis of these observations it has been suggested that cholecystectomy, by favouring a higher concentration of deoxycholic acid in the colonic lumen, may play a role, which should not be ignored, in the genesis of colorectal neoplasms[9]. Nevertheless, the foregoing observations do not seem to be confirmed in practice.

CLINICAL AND EPIDEMIOLOGICAL STUDIES

The incidence of colorectal neoplasia in patients with a previous cholecystectomy varies from 1 %[10], to 19.1 %[11], with an average of 8–9 %[12,13]. Periodic follow-up of cholecystectomized patients, usually for cholelithiasis, found colorectal cancer in only 0.7 %[14], 2 %[9] and 3 % of cases[13]. Comparisons between healthy patients, or at least those without neoplastic diseases, have not demonstrated significant or decisive differences, either in retrospective or prospective studies. However, if the sex factor alone is taken into account, some studies[9,12,15,16] do report a greater risk of colon cancer in females ($RR = 1.7$, $p < 0.05$) after cholecystectomy, especially 8–15 years after the operation.

The possible influence of a previous cholecystectomy on the exact colonic location of the neoplasia has also been investigated, with conflicting results. The right colon appears to be most often involved[9,17], although a significant correlation has also been noted for the rectum[12]. Certain other authors[15,18,19] found no particular colonic segment to be favoured.

In our own experience no significant correlation between a previous cholecystectomy and the appearance of a colonic neoplasm has emerged, even taking into account the sex factor and the site of the cancer itself. We reviewed the records of 250 patients who had undergone intestinal resection for colorectal cancer, in the 6th Surgical Clinic of the University 'La Sapienza' of Rome, between 1975 and 1983 (Table 2). The patients were also contacted by telephone, to confirm and/or obtain further information regarding biliary diseases.

As control group we selected 250 subjects matched for sex and age, with diseases which were neither gastroenterological nor neoplastic (Table 3). A previous cholecystectomy, performed at least 2 years before the diagnosis of colorectal cancer, was recorded in 9.3 % of subjects in the study group. This rate is within the average range reported by other workers and is not

Table 2 Colorectal cancer group: 250 cases (1975–83)

Sex	M=129; F=121		
Age	29–85 years (63 years average)		
Site	Right colon	43 cases	17%
	Left colon	38 cases	15%
	Sigmoid colon	68 cases	27%
	Rectum	101 cases	41%

Table 3 Control matched group: 250 cases

Sex	M=129; F=121	
Age	29–85 years (63 years average)	
Diseases	Varicose veins	75 cases
	Groin hernias	50 cases
	Breast cystic hyperplasia	63 cases
	Nodular goitres	62 cases

significantly different ($\chi^2=1$; $p=0.2$) from that of the control group (Table 4), even considering the sex factor (Table 5).

In the cholecystectomized patients the right colon was not favoured by neoplasias when compared either to the left colon or to the rectum (Table 6). Our retrospective study also failed to find any correlation between the incidence of colorectal cancer and the presence of cholelithiasis, even in those cases diagnosed during intestinal resection for cancer.

We also followed up 200 patients (80 men, 120 women) whose ages ranged from 19 to 70 years, at from 10 to 20 years (median 16) following cholecystectomy for cholelithiasis. Only one patient, a woman, had developed a sigmoid carcinoma, 12 years after removal of the gallbladder, at the age of 62.

Table 4 Incidence of cholecystectomy in patients with colorectal cancer and in control group

		Incidence of cholecystectomy	
	No. of cases	*No. of cases*	*Percentage*
Cancer group	250	23	9.2
Control group	250	31	12.4

$\chi^2=1$; $p=0.2$

Table 5 Incidence of cholecystectomy in patients with colorectal cancer by sex

		Incidence of cholecystectomy	
Cancer group	*No. of cases*	*No. of cases*	*Percentage*
Males	129	9	6.9
Females	121	14	11.5

$\chi^2=1.3$; $p=0.2$

Table 6 Incidence of cholecystectomy in patients with colorectal cancer by colonic site

Colonic site	No. of cases	Incidence of cholecystectomy: No. of cases	Percentage
Right colon (RC)	43	6	13.9
Left colon (LC)	32	2	6.2
Sigmoid colon (SC)	74	4	5.4
Rectum (R)	101	12	11.8

RC–LF: $\chi^2=1$, $p=0.2$ RC–SC: $\chi^2=2.6$, $p=0.1$ RC–R: $\chi^2=1.3$, $p=0.2$

DISCUSSION

Reviewing the results of the relevant pathophysiological and clinico-epidemiological studies, one can appreciate how difficult it is to confirm or deny the suspected carcinogenic action of gallbladder removal. The real problem in comparing or interpreting the many works on this subject is their lack of homogeneity. This arises because of the multiple confounding variables, factors which may be analysed in different ways: the selection, number and type of patients included, their sex and age, the length of follow-up, and, to complicate matters further, all within the context of prospective and/or retrospective studies.

As regards the number of cases examined, it is worth noting that the study with the largest numbers to date[14] did not find any correlation between cholecystectomy and colorectal cancer, whereas the studies using smaller numbers did[9]. In epidemiological studies conducted on total populations over a vast area, the results were still contradictory[11,17].

The risk of colon cancer after cholecystectomy is not always assessed in the same study, and to ensure greater statistical significance, by a double comparison between two groups of patients – one with colorectal neoplasias and one with previous cholecystectomy[13]. Most of this research reviews only patients who had undergone cholecystectomy[9,14] or only those operated on for colorectal cancer[11,12,17,19]. Moreover some studies refer to autopsied series, even with selected cases[15,16,18]. The sex factor further complicates an already tricky problem. We find studies including females only[11] or males as well. Nevertheless the findings here contrast all the same[9,14]. The high incidence of previous cholecystectomy in female patients with colorectal cancer[9,12,15–17,19] could, on the other hand, be explained by their natural predisposition to biliary lithiasis[20,21], hence the greater number of cholecystectomies. The hypothesis that female sex might mediate in the carcinogenic effect of cholecystectomy would seem to be also confirmed by the finding of oestrogen receptors in neoplastic tissue[22]. However, these receptors have not been found in adenomatous polyps[23], which degenerate more often in females[24].

Age may be a variable to be considered. Results which appear to confirm the influence of age are those from patients over the fourth decade. The incidence of colorectal cancer is significantly higher in this age group[25]. Colonic neoplasms usually arise at an average of 13–18 years after gallbladder removal[12,13]. So a follow-up of these patients, long enough to include this period in the various studies[9,13,14] would not seem to be an important variable.

To achieve greater statistical significance, cholecystectomies performed in the 2 years before the diagnosis of the neoplasms were not generally included in these studies. Even though not then diagnosed, the tumour may well have been already present.

Contradictory results in cholecystectomized patients could also be explained by the presence or absence of further carcinogenic factors, other than the secondary bile acids already mentioned. Even the role played by these acids is questionable[26–28], and carcinogenic properties have been noted also for the primary bile acid chenodeoxycholic[29]. Increased faecal excretion of primary, rather than secondary, bile acid was recently observed in patients with colorectal neoplasms, although this was in a Japanese population[30] who are at low risk for this cancer. Besides, insignificant amounts of bile acids, in particular deoxycholic acid, have been found in the homogenate of colonic neoplasms, with no relationship to the size of the cancer itself or even to the surrounding uninvolved tissue[31]. On the other hand, colorectal neoplasias might be linked, by dietary factors, more to the gallstones than to the cholecystectomy itself. A diet rich in animal fat, which notoriously influences the appearance of gallstones, may facilitate and/or accelerate carcinogenesis in the colon[4,32]. However, this hypothesis does not seem to be borne out in experimental clinical studies[33], or epidemiological studies[34,35].

Lastly, one should note that the highest risk of colorectal cancer post-cholecystectomy has been reported mainly in North America[9,17], Sweden[16] and New Zealand[12], countries which, for various reasons quite apart from biliary disease, already have a higher incidence of large bowel cancer[4]. Similar findings have not been reported with any significance in populations with a lower risk of cancer[35–37].

CONCLUSION

In conclusion, one can clearly see how hard it is, in view of the many clinical and epidemiological variables, to confirm or deny a link between previous cholecystectomy and colorectal cancer. The most useful direction for future studies might be a clinical and instrumental follow-up of cholecystectomized patients under 40 years of age, in a population at low risk for cholelithiasis and colorectal cancer. This approach would also help to broaden our knowledge of the aetiology of the cancer itself. Meanwhile, until research confirms or refutes the increased risk of colorectal cancer in cholecystectomized patients, the most practical course would be to follow at least the women at risk, over 40 years of age.

References

1. Pomare, E. W. and Heaton, K. W. (1973). The effect of cholecystectomy on bile salt metabolism. *Gut*, **14**, 753–762
2. Hill, M. J. (1975). The role of colon anaerobes in the metabolism of bile acids and steroids, and its relation to colon cancer. *Cancer*, **36**, 2387–2400
3. Hepner, G. W., Hofmann, A. F., Malageda, J. R., Szczepanik, P. A. and Klein, P. D. (1974).

Increased bacterial degradation of bile acids in cholecystectomized patients. *Gastroenterology*, **66**, 556–564
4. Stubbs, R. S. (1983). The aetiology of colorectal cancer. *Br. J. Surg.*, **70**, 313–316
5. Narisawa, T., Magadia, N. E., Weisburger, J. H. and Wynder, E. L. (1974). Promoting effect of bile acids on colon carcinogenesis after intrarectal instillations of N-methyl-N-nitro-N-nitrosoguanidine in rats. *J. Natl. Cancer Inst.*, **53**, 1093–1097
6. Reddy, B. S., Narisawa, T., Weisburger, J. H. and Wynder, E. L. (1976). Promoting effect of sodium deoxycholate on colon adenocarcinomas in germ free rats. *J. Natl. Cancer Inst.*, **56**, 441–442
7. Hill, M. J., Drasar, B. S., Williams, R. E. O., Meade, T. W., Cox, A. G., Simpson, J. E. P. and Morson, B. C. (1975) Faecal bile acids and clostridia in patient with cancer of the large bowel. *Lancet*, **1**, 535–539
8. Reddy, B. S. and Wynder, E. L. (1973). Large bowel carcinogenesis: faecal constituents of population with diverse incidence rates of colon cancer, *J. Natl. Cancer Inst.*, **50**, 1437–1442
9. Linos, D. A., O'Fallon, W. M., Beart, R. W. Jr, Beard, C. M., Dockerty, M. B. and Kurland, L. T. (1981). Cholecystectomy and carcinoma of the colon. *Lancet*, **2**, 379–381
10. Hare, A. M. (1974). Carcinoma of the colon and cholecystectomy. *Lancet*, **2**, 1395
11. Weiss, N. S., Daling, J. R. and Chow, W. H. (1982). Cholecystectomy and the incidence of cancer of the large bowel. *Cancer*, **49**, 1713–1715
12. Turnbull, P. R. G., Smith, A. H. and Isbister, W. H. (1981). Cholecystectomy and cancer of the large bowel. *Br. J. Surg.*, **68**, 551–553
13. Abrams, J. S., Anton, J. R. and Dreyfuss, D. C. (1983). The absence of a relationship between cholecystectomy and the subsequent occurrence of cancer of the proximal colon. *Dis. Col. Rect.*, **26**, 141–144
14. Adami, H. O., Meirik, O., Gustavsson, S., Nyren, O. and Krusemo, U. B. (1983). Colo-rectal cancer after cholecystectomy: absence of risk increase within 11–14 years. *Gastroenterology*, **85**, 859–865
15. Capron, J. P., Delamarre, J., Canarelli, J. P., Brousse, N. and Dupas, J. L. (1978). La cholécystectomie favorise-t-elle l'apparition du cancer rectocolique? *Gastroenterol. Clin. Biol.*, **2**, 383–389
16. Lowenfels, A. B., Domellof, L., Lindstrom, C. G., Bergman, F., Monk, M. A. and Sternby, N. Y. (1982). Cholelithiasis, cholecystectomy and cancer: a case control study in Sweden. *Gastroenterology*, **83**, 672–676
17. Vernick, L. J. and Kuller, L. H. (1981). Cholecystectomy and right-sided colon cancer: an epidemiological study. *Lancet*, **2**, 381–383
18. Turunen, M. J. and Kivilaakso, E. (1981). Increased risk of colorectal cancer after cholecystectomy. *Ann. Surg.*, **194**, 639–641
19. Markman, M. (1982). Cholecystectomy and carcinoma of the colon. *Lancet*, **2**, 47
20. Lindstrom, C. G. (1977). Frequency of gallstone disease in a well defined Swedish population. *Scand. J. Gastroenterol.*, **12**, 341–346
21. Schottenfeld, D. and Winawer, S. J. (1983). Cholecystectomy and colorectal cancer. *Gastroenterology*, **85**, 966–967
22. McClendon, J. E., Appleby, D., Claudon, D. B., Donegan, W. L. and De Cosse, J. J. (1977). Colonic neoplasms: tissue estrogen receptor and carcinoembryonic antigen. *Arch. Surg.*, **112**, 240–241
23. Agrez, M. V. and Spencer, R. J. (1982). Estrogen receptor protein in adenomas of the large bowel. *Dis. Col. Rect.*, **25**, 348–350
24. Muto, T., Kamiya, J., Sawada, T., Susama, S., Itai, Y., Ikenega, T., Yamashiro, M., Hino, Y. and Yamaguchi, S. (1980). Colonoscopic polypectomy in diagnosis and treatment of early carcinoma of the large intestine. *Dis. Col. Rect.*, **23**, 68–75
25. Stefanini, P., Speranza, V., Carboni, M., Benedetti-Valentini, F. B. and Gentileschi, E. (1970). *Il cancro del grosso intestino*. 1st Edn. (Rome: Carlo Erba)
26. Moskovitz, M., White, C., Barnett, R. N., Stevens, S., Russel, E., Vargo, D. and Floch, M. (1979). Diet, fecal bile acids and neutral sterols in carcinoma of the colon. *Dig. Dis. Sci.*, **24**, 746–751
27. Mudd, D. G., McKelvey, S. T. D., Norwood, W., Elmore, D. T. and Roy, A. D. (1980). Faecal bile acid concentrations of patients with carcinoma or increased risk of carcinoma in the large bowel. *Gut*, **21**, 587–590

28. Brydon, W. G., McRoss, A. H., Anderson, J. R. and Douglas, S. (1982). Diet and faecal lipids following cholecystectomy in men. *Digestion*, **25**, 248–252
29. Czygan, P., Seitz, H., Waldher, R., Stiehl, A., Raedsch, R. and Kommerell, B. (1983). Chenodeoxycholic acid but not ursodeoxycholic acid enhances colonic carcinogenesis in the rat. *Gastroenterology*, **84**, 1132
30. Kaibara, N., Sasaki, T., Ikeguchi, M., Kuga, S. and Ikaka, S. (1983). Fecal bile acids and neutral sterols in Japanese with large bowel cancer. *Oncology*, **40**, 255–258
31. Gelb, A. M., McSherry, C. K., Sadowsky, J. R. and Mosbach, E. H. (1982). Tissue bile acids in patients with colon cancer and colonic polyps. *Am. J. Gastroenterol.*, **77**, 314–317
32. Cruse, J. P., Lewin, M. R. and Clark, C. G. (1982). Dietary cholesterol deprivation improves survival and reduces incidence of metastatic colon cancer in dimethylhydrazine-pretreated rats. *Gut*, **23**, 594–599
33. Caprilli, R., Pietroiusti, A., Giuliano, M., Fanucci, A., Cerro, P., Prantera, C. and Mangiarotti, R. (1983). Dieta, colecistectomia e cancro del colon. Studio caso-controllo. *Sett. Ital. Mal. Digest.* (SIMAD 3), Vol. 1, p. A68 (Bari)
34. Linos, D. A., O'Fallon, W. M., Thistle, J. L. and Kurland, L. T. (1982). Cholelithiasis and carcinoma of the colon. *Cancer*, **50**, 1015–1019
35. Narisawa, T., Sano, M., Sato, H., Takahashi, T. and Arakawa, H. (1983). Relationship between cholecystectomy and colonic cancer in low-risk Japanese population. *Dis. Col. Rect.*, **26**, 512–515
36. Sama, C., Morselli Labate, A. M., Taroni, F., Roda, E., Chiodarelli, C., Serra, S., Gozzetti, G. and Barbara, L. (1983). La colecistectomia come possibile fattore di rischio per il cancro del colon: uno studio caso-controllo. *Sett. Ital. Mal. Dig.* (SIMAD 3), Vol. 1, p. A67 (Bari)
37. Caprilli, R., Pietroiusti, A., Chierchini, P., Giuliano, M., Andreoli, A. and Prantera, C. (1981). Cholecystectomy and colorectal cancer. A retrospective study. *Ital. J. Gastroenterol.*, **13**, 46–47

23
Dietary habits and cholelithiasis

A. F. ATTILI and the GREPCO Group*

Evidence exists that dietary factors play a regulatory role in plasma lipid levels[1], biliary lipid composition[2-4] and bile acid kinetics[5-7]. Dietary habits of gallstone subjects have been compared with those of matched controls[8-11]. Studies from France[8,9] showed a higher caloric intake in gallstone subjects than in controls; studies from Australia showed that caloric intake was similar[10] in the two groups, or lower[11] in gallstone than in control subjects. As far as concerns epidemiological studies, data on eating habits reported in the Framingham study[12] failed to reveal an association between presence of clinically diagnosed cases of gallbladder disease and daily intake of fat, protein and cholesterol. This paper deals with the eating habits as recorded during an epidemiological survey aimed primarily at investigating the prevalence of gallstone disease in a free-living population.

MATERIALS AND METHODS

This study is part of a large cross-sectional survey on gallbladder disease in a population of female civil servants. Details of the protocol have been published elsewhere[13]. Only data obtained in 60 gallstone women and in 917 women without gallstones who answered the part of the questionnaire devoted to dietary habits are referred to here.

Quantitative daily consumption

Four food items (bread, pasta, meat and cheese) were considered as those with the highest daily consumption in Italy and it was requested that their use be indicated in terms of g/day. Daily consumption of sugar (g/day) was calculated by multiplying the indicated number of consumed teaspoonfuls by a factor of 5.

* For the composition of the Group see p. xi

Frequency of consumption and consumption score

Consumption of other less common foods was recorded by the method of frequency of consumption. The possible answers to be given were as follows: (a) never (consumed); (b) rarely; (c) once or twice a month; (d) one to four times a week; (e) five to seven times a week; (f) more than once a day. For analysis of the data subjects who gave answers (a), (b) and (c) were given a consumption score 0; a consumption score 1 was attributed to subjects who gave the (d) answer and a consumption score 2 to those who gave answers (e) and (f).

The effect on food consumption of (a) increasing age, (b) presence of biliary colic and (c) awareness of having gallstones was investigated by comparing the results obtained in (a) four different age classes (20–29, 30–39, 40–49, 50–64 years); (b) women with or without presence of at least one episode of biliary colic in the past 5 years, (c) gallstone women aware or unaware of having gallstones.

Wine

Daily wine consumption was assessed by a quantitative questionnaire. The following five classes were considered: (a) no wine; (b) less than ½ litre; (c) about ½ litre; (d) about 1 litre and (e) more than 1 litre.

Dietary fat

Habitual consumption of different cooking and seasoning fats was assessed on the basis of a semiquantitative questionnaire using a score ranging from 0 (nil) to 8 (high quantity for both cooking and seasoning). Information on the type of dietary fat was also obtained by analysing erythrocyte fatty acid composition by gas–liquid chromatography (GLC) as described elsewhere[14].

Frequency of meals and slimming diets

Subjects were also asked to indicate: (1) whether they were used to having breakfast; (2) which was their main meal; (3) whether they were used to having a snack between meals; (4) whether they had ever tried a slimming diet and how many kilograms did they lose.

The association of dietary habits to gallstones was studied by a stepwise logistic regression analysis according to the method described in the appendix of this volume. Analysis included 55 variables. Age, presence of biliary colic and awareness of having gallstones were taken into account as possible confounders. Student's *t*-test for unpaired data and Fisher's Z exact test were used where appropriate.

RESULTS

Mean daily consumption of bread, pasta, meat, cheese and sugar are given in Table 1. Prevalence of gallstone women according to frequency of food

Table 1 Mean (±SD) daily consumption (g/day) of some common Italian foods and effect of age, biliary symptoms and awareness of having gallstones on food consumption

Food	Gallstone females	Non-gallstone females	p	Effect of Age	Effect of Symptoms	Effect of Awareness
Bread	102.4±54.3	120.5±75.5	<0.05	(+)	N	(−)
Pasta	54.8±39.0	60.9±44.6	n.s.	+	N	+
Meat	104.2±28.1	112.2±49.8	<0.05	−	N	N
Cheese	68.4±36.5	85.8±51.9	<0.001	N	N	N
Sugar	11.6± 8.3	15.8±13.2	<0.001	−	N	(+)

n.s. = not significant; N = no significant change; + = significant increase; − = significant decrease in mean daily food consumption. Symbols are indicated between parentheses when a trend is evident but does not reach statistical significance

consumption is indicated in Table 2. These tables also show the effects on food consumption of (a) increasing age, (b) presence of biliary colic and (c) awareness of having gallstones.

Prevalence of gallstones according to classes of wine consumption is shown in Fig. 1. Women with a higher daily wine consumption showed a higher, although not significant, prevalence of gallstones than women with low or no consumption of wine.

Frequency of use of different seasoning and cooking fats did not differ between women with or without gallstones. GLC analysis of erythrocyte fatty acids (Fig. 2) failed to reveal any difference between subjects with or without gallstones.

Seventy-nine and 80% of subjects with and without gallstones, respectively, were used to having a breakfast. No difference was observed as far as

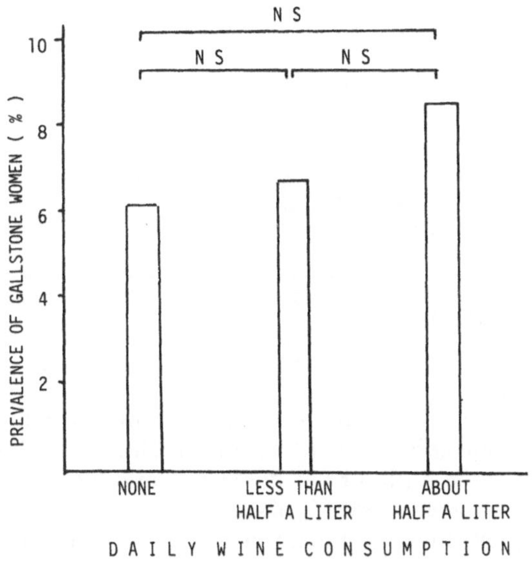

Figure 1 Prevalence of gallstone women according to three different classes of daily wine consumption

Table 2 Prevalence (%) of gallstone women according to frequency of consumption of various foodstuffs and effect of age, presence of biliary symptoms and awareness of having gallstones on food consumption

	*Consumption score**					*Effect of*		
Food	*0*	*1*	*2*		*p*	*Age*	*Symptoms*	*Awareness*
Sweetstuffs	6.5	7.0	1.9	%	n.s.	–	N	N
	557	313	107	S				
Bread sticks	5.9	7.8	7.2	%	n.s.	N	N	N
	830	64	83	S				
Lean meat	4.1	6.5	6.6	%	n.s.	N	N	N
	170	400	407	S				
Fat meat	6.6	4.0	6.7	%	n.s.	–	N	N
	715	173	89	S				
Pork meat	6.4	4.6	0.0	%	n.s.	N	–	(–)
	865	108	4	S				
Poultry	7.0	4.8	2.6	%	n.s.	N	(+)	N
	629	310	38	S				
Rabbit	6.1	8.8	0.0	%	n.s.	N	N	N
	940	34	3	S				
Pressed meat	7.2	3.7	5.5	%	<0.05	–	–	(–)
	649	273	55	S				
Lean ham	5.9	6.1	7.4	%	n.s.	N	N	N
	424	445	108	S				
Fatty ham	6.5	5.3	2.6	%	n.s.	–	–	N
	749	189	39	S				
Sausages	6.5	0.0	33.3	%	<0.05	N	–	N
	911	63	3	S				
Meat broth	6.6	4.8	0.0	%	n.s.	–	N	N
	755	208	14	S				
Fish	7.4	5.0	0.0	%	n.s.	(+)	N	(+)
	530	424	23	S				
Milk	6.4	11.8	4.9	%	n.s.	–	N	(+)
	313	110	554	S				
Eggs	11.2	4.9	4.7	%	<0.05	–	N	–
	197	674	106	S				
Chocolate	6.5	3.2	6.5	%	n.s.	–	N	N
	851	95	31	S				
Legumes	7.1	4.3	4.5	%	n.s.	–	N	(–)
	633	300	44	S				
Vegetables	8.8	6.4	5.8	%	n.s.	N	N	N
	57	313	607	S				
Fresh fruit	4.0	10.6	5.8	%	n.s.	N	N	N
	50	94	833	S				

* = See methods; % = prevalence of gallstone women; S = number of subjects. Other abbreviations and symbols as in Table 1

concerns the indication of the main meal. A significantly lower percentage ($p<0.05$) of gallstone subjects were used to having a snack between meals with respect to women without gallstones (11 and 23 %, respectively).

As regards slimming diets, 34.8 % of subjects with gallstones and 36.1 % of women without gallstones presented this history; mean kg lost did not differ between the two groups (6.3 and 6.4, respectively).

Using the stepwise logistic function analysis, three variables were found to

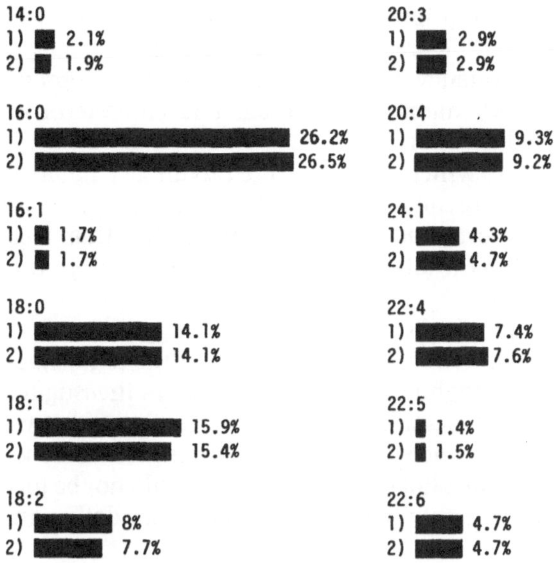

Figure 2 Erythrocyte fatty acid pattern (%) in (1) women without gallstones and (2) women with gallstones

be significantly and inversely related to the presence of gallstones, i.e. quantitative daily consumption of sugar ($t = -2.89$; $p < 0.01$) and cheese ($t = -2.15$; $p < 0.05$) and frequency of consumption of fish ($t = -2.08$; $p < 0.05$). No association was observed with the other variables including body mass index and physical activity.

DISCUSSION

The questionnaire interview method used here for recording dietary habits does not permit calculation of daily intake of calories. Nevertheless it is noteworthy that, in our study, women with gallstones consumed per day less bread, meat, cheese and sugar and less often ate fatty meals and eggs than women without gallstones. Interpretation of these findings, which are in contrast with the common opinion that gallstone disease is associated with a high caloric intake, should, however, take into account some factors which can greatly influence dietary habits. Traditionally, patients who are found to have gallstones are advised to restrict their intake of fatty foods in order to reduce gallbladder contraction and frequency of biliary colic. Presence of biliary colic could be *per se* an important diet-modifying factor. On the other hand, in our epidemiological study gallstone subjects were older than those without gallstones and increasing age may well be associated with modifications in eating habits.

It is evident from Tables 1 and 2 that most of the observed differences in food consumption are due to the effect of (a) increasing age, (b) presence of biliary colic and (c) awareness of having gallstones. In fact, after controlling for these three variables in a multiple logistic function analysis, only a weak negative association between the presence of gallstones and the daily intake of sugar and cheese and frequency of consumption of fish was observed. Also in the Framingham study[12] dietary fat, protein and cholesterol intake were not related to gallbladder disease.

Two other factors which may be related to dietary habits, i.e. obesity and physical activity, were not systematically investigated with regard to dietary habits because the former is more probably an effect than a cause of changes in dietary habits and the latter did not differ between subjects with or without gallstones.

A slight, though not significant, trend suggesting that persons who consumed less alcohol ran a higher risk of subsequent gallbladder disease was observed in the Framingham study[12]. In the present investigation we observed a slight though not significant positive association between daily wine consumption and presence of gallstones. Although in Italy wine is the most important source of alcohol consumption, it should not be forgotten that our population comprised only women and their mean daily wine consumption was rather low.

Studies on diets high or low in bran content demonstrated a reduction in cholesterol saturation of bile in patients with gallstones[3] but no effect on bile composition in normal persons[15]. Very little effect on the overall metabolism of cholesterol in man has been demonstrated[16]. Biliary lipid composition and biliary bile acid composition are not modified by a vegetarian diet in man[17]. In our study no significant association was observed between frequency of consumption of legumes, vegetables or fruits and presence of gallstones.

Substituting polyunsaturated for saturated fat in the American diet has been reported to increase the incidence of gallstones[18]. This finding was not confirmed by another study in similar groups of patients[19]. In our study no association was observed between presence of gallstones and frequency of consumption of different seasoning and cooking fats. Percentage composition of erythrocyte fatty acids, which is an objective index of the short- and long-term changes in dietary lipids[20,21], was not different between subjects with or without gallstones. This observation, however, deserves a deeper statistical evaluation and will be published elsewhere.

Increased biliary cholesterol saturation has been demonstrated during fasting[22], while gallbladder stimulation has an opposite effect. Low frequency of snack between meals, which could mean low gallbladder stimulation and contraction, has been shown in gallstone subjects in the present investigation. Although this observation needs further confirmation and better definition, decreased meal frequency should be regarded as a possible risk factor for the development of gallstones in man.

References

1. Truswell, A. S. (1978). Diet and plasma lipids – a reappraisal. *Am. J. Clin. Nutr.*, **31**, 977–989
2. DenBesten, L., Connor, W. E. and Bell, S. (1973). The effect of dietary cholesterol on the composition of human bile. *Surgery*, **73**, 266–273

3. Pomare, E. W., Heaton, K. W., Low-Beer, T. S. and Espiner, H. J. (1976). The effect of wheat bran upon bile salt metabolism and upon the lipid composition. *Am. J. Dig. Dis.*, **21**, 521–526
4. Sarles, H., Chabert, C., Pommeau, Y., Save, E., Mouret, H. and Gerolami, A. (1969). Diet and cholesterol gallstones. *Am. J. Dig. Dis.*, **14**, 531–537
5. McDougall, R. M., Yakymyshyn, L., Walker, K. and Thurston, O. L. (1978). Effect of wheat bran on serum lipoproteins and biliary lipids. *Can. J. Surg.*, **21**, 433–435
6. Low-Beer, T. S. (1977). Diet and bile acid metabolism. *Clin. Gastroenterol.*, **6**, 165–178
7. Cummings, J. H., Wiggins, H. S., Jenkins, D. J. A., Houston, H., Jivraj, T., Drasar, B. S. and Hill, M. J., (1978). Influence of diets high and low in animal fat on bowel habit, gastrointestinal transit time, fecal microflora, bile acid and fat excretion. *J. Clin. Invest.*, **61**, 953–963
8. Sarles, H., Chalvet, H., Ambrosi, L., Gazeix, N. and D'Ortoli, G. (1957). Etude statistique des facteurs diététiques dans la pathologie de la lithiase biliaire humaine. *Sem. Hôp. Paris*, **33**, 3424–3438
9. Sarles, H., Chabert, C., Pommeau, Y., Save, E., Mouret, H. and Gerolami, A. (1969). Diet and cholesterol gallstones. A study of 101 patients with cholelithiasis compared to 101 matched controls. *Am. J. Dig. Dis.*, **14**, 531–534
10. Wheeler, M., Hills, L. L. and Laby, B. (1970). Cholelithiasis, a clinical and dietary survey. *Gut*, **11**, 430–437
11. Burnett, W. (1971). The epidemiology of gallstones. *Tijdschrift voor Gastroenterologie*, **14**, 79–89
12. Friedman, G. D., Kannel, W. B. and Dawber, T. R. (1966). The epidemiology of gallstone disease: observations in the Framingham study. *J. Chron. Dis.*, **19**, 273–292
13. The Rome Group for the Epidemiology and Prevention of Cholelithiasis (GREPCO) (1984). Prevalence of gallstone disease in an Italian adult female population. *Am. J. Epidemiol.* (In press)
14. Angelico, F., Amodeo, P., Borgogelli, C., Montali, A., Ricci, G. and Cantafora, A. (1980). Red blood cell fatty acid composition in a sample of middle aged men on free diet. *Nutr. Metab.*, **24**, 148–153
15. Bennion, L. J. and Scott, M. G. (1978). Risk factors for the development of cholelithiasis in man (second of two parts). *N. Engl. J. Med.*, **299**, 1221–1227
16. Raymond, T. L., Connor, W. E. and Lin, D. S. (1977). The interaction of dietary fibers and cholesterol upon the plasma lipids and lipoproteins, sterol balance, and bowel function in human subjects. *J. Clin. Invest.*, **60**, 1429–1437
17. Huijbregts, A. W. M., Van Schaik, A., Van Berge-Henegouwen, G. P. and Van Der Werf, S. D. J. (1980). Serum lipids, biliary lipid composition and bile acid metabolism in vegetarians as compared to normal controls. *Eur. J. Clin. Invest.*, **10**, 443–449
18. Sturdevant, R. A. L., Pearce, M. L. and Dayton, S. (1973). Increased prevalence of cholelithiasis in men ingesting a serum cholesterol lowering diet. *N. Engl. J. Med.*, **288**, 24–27
19. Miettinen, M., Turpeinen, O., Karvonen, M. J. *et al.* (1976). Prevalence of cholelithiasis in men and women ingesting a serum cholesterol lowering diet. *Ann. Clin. Res.*, **8**, 111–116
20. Farquhar, J. W. and Ahrens, E. H. Jr. (1963). Effects of dietary fats on human erythrocyte fatty acid pattern. *J. Clin. Invest.*, **42**, 657–686
21. Angelico, F., Arca, M., Calvieri, A., Cantafora, A., Guccione, P., Monini, P., Montali, A. and Ricci, G. (1983). Plasma and erythrocyte fatty acids: a methodology for evaluation of hypocholesterolemic dietary interventions. *Prev. Med.*, **12**, 124–127
22. Williams, C. N., Morse, J. W. I., MacDonald, I. A., Kotoor, R. and Riding, M. (1977). Increased lithogenicity of bile on fasting in normal subjects. *Am. J. Dig. Dis.*, **22**, 189–193

PART 4
PREVENTION OF GALLSTONE DISEASE: PRESENT STATUS

Chairmen: G. RICCI and J. STAMLER

24
Factors associated with gallstone disease: observations in the GREPCO study

F. ANGELICO and the GREPCO Group*

INTRODUCTION

Gallstone disease, and particularly cholesterol gallstones, is a common disease in most developed countries. The overall impression is that of increasing prevalence in Europe, North America and in the affluent countries. However, the understanding of factors predisposing to the disease has progressed slowly and information still derives primarily from clinical observations and autopsy series.

The study of risk factors for gallstone disease has been undertaken in few epidemiological prospective investigations, where the risk of development of the disease has been related to the level of putative risk factors determined at entry into the studies[1,2]. Very few studies are based on statistically valid random samples of the general population. In fact, the current knowledge on associated factors derives mainly from studies carried out on selected groups of individuals or on population samples known to be at high risk for gallstones for possible genetic factors[3–6].

Most of the reported epidemiological associations have been established by studies not primarily devoted to gallstone disease, where cases were mainly represented by cholecystectomies, and no attempt was made to identify silent gallstones. Therefore, the failure to identify silent stones may have either obscured possible associations or resulted in false associations. In fact, approximately half the cases of gallstones are silent and the accurate assessment of associated factors necessarily implies that one is able to determine who in the population under study has the disease and who has not. Because of these selection and diagnostic problems, the reported associations are difficult to generalize, and conflicting results have been frequently described.

The relation of gallstone disease to the suggested aetiological factors has

* For the composition of the Group, see p. xi

been examined at the baseline examination of a sample of 1081 female civil servants, enrolled into a prospective epidemiological study of gallstone disease based on ultrasonography[7].

METHODS

This study is part of an extensive survey on the epidemiology of gallstone disease and related factors. The general aims, methodological details and prevalence data of this study are given in Chapter 3 of this book, and have been reported elsewhere[7].

Body mass index (barefoot and without overcoat) was calculated dividing weight (kg) by height (m).

Blood pressure was measured with a mercury sphygmomanometer at the right arm in the sitting position after 5 min rest, by doctors trained with the tapes of the London School of Hygiene. The mean values of two consecutive measurements (made 1 min apart) were taken into account. The fifth Korotkoff phase was taken to define diastolic pressure.

Women participating in the study completed a questionnaire which was subsequently checked jointly with a member of the clinical staff. A section of the questionnaire concerned habitual physical activity, which was recorded according to the following scores: (a) time spent walking to/from working place (1 = 1–9 min; 2 = 10–19 min; 3 = 20–29 min; 4 = more than 30 min); (b) time spent walking other than above (1 = less than 30 min; 2 = 30–60 min; 3 = more than 60 min); (c) physical activity at work (1 = light; 2 = moderate; 4 = heavy); (d) habitual physical activity at leisure (1 = sedentary; 2 = walking, gardening etc.; 5 = regular sports).

As far as smoking habits were concerned, women were asked whether they were smokers and how many cigarettes they smoked per day.

Other sections of the questionnaire concerned family history of gallstones, use of oral contraceptives and lipid-lowering drugs, parity, menopause and previous slimming diets (kg lost).

Data were statistically evaluated by the Student's unpaired *t*-test, χ^2 test[8] and the multiple logistic function analysis[9,10]. Age standardization was performed by the direct method, taking the whole sample examined as reference population.

RESULTS

The results of the present study refer to 66 women with evidence of gallstones, 36 women with history of cholecystectomy, and 979 women shown to be free from gallstones.

The prevalence of gallstones and cholecystectomies in different age groups and the relations of serum lipids to gallstone disease are discussed in detail in other chapters of this book.

Mean body mass index was significantly higher ($p < 0.01$) in women with gallstones, as compared with those without gallstones, whereas cholecystectomized women showed intermediate values (Table 1). The prevalence of both

Table 1 Age-adjusted mean values of some variables and prevalence of smokers in women with and without gallstones, and in cholecystectomized women

Variables	*Women without gallstones (n=979)*	*Women with gallstones (n=66)*	*Cholecystectomized women (n=36)*
Body mass index (kg/m^2)	23.9+3.4	25.3+5.2**	24.8+3.3
Systolic blood pressure (mmHg)	121.2+16.2	124.1+15.3	122.6+15.7
Diastolic blood pressure (mmHg)	76.5+9.9	79.2+9.4*	78.1+9.1
Fasting blood glucose (mg/dl)	85.7+12.1	87.1+11.1	91.2+10.3*
Cigarettes/day	5.3+8.0	4.3+7.7	5.7+9.9
Prevalence of smokers (%)	42.4	37.9	47.2

* $p<0.05$; ** $p<0.01$.

gallstones and cholecystectomies was significantly higher in the two upper quartiles of body mass index distribution, as compared to the two bottom quartiles (Fig. 1).

Mean age-adjusted diastolic blood pressure was significantly higher ($p<0.05$) in women with gallstones; here again, cholecystectomized females showed intermediate values. The same trend was found for systolic blood pressure, although the differences were not significant (Table 1).

Smoking habits, defined as number of cigarettes smoked per day, as well as prevalence of smokers, were found to be slightly lower in women with gallstones, as compared to the other two groups, although not to a statistically significant extent (Table 1).

The level of the habitual physical activity, expressed in terms of different types of physical activity, was not statistically different between the three

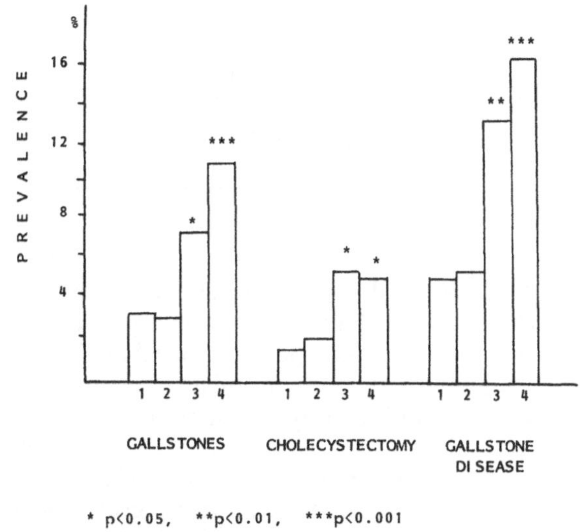

Figure 1 Distribution of women with and without gallstones, and of cholecystectomized women according to quartiles of body mass index

groups considered, although women free from gallstones tended to be slightly more active (Table 2).

Women who had had three or more pregnancies showed a significantly higher crude prevalence of both gallstones and cholecystectomies than nulliparous and those with parity 1 or 2 (Table 3). No significant association was observed between gallstone disease and the other sex-specific factors, including age at menopause, prevalence of oral contraceptive users, duration and frequency of menstrual cycle.

Age-adjusted mean fasting blood glucose was significantly higher in cholecystectomized women ($p<0.05$) (Table 1). Accordingly, the prevalence of cholecystectomized women was significantly higher in the two upper quartiles of fasting blood glucose distribution (Fig. 2). The relatively low proportion of diabetics in our population did not permit assessment of the association of gallstone disease with diabetes mellitus.

Table 2 Age-adjusted mean levels of physical activity in women with and without gallstones and in cholecystectomized women (criteria for the evaluation of physical activity are given in the paragraph on methods)

Physical activity	*Women without gallstones* ($n=979$)	*Women with gallstones* ($n=66$)	*Cholecystectomized women* ($n=36$)
Time spent walking to/from working site	2.39+1.07	2.31+0.94	2.14+0.86
Time spent walking other than above	1.92+0.74	1.87+0.71	1.71+0.92
Physical activity at work	1.07+0.30	1.09+0.32	1.16+0.51
Physical activity at leisure	1.98+0.79	1.91+0.61	1.84+0.39

Table 3 Prevalence of gallstone and cholecystectomized women according to number of pregnancies

Number of pregnancies	*n*	*Gallstone women* (%)	*Cholecystectomized women* (%)
0	336	4.5**	3.9
1–2	620	6.0*	2.2***
≥3	125	11.2	7.2

* $p<0.05$; ** $p<0.02$; *** $p<0.01$

The relations of gallstone disease with 19 independent variables were assessed by separate multiple logistic function analyses, including either gallstones or cholecystectomies as dependent variables. The 19 independent variables were: age, body mass index, number of pregnancies, menopause, oral contraceptive use, habitual physical activity, smoking habits, lipid-lowering drugs, family history for gallstone disease, alcohol consumption, previous slimming diets, butter, olive oil and corn oil intakes, total and HDL cholesterol, total to HDL-cholesterol ratio, triglycerides, and fasting blood glucose. The variables contributing significantly to the fit of the observation were selected through a discriminant stepwise procedure. Table 4 shows the

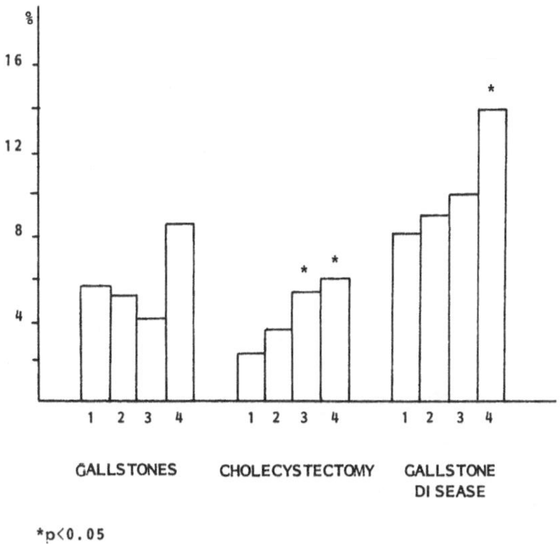

Figure 2 Distribution of women with and without gallstones, and of cholecystectomized women according to quartiles of fasting blood glucose

Table 4 Relation between gallstones ($n=66$) and 19 variables in 993 women

Variables	*Coefficients*	*S.E.*	*t*
Age	0.063	0.015	4.11**
Body mass index	0.077	0.031	2.52*
No. of pregnancies	0.205	0.115	1.78
Total cholesterol	−0.009	0.004	−2.58*
Triglycerides	0.007	0.003	2.38*

* $p<0.05$; ** $p<0.001$

BMPD multiple logistic function analysis: last equation of stepwise procedure

last equation of the stepwise analysis with gallstones as dependent variable. The variables selected out of the initial 19 were age, body mass index, parity, and triglycerides, all positively related to gallstones, and total cholesterol, negatively related.

Figure 3 shows the regression curve between gallstones and body mass index derived from the multivariate analysis.

In the final equation of the multivariate stepwise analysis the relation between parity and gallstones did not reach a statistically significant level. To better understand this association, further multiple logistic function analyses were performed, introducing second-degree terms of the variables showing coefficients with a p-value <0.1. A significant negative interaction between parity and age was demonstrated, indicating that the increase in the relative risk for gallstones due to pregnancies is higher among younger than among older women (Table 5).

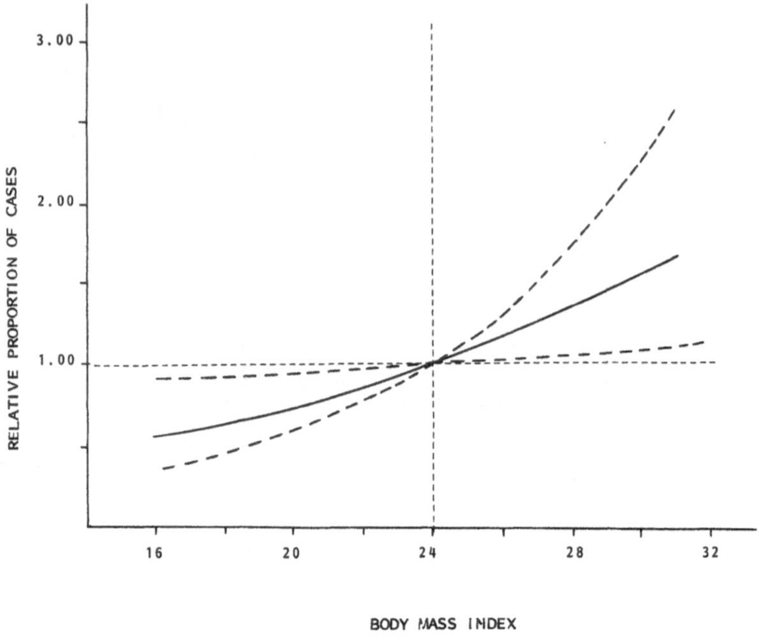

Figure 3 Correlation between body mass index and the risk for gallstones (as relative proportion of cases) derived from a multiple logistic analysis including 19 independent variables. Dotted lines indicate 95 % confidence limits

In the last equation of the discriminant stepwise procedure including cholecystectomy as dependent variable, out of the initial 19 variables the most useful in discriminating between cases and non-cases were age, serum triglycerides and fasting blood glucose, all positively related to cholecystectomy.

DISCUSSION

The approach of the present study was to assess factors associated to gallstone disease in a female free-living population screened for gallstones and cholecystectomy. In our survey 43 % of all cases of gallstone disease were represented by women unaware of their condition; only 35 % had been cholecystectomized[7].

Gallstone disease was positively and independently related with age, body mass index, parity and serum triglycerides, while a negative association was observed with total serum cholesterol.

In agreement with previous reports[1-3,5], obesity was strongly associated with gallstones. The relative risk for gallstones showed a steady increase with increasing body mass index levels, confirming the clinical observations suggesting fatness as a possible predisposing factor for gallstones. These epidemiological findings are also in agreement with the results of metabolic studies of obese people, which have demonstrated significantly higher bile cholesterol saturation in the former than in non-obese controls[11]. Differences

Table 5 Relative proportion of cases of gallstones according to number of pregnancies and different ages

No. of pregnancies	Relative proportion of cases (years)			
	25	30	40	50
0	1.00	1.00	1.00	1.00
1	2.25	1.94	1.44	1.07
2	5.05	3.75	2.07	1.14
3	11.36	7.27	2.98	1.22

Data have been obtained by a multiple logistic regression analysis with 19 independent variables, introducing second-degree terms (see text and Appendix of this book)

in body mass index between women with and without gallstones may well explain the mean higher diastolic blood pressure observed in the group of women who were found to have gallstones.

In agreement with previous findings[1,3], parity appeared to play a major role, the prevalence of women with gallstones showing an evident increase in women who had had more than two pregnancies. A multivariate analysis including 19 variables showed the association between parity and gallstones to be highly dependent on age. In fact, parity appeared to play a major role particularly among younger women, in whom each additional pregnancy increased the relative risk for gallstones by several times. Thus, the relative risk of a 25-year-old woman with three pregnancies was almost 12 times higher than that of a nulliparous one of the same age, while the relative risk of a 40-year-old woman of the same parity was only four times as high. However, a question which cannot be answered by our cross-sectional study is whether the observed effect of parity is simply to precipitate symptoms in a patient who already has a silent gallstone, or rather to induce gallstone formation.

No independent association was demonstrated between either gallstones or cholecystectomy and the following variables: habitual physical activity, smoking habits, age at menopause, alcohol intake, cooking and seasoning fat consumption, slimming diets, family history for gallstones. In agreement with two recent reports[3,4], no significant association was found with oral contraceptive use.

Cholecystectomy was positively and independently related to age, serum triglycerides and fasting blood glucose, suggesting that in studies of associated factors it should be regarded as a separate condition. No apparent explanation can be given to the independent association of cholecystectomy with fasting blood glucose.

How many of the observed associations are aetiological associations? On the basis of our prevalence data it is impossible to say whether a putative risk factor arose before or after the diagnosis of gallstones. Associated factors identified in such studies could, in fact, be sequelae rather than causes of the disease. Therefore, the only certain way to eliminate bias in the study of associated factors and to obtain information on the risk factors for the disease is: (1) to undertake screenings on representative population groups; (2) to identify individuals with pre-existing gallstone disease; (3) to follow the remainder with regular examinations thereafter. All this is necessary to detect new cases and to relate the risk of subsequent disease development to the levels of the putative risk factors observed at entry into the study. Such a study on risk factors seems particularly important now that an effective medical treatment of cholesterol gallstones has become available. The identification of high-risk groups also represents a necessary step towards the prevention of the disease.

The ongoing follow-up of our population group will probably add new insight in the evaluation of the causal role of the observed cross-sectional associations.

References

1. Friedman, G. D., Kannel, W. B. and Dawber, T. R. (1966). The epidemiology of gallbladder disease: observations in the Framingham Study. *J. Chron. Dis.*, **19**, 273–292
2. The Coronary Drug Protection Research Group (1977). Gallbladder disease as a side effect of drugs influencing lipid metabolism. Experience in the Coronary Drug Project. *N. Engl. J. Med.*, **296**, 1185–1190
3. Layde, P. M., Vessey, M. P. and Yeates, D. (1982). Risk factors for gallbladder disease: a cohort study of young women attending family planning clinics. *J. Epidemiol. Community Med.*, **36**, 274–278
4. Royal College of General Practitioners (1982). Oral contraceptives and gallbladder disease. *Lancet*, **2**, 957–959
5. Petitti, D. B., Friedman, G. D. and Klatsky, A. L. (1981). Association of a history of gallbladder disease with a reduced concentration of high-density-lipoprotein cholesterol. *N. Engl. J. Med.*, **304**, 1396–1398
6. Sampliner, R. E., Bennet, P. H., Comess, L. J., Rose, F. A. and Burch, T. A. (1970). Gallbladder disease in Pima Indians. Demonstration of high prevalence and early onset by cholecystography. *N. Engl. J. Med.*, **283**, 1358–1364
7. Rome Group for Epidemiology and Prevention of Cholelithiasis (GREPCO) (1984). Prevalence of gallstone disease in an Italian adult female population. *Am. J. Epidemiol.* (In press)
8. Remington, R. D. and Schark, M. A. (1970). *Statistics with Applications to the Biological and Health Sciences.* (Englewood Cliffs, NJ: Prentice-Hall)
9. Walker, S. H. and Duncan, O. B. (1967). Estimation of probability of an event as a function of several independent variables. *Biometrika*, **54**, 167–179
10. Capocaccia, R., Rome Group for Epidemiology and Prevention of Cholelithiasis (GREPCO). Biostatistical methods in Epidemiological Surveys. See Appendix, this volume
11. Bennion, L. J. and Grundy, S. M. (1975). Effects of obesity and calorie intake on biliary lipid metabolism in man. *J. Clin. Invest.*, **57**, 473–477

25
Prevention of coronary heart disease and risk of cholelithiasis

G. C. URBINATI and the GREPCO Group*

Certain clinical and experimental observations appear to indicate that dietary[1–3] and/or pharmacological[4,5] measures aimed at reducing metabolic risk factors of coronary heart disease (first and foremost cholesterolaemia) may alter bile composition thus favouring gallstone formation. Epidemiological data, too, seem to point in this direction although they are not univocal[6–10].

The Rome Group for the Epidemiology and Prevention of Cholelithiasis (GREPCO) has approached this problem from an epidemiological point of view by examining with an echographic method two groups of a male working population that had 3 years previously concluded a controlled trial of primary prevention of coronary heart disease within the framework of the Rome Project of Coronary Heart Disease Prevention (PPCC).

PPCC is a controlled trial of primary prevention of coronary heart disease, performed in Rome from 1973 to 1981; it represents the Italian section of the WHO European Multifactor Preventive Trial of CHD which was conducted simultaneously, apart from Italy, also in the United Kingdom (London), Belgium (Brussels–Ghent), Poland (Warsaw–Cracow), and Spain (Barcelona) under the coordination of the Regional Office for Europe of the WHO (Copenhagen)[11,12]. Principal investigators of the Italian section are: Prof. G. Ricci and Prof. G. C. Urbinati (Institute of Systematic Medical Therapy, University of Rome "La Sapienza"), and Prof. A. Menotti (National Health Institute).

The trial was intended to assess if, and to what extent, it is possible to modify the main coronary risk factors in working population samples and, in case such a possibility exists, to evaluate the effects of these changes on the incidence and mortality for CHD and on total mortality.

As for the structure of the project, the statistical units were represented by pairs of working groups ('factories') including men whose age at entry ranged

* For the composition of the Group see p. xi

between 40 and 59 years; these groups were randomly allocated to treatment and control.

In treatment 'factories' the first step was an initial screening for the assessment of certain major coronary risk factors; this was offered to all members of the groups. In control 'factories' initial screening was offered only to a limited subsample (in Rome, 10–25 %). By this initial examination the treatment and control populations could be compared and a baseline obtained. In addition, the subjects of the treatment groups (and of the control groups, limited to the subsamples) could be classified according to various levels of coronary risk at baseline.

Those found to be in the upper 20 % of a risk score (according to an additive point system suggested by the European Collaborative Group) were arbitrarily defined as high-risk subjects[11]. Factors considered for the 'risk score' were age, systolic blood pressure, serum cholesterol level, degree of physical activity at work, and cigarette consumption.

Subjects defined as high-risk were exposed to an individual preventive intervention. Other categories of subjects in the treatment 'factories' were also exposed to this programme, viz. those who, without falling into the upper 20 % of the 'risk score', satisfied one of the following conditions: (1) they fell into the upper 20 % of a risk rating elaborated by applying two different solutions of the multiple logistic function derived from a previous independent longitudinal observation study[13]; (2) were hypertensive; (3) were dyslipidaemic according to an arbitrary definition (serum cholesterol level ≥250 mg/dl and/or serum triglyceride level ≥200 mg/dl). The total of individually treated subjects amounted therefore to over 30 % of the entire study population.

The remaining population of the treatment 'factories' was exposed only to a collective programme of health education which also benefited the subjects submitted to individual treatment.

In the control 'factories', obviously no form of treatment, either individual or collective, was contemplated. Subjects examined at the initial screening were referred to the existing health service.

Every year (for 5 years) a re-screening was performed for the assessment of risk factors in a random 10 % sample of the treatment 'factories' and on all high-risk subjects as well as all those exposed to individual treatment programme – always limited to the treatment 'factories'.

Every 2 years (i.e. 2 and 4 years after the initial screening), re-screening was performed in the control 'factories' in order to assess risk factors in the same random subsample already tested at time 0. In addition, it was planned to re-screen at the end of the 6th year all the survivors both in treatment and control 'factories' in order to assess the risk factors.

Already from the start of the trial, a monitoring system for fatal and non-fatal coronary and cerebrovascular events and for deaths from all causes was carried out both in the treatment and control groups. As for individual preventive intervention, this was preferentially done by hygienic–dietary measures but also by drug treatment, where necessary (in hypertensives and certain other categories). Guidelines for reducing (or keeping at a low level) blood cholesterol are illustrated in Table 1.

Table 1 PPCC, Rome. Guidelines for individual treatment

Serum cholesterol (any level)	*Diet*
	Low total fat
	Low saturated fat
	Relatively high polyunsaturated fat
	Low cholesterol
	Low refined carbohydrates
	Low calories (in case of overweight)
	High fibres
	Drugs (in selected cases only)

As already pointed out, the trial lasted 6 years and has yielded positive results both in terms of efficiency and efficacy, the latter being statistically significant for some of the main end-points.

Over the 6 years of follow-up the mean reduction in the mean levels of the main coronary risk factors in treated groups, as compared to controls, was as follows: serum cholesterol 4.8 %; systolic blood pressure 4.6 %; number of cigarettes per day 8.7 %; body weight 2.4 %; estimated coronary risk 38.9 %.

At the end of the 6 years of observation, mortality for all causes was lower by 6.0–10.7 % in treated groups than in controls; mortality for coronary heart disease was also lower (by 25.4 %). Differences concerning coronary mortality and coronary incidence – hard criteria – are statistically significant[14].

On the occasion of the final examination carried out by the PPCC Research Group at the end of the 6-year trial, a special study was carried out on consumption of lipid-lowering drugs and dietary changes in the two groups and this was done on the basis of anamnestic data collected.

The results of this study are shown in Tables 2 and 3, from which it will be seen that consumption of lipid-lowering drugs and changes in dietary habits were more frequent in the group exposed to direct treatment by the PPCC Research Group compared to the group referred to the existing health service (19 % more as concerned drug consumption, and 58 % more as concerned diet in group DPE).

Three years after the end of the PPCC, a study aimed at detecting gallstone disease has been planned. This ongoing study will be carried out in all men belonging to the treatment factory and in about 25 % of men belonging to the

Table 2 PPCC, Rome. Consumption of lipid-lowering drugs during thè trial. Evaluation at final examination based on personal history

	DPE (*treatment*) (n=466)	*MT* (*control*) (n=895)
Total of months	1107	1791
Person-years	0.0330	0.0278
Number of subjects treated with lipid-lowering drugs for at least 6 months in the 6-year period	40 (=8.6 %)	83 (=9.3 %)
	DPE/MT = 1.19	

Table 3 PPCC, Rome. Dietary changes during the trial. Evaluation at final examination based on personal history

	DPE (treatment) ($n=466$)	*MT (control)* ($n=895$)
Total of months	5843	7115
Person-years	0.1741	0.1104
Number of subjects who modified their diet for at least 12 months in the 6-year period	150 (=32.2 %)	252 (=28.2 %)
	DPE/MT = 1.58	

control factory. Gallstone disease will be detected by ultrasound examination of the gallbladder using the same diagnostic criteria employed in a previous epidemiological study run by GREPCO[15].

Table 4 shows the distribution of cholelithiasis, cholecystectomy and gallstone disease in the 5-year age groups of the subjects so far examined.

The age-standardized prevalence of gallstone disease (cholelithiasis plus cholecystectomy) was fairly similar in the two groups, i.e. 15.80 % in group DPE and 13.69 % in group MT, with a relative risk of 1.15 (Fig. 1). A statistically significant difference was found between treated and controls as far as previous cholecystectomy was concerned (8.72 % vs. 3.91 %; chi-square test $p<0.05$).

Table 4 Distribution of cholelithiasis, cholecystectomy and gallstone disease in the subjects belonging to the two population groups examined 3 years after the end of the PPCC (DPE: treatment; MT: control). GREPCO, 1983: preliminary results

Factory	*Age*	*n*	*Cholelithiasis*	*Cholecystectomy*	*Gallstone disease*
DPE	49–53	79	5	7	12
	54–58	98	3	10	13
	59–63	114	9	7	16
	64–68	76	9	8	17
	49–68	367	26	32	58
MT	49–53	63	2	3	5
	54–58	74	9	3	12
	59–63	141	15	3	18
	64–68	80	9	5	14
	49–68	358	35	14	49

However, we were able to ascertain in cholecystectomized subjects whether surgery had been performed before or after their enrolment in PPCC. Seventeen subjects of the DPE sample and 14 of the MT sample had been cholecystectomized before. These subjects being excluded from the comparison between the two groups, the difference is no more significant.

The preliminary findings of this ongoing study jointly carried out by the research groups of PPCC and GREPCO in two samples of Roman working population intended to come to a better understanding of the presumed

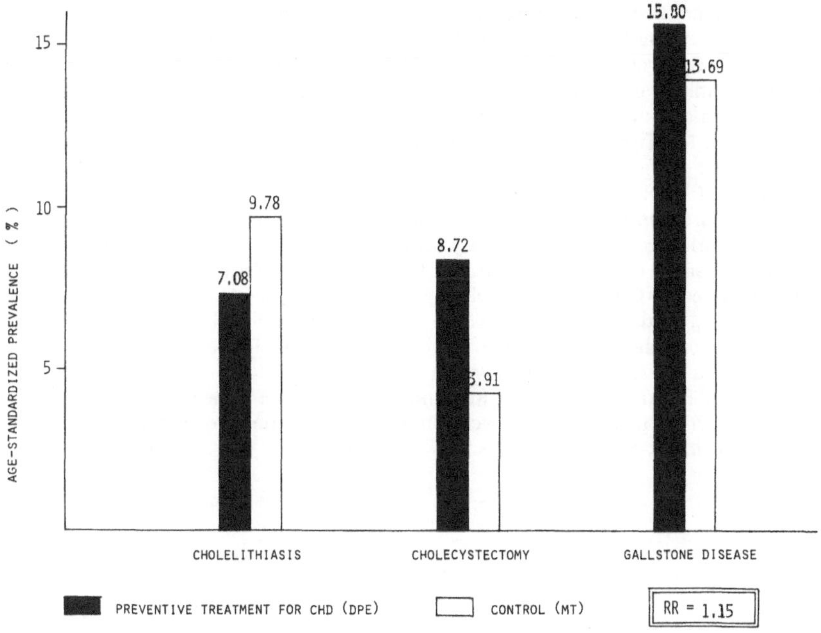

Figure 1 Age-standardized prevalence (%) of cholelithiasis, cholecystectomy and gallstone disease in treatment and control groups of the PPCC. GREPCO, 1983: preliminary results

lithogenic effect of dietary and/or drug treatments aiming at lowering serum lipid levels and especially cholesterol level, appear to suggest the efficacy of the multifactorial intervention on the prevention of coronary heart disease and the absence of a significant increase in the risk of gallstone formation.

It is therefore desirable that primary prevention of coronary heart disease be extended to the population at large, at the same time perhaps intensifying the surveillance for biliary complications, keeping in mind the possibilities offered by echography.

References

1. Grundy, S. M. (1975). Effects of polyunsaturated fats on lipid metabolism in patients with hypertriglyceridemia. *J. Clin. Invest.*, **51**, 273–292
2. Lewis, B. (1958). Effect of certain dietary oils on bile-acid secretion and serum-cholesterol. *Lancet*, **1**, 1090–1092
3. Lindstedt, S., Avigan, J., Goodman, D. S., Sjovall, J. and Steinberg, D. (1965). The effect of dietary fat on the turnover of cholic acid and on the composition of the biliary bile acids in man. *J. Clin. Invest.*, **44**, 1754–1765
4. Pertsemlidis, D., Panveliwalla, D. and Ahrens, E. H. Jr. (1974). Effects of clofibrate and of an estrogen-progestin combination on fasting biliary lipids and cholic acid kinetics in man. *Gastroenterology*, **66**, 565–573
5. Angelin, B., Einarsson, K. and Leijd, B. (1979). Biliary lipid composition during treatment with different hypolipidaemic drugs. *Eur. J. Clin. Invest.*, **9**, 185–190
6. Sturdevant, R. A. L., Pearce, M. L. and Dayton, S. (1973). Increased prevalence of cholelithiasis in men ingesting a serum-cholesterol-lowering diet. *N. Engl. J. Med.*, **288**, 24–27

7. The Coronary Drug Project Research Group (1977). Gallbladder disease as a side effect of drugs influencing lipid metabolism. *N. Engl. J. Med.*, **296**, 1185–1190
8. Cooper, J., Geizerova, H. and Oliver, M. F. (1975). Clofibrate and gallstones. *Lancet*, **1**, 1083
9. The Committee of Principal Investigators (1978). A co-operative trial in the primary prevention of ischaemic heart disease using clofibrate. *Br. Heart J.*, **40**, 1069–1118
10. Miettinen, M., Turpeinen, O., Karvonen, M. J., Paavilainen, E. and Elosuo, R. (1976). Prevalence of cholelithiasis in men and women ingesting a serum-cholesterol-lowering diet. *Ann. Clin. Res.*, **8**, 111–116
11. W.H.O. European Collaborative Group (1974). An international controlled trial in the multifactorial prevention of coronary heart disease. *Int. J. Epidemiol.*, **3**, 219–224
12. Research Group of the Rome Project of Coronary Heart Disease Prevention (1976). The Rome Project of Coronary Heart Disease Prevention. *Ann. Ist. Sup. Sanit.*, **12**, 316–330
13. Mariotti, S., Verdecchia, A., Capocaccia, R., Conti, S., Farchi, G. and Menotti, A. (1977). Identificazione di soggetti ad alto rischio nel Progetto Romano di Prevenzione della Cardiopatia Coronarica. *G. Ital. Cardiol.*, **7**, 141–146
14. Gruppo di Ricerca del Progetto Romano di Prevenzione della Cardiopatia Coronarica (1982). Il Progetto Romano di Prevenzione della Cardiopatia Coronarica. Risultati finali. *G. Ital. Cardiol.*, **12**, 541–554.

26
Long-term natural history of silent gallstones: implications for secondary prevention

D. F. RANSOHOFF

INTRODUCTION

Approximately 15 million Americans have gallstones[1]. The majority of these gallstones are silent[2,3]. The question of how to manage silent gallstone disease has received considerable attention in recent years for two reasons. First, ultrasonographic examination of the abdomen now causes gallstones to be identified more frequently as 'incidental findings'. Second, medical dissolution therapy is likely to become available as a possible option for management of cholesterol gallstones.

The question about whether to treat silent gallstones at all – either surgically or medically – is not clear-cut[4]. Concerning prophylactic cholecystectomy, recent recommendations vary from advice that it be done 'routinely'[5] to advice that it be done only in persons under age 50[6] or age 40[7]. An important consideration in the decision about treatment is the natural history of silent gallstones. In the past many textbooks have indicated that up to 50% of persons with silent gallstones will develop biliary pain or complications over 10–20 years. The belief that silent gallstones commonly cause problems has been responsible, in part, for recommendations to treat silent gallstones with prophylactic cholecystectomy.

In this chapter the following questions will be addressed:

(1) What is a silent gallstone? This question is important because 'non-silent' gallstones may have a different natural history compared to silent stones; thus we must consider what a 'silent' gallstone is.
(2) What is the natural history of silent gallstones? The major reports concerning natural history will be reviewed.
(3) What are reasonable recommendations about how to manage silent gallstones?

WHAT IS A SILENT GALLSTONE?

A silent gallstone is a gallstone that has not caused biliary pain or a biliary complication such as acute cholecystitis. In the past it was believed that gallstones caused symptoms such as flatulence, belching, and fatty food intolerance; several studies, however, have challenged that idea[8–10]. Thus persons with 'non-specific' symptoms, and without episodes of biliary pain, should be considered to have silent gallstones.

NATURAL HISTORY STUDIES – WHAT DO WE WANT THEM TO TELL US?

As we review the major reports about the natural history of silent gallstones, what are the clinical questions we want to answer? First, we would like to know how often a biliary problem (i.e. biliary pain, or a biliary complication such as acute cholecystitis) occurs. If the rate to develop biliary problems is high, then we would tend to favour prophylactic cholecystectomy. In other words if an operation is required sooner or later, it is better to operate sooner while a patient is young and still in good health. On the other hand, if the rate to develop biliary problems is low, then we would tend to favour expectant management. Second, we would like to know how often the presenting biliary problem is pain (which would permit a lower-risk elective operation) and how often it is a biliary complication (which would require a higher-risk operation). If the presenting biliary problem frequently is a complication, we would tend to favour prophylactic cholecystectomy.

NATURAL HISTORY STUDIES – WHAT DO THEY SHOW?

Among the natural history studies of silent gallstone disease, the ones to be discussed here are the largest or most commonly cited (see Table 1). Additional studies are noted briefly here, and in more detail elsewhere[11].

Comfort *et al.*[12]

One major study about natural history, reported in 1948, is a retrospective review performed at the Mayo Clinic between the years 1925 and 1934. Nine hundred and ninety-eight patients whose gallstones were 'found incidentally during the course of some other abdominal operation' were considered for inclusion in this study. Approximately half the group was excluded because the operation was for cancer. Other persons had intra-abdominal problems such as duodenal ulcer disease which might cause confusion with symptoms of gallbladder disease. Letters were sent to 184 non-excluded patients. One hundred and fifteen replied, and 112 were considered to have silent gallstones: that is, no indigestion or colic. These 112 persons were then said to be followed for a period of 10–20 years. Over that time, 61 persons remained asymptomatic while 51 persons developed symptoms of indigestion ('gaseous indigestion, intolerance to certain foods, and heartburn') (30 persons), colic

Table 1 Studies on the natural history of silent gallstones

				Outcome		
				Rate to develop biliary pain or a biliary complication		Comment
Reference and date	*Location*	*No. of subjects*	*Years of follow-up*	*Overall crude rate*	*Yearly incidence rate*	
Comfort *et al.*, 1948	Minnesota	112	10–20	21 (19 %)	n.a.	
Lund, 1960	Denmark	34	5–20	18 (53 %)	*	
Newman *et al.*, 1968	New York	191	2–22	n.a.	'2.2 % per year'	a
Gracie and Ransohoff, 1982	Michigan	123	11–24	16 (13 %)	2 % per year, 0–4 years 1 % per year, 5–9 years 0.5 % per year, 10–14 years 0 % per year, thereafter	b

n.a. = not available

a = The data on which the 2.2 % figure is based are not presented in detail

b = As of 1980, 42 persons were still at risk of developing biliary problems

* = Lund states that 'previously asymptomatic stones . . . induced symptoms, in the majority of cases, within the first five years, if they did give rise to symptoms'. However, the data on which this statement is based are not presented

(16 persons), and jaundice and colic (5 persons). In 4 of the 5 persons with jaundice and colic the jaundice was 'slight' and 'followed an attack of colic and was transient only'.

Comfort concluded that in 51 of 112 persons, about 50%, symptoms or complications developed over 10–20 years. This report – and the 50% figure – have been cited frequently in the medical literature.

Let us consider the clinical questions we asked initially. First, how often did stones become symptomatic? The answer would appear to be in 51 of 112 cases, or about 50%. However, if we consider only colic and jaundice as being symptoms attributable to gallstone disease, then the answer would be 21 of 112, or 19%. Second, how often was the presenting problem a complication? We are uncertain, but the rate appears to be low: in only one of the five patients with jaundice was the jaundice non-transient.

Lund[13]

Another major report was published in 1960. Considered for inclusion in this study were 526 patients admitted to the Copenhagen County Hospital from 1936 to 1950 who were diagnosed as having gallstone disease but who did not have a cholecystectomy. The diagnosis was based on non-visualization of the gallbladder and the clinical history of 366 persons, gallstones seen on a plain abdominal X-ray in 118 persons, and a negative stone shadow on oral cholecystography in 42 persons. Many persons were symptomatic. In about 100 cases 'the gallstones were chance findings in X-rays of the abdomen'. After questioning, 34 persons were considered to have silent gallstones and were then said to be followed for 5–20 years over which time 'one-third' (about 11 persons) developed 'severe or frequent attacks of pain', while 'one-fifth' (about 7 persons) developed complications probably consisting of acute cholecystitis, jaundice, and pancreatitis. Lund comments that the 'previously asymptomatic stones . . . induced symptoms, in the majority of cases, within the first five years, if they did give rise to symptoms'.

Considering our clinical questions: first, how often did stones become symptomatic? The answer is in 18 of 34, or 53%. Second, how often was the presenting problem a complication? We do not know whether the complication was the initial problem.

Gracie and Ransohoff[14]

Considered for inclusion in this study, reported in 1982, were approximately 4300 faculty members at the University of Michigan. The subjects – almost all men – were offered comprehensive screening examinations, routinely including an oral cholecystogram, at the Periodic Health Appraisal Unit between 1956 and 1969[15]. An initial evaluation was performed on 3326 persons, and 1545 persons had at least one subsequent routine evaluation. These evaluations identified 123 persons with silent gallstones. All 123 persons were followed for up to 24 years to determine whether biliary pain or a complication had occurred, whether a cholecystectomy had even been done, and whether a person had died. Biliary pain developed in 16 persons; three of these persons subsequently developed a biliary complication – acute cholecystitis in two and pancreatitis in one. All three had an uneventful cholecystectomy. No persons died because of gallstone disease. Assessment of the results by life-table analysis indicates that the cumulative probability to develop biliary pain was 10% at 5 years, 15% at 10 years, and 18% at 15 and at 20 years. The yearly risk to develop biliary pain appears to decrease with the passage of time.

Concerning the clinical questions: first, how often did stones become symptomatic? The answer is in 18 % at 15 and at 20 years. Second, how often was the presenting problem a complication? The answer is that all three persons having a complication had had a prior episode of biliary pain. Clearly, however, the number of complications was small, and from this study we cannot conclude that persons will usually have a warning biliary symptom before having a biliary complication.

Other studies[16–18]

Newman *et al.*[16] identified 191 persons with painless gallstone disease and reported that 'Approximately 2.2 % of cases with painless gallstones develop pain each year.' It is not clear how many persons presented with complications. Ralston and Smith[17] identified 14 persons with asymptomatic gallstones, and of four patients who developed symptoms 'two required surgical treatment eventually' after 15 or more years. It is not clear whether complications occurred. Wenckert and Robertson[18] reported a study that is often cited with regard to silent gallstones, however the study was actually 'a series in which cholecystography had confirmed the presence of clinically suspected gallstone disease' and thus is about patients who had symptomatic and not silent gallstones.

Each of these studies about natural history has limitations. Nevertheless, these studies constitute most of the 'body of knowledge' available to make management decisions about silent gallstone disease. What can we conclude from these studies? What questions are still unanswered?

What these studies do tell us, I think, is that the natural history of silent gallstones is generally 'benign'. If one reinterprets Comfort's data to exclude painless dyspepsia as a symptom attributable to gallstone disease, then the results of that study are quite similar to those more recently reported[14]. Perhaps then it is roughly 18 or 20 % of persons who will develop biliary problems in 15–20 years, at least in the USA. The results of Lund from Copenhagen are different. Perhaps the difference can be explained by the fact that the persons reported in that study had been hospitalized on a surgical service and that plain abdominal X-rays had revealed many of the gallstones. Or one can speculate that genetic or demographic features may account for a difference in natural history[14].

NATURAL HISTORY STUDIES – WHAT QUESTIONS ARE UNANSWERED?

Some potentially important questions about natural history remain unanswered[4,11,14,19]. Do silent gallstones have a different natural history in women compared to men? Or in older persons compared to younger persons (or vice-versa)? Or in persons with a 'non-functioning' gallbladder? Or in persons with a single large gallstone? Because of the small number of natural history studies, the small number of subjects, and the small number of biliary problems that occur in any one study, these questions cannot be answered with certainty. We do not know whether *any* of these groups has a particularly high (or low) risk of developing pain or complications. Indeed, very little is understood about the pathogenesis of pain and complications and why problems occur in some people and not in others. To identify predictors of natural history we would like to follow a large number of patients for a long period of time. However, such a study would be prohibitively expensive and time-consuming. So these are unanswered questions about *which* persons with silent gallstones develop problems.

How important are these uncertainties? How important is it to know precisely what the natural history of silent gallstones is? While natural history may be important, we must remember that natural history is only one of several issues that clinicians must consider in making a decision about therapy. Other issues include these: What is the mortality rate for a prophylactic cholecystectomy? What is the mortality rate for a cholecystectomy done at an older age after a person develops pain? What is the mortality rate for a cholecystectomy after a biliary complication? How many years of life will be lost by a young person (who may die after a prophylactic cholecystectomy) compared to an older person (who may die if a cholecystectomy is required in expectant management)?

The point is that natural history, while clearly an important issue, is only *one* of several issues that must be considered in a quantitative assessment to choose whether to treat with a prophylactic cholecystectomy (or with medical dissolution). These issues can be handled quantitatively in a technique called 'decision analysis'[20].

A DECISION ANALYSIS APPROACH

Conceptually a decision analysis is a 'hypothetical' clinical trial which uses data about probabilities (e.g. the probability of developing biliary pain, or the probability of dying at operation) from the medical literature. In a decision analysis, groups of persons with silent gallstones can be 'managed' with prophylactic cholecystectomy or with expectant management and followed over time; the outcome events of interest can be counted (e.g. the numbers of persons who develop biliary pain or a biliary complication and who die from cholecystectomy); and the strategies can then be compared so that a choice can be made. While a full description of decision analysis is beyond the scope of this essay and is covered elsewhere[20], some results of such a hypothetical clinical trial are presented in Table 2. Life expectancy is *decreased* by 4 days for a 30-year-old man who chooses prophylactic cholecystectomy instead of

Table 2 Results of a decision analysis: prophylactic cholecystectomy vs. expectant management for a 30-year-old man with silent gallstone disease*

	Prophylactic cholecystectomy	*Expectant management*
Likelihood of operation	100 %	26.1 %
Likelihood of developing biliary pain	0 %	23.6 %
Likelihood of developing a biliary complication	0 %	2.6 %
Case fatality rate from gallstone disease	0.1 %	0.3 %
Life expectancy decrease due to gallstone disease	11 days†	7 days
Average cost of gallstone surgery, per person	$4000	$1150

* *Assumptions:*

(a) *Operative mortality rate*

prophylactic (or elective) cholecystectomy:	age 30:	0.107 %
cholecystectomy for complication:	age 30:	0.427 %
	age 50:	2.160 %
	age 70:	10.935 %

(b) *Yearly incidence rate to develop a biliary problem*

0–4 years:	2 %	per year
5–9 years:	1 %	per year
after 10 years:	0.5 %	per year

(c) The presenting biliary problem is pain in 9 out of 10 persons and is a complication in 1 out of 10 persons

† A person choosing prophylactic cholecystectomy loses, on average, 4 more days of life (11 − 7 = 4) than the person choosing expectant management because death due to cholecystectomy for prophylaxis occurs at a younger age compared to death due to cholecystectomy in expectant management

expectant management. In additional analyses, even if one were to suppose a very 'pessimistic' view of the natural history of silent gallstones, for example a 6 % per year rate to develop biliary pain or complications, still only a small gain in life expectancy would occur (11 days) for a 30-year-old man who chooses prophylactic cholecystectomy instead of expectant management.

CONCLUSION AND RECOMMENDATIONS

In conclusion, recently published data and reinterpretation of older data suggest that the natural history of silent gallstones is more benign than we have believed in the past. For persons with silent stones the cumulative probability of developing biliary problems appears to be approximately 18 % after 20 years. Some questions about natural history may remain unanswered because of the difficulties in gathering data. However, decision analysis suggests that the importance of many of these uncertainties is small. A person's life expectancy is not, in general, increased by a policy of prophylactic cholecystectomy. Thus silent gallstones should, in general, be left to rest in peace.

References

1. Ingelfinger, F. J. (1968). Digestive disease as a national problem. V. Gallstones. *Gastroenterology*, **55**, 102–104

2. Wilbur, R. S. and Bolt, R. J. (1959). Incidence of gall bladder disease in 'normal' men. *Gastroenterology*, **36**, 251–255
3. Bainton, D., Davies, G. T., Evans, K. T. and Gravelle, I. H. (1976). Gallbladder disease: prevalence in a South Wales industrial town. *N. Engl. J. Med.*, **294**, 1147–1149
4. Donaldson, R. M. Jr. (1982). Advice for the patient with 'silent' gallstones. *N. Engl. J. Med.*, **307**, 815–817
5. Tan, E. G. C. and Warren, K. W. (1982). Diseases of the gallbladder and bile ducts. In Schiff, L. and Schiff, E. R. (eds.) *Diseases of the Liver*. 5th Edn. pp. 1507–1559. (Philadelphia: J. B. Lippincott)
6. Schoenfield, L. J. (1980). Diseases of the gallbladder and bile ducts. In Isselbacher, K. J., Adams, R. A., Braunwald, E., Petersdorf, R. G. and Wilson, J. D. (eds.) *Harrison's Principles of Internal Medicine*. 9th Edn. pp. 1489–1498. (New York: McGraw-Hill)
7. Spiro, H. M. (1977). *Clinical Gastroenterology*. 2nd Edn. p. 926. (New York: Macmillan)
8. Price, W. H. (1963). Gall-bladder dyspepsia. *Br. Med. J.*, **2**, 138–141
9. Koch, J. P. and Donaldson, R. M. Jr. (1964). A survey of food intolerances in hospitalized patients. *N. Engl. J. Med.*, **271**, 657–660
10. Taggart, D. and Billington, B. P. (1966). Fatty foods and dyspepsia. *Lancet*, **2**, 464–466
11. Gracie, W. A. and Ransohoff, D. F. Natural history and expectant management of gallstone disease. In Cohen, S. and Soloway, R. D. (eds.) *Gallstones*. (New York: Churchill Livingstone) (In press)
12. Comfort, M. W., Gray, H. K. and Wilson, J. M. (1948). The silent gallstone: a ten to twenty year follow-up study of 112 cases. *Ann. Surg.*, **128**, 931–937
13. Lund, J. (1960). Surgical indications in cholelithiasis: prophylactic cholecystectomy elucidated on the basis of long-term follow up on 526 non-operated cases. *Ann. Surg.*, **151**, 153–162
14. Gracie, W. A. and Ransohoff, D. F. (1982). The natural history of silent gallstones: the innocent gallstone is not a myth. *N. Engl. J. Med.*, **307**, 798–800
15. Tupper, C. J. and Beckett, M. B. (1958). Faculty health appraisal, University of Michigan. *Univ. Mich. Med. Bull.*, **24**, 35–43
16. Newman, H. F., Northup, J. D., Rosenblum, M. and Abrams, H. (1968). Complications of cholelithiasis. *Am. J. Gastroenterol.*, **50**, 476–496
17. Ralston, D. E. and Smith, L. A. (1965). The natural history of cholelithiasis: a 15 to 30-year follow-up of 116 patients. *Minn. Med.*, **48**, 327–332
18. Wenckert, A. and Robertson, B. (1966). The natural course of gallstone disease: eleven-year review of 781 nonoperated cases. *Gastroenterology*, **50**, 376–381
19. Gracie, W. A. and Ransohoff, D. F. (1983). The silent gallstone: requiescat in pace. In Delany, J. P. and Varco, R. L. (eds.) *Controversies in Surgery*. II. pp. 361–372. (Philadelphia: W. B. Saunders)
20. Ransohoff, D. F., Gracie, W. A., Wolfenson, L. B. and Neuhauser, D. (1983). Prophylactic cholecystectomy or expectant management for persons with silent gallstones: a decision analysis to assess survival. *Ann. Intern. Med.*, **99**, 199–204

27
Factors associated with gallstone disease: observations in the 'Sirmione Study'

E. RODA for the 'Progetto Sirmione'*

Although many factors have been considered in the past as possible predisposing factors to the formation of gallstones[6], the actual knowledge about the epidemiology of gallstone disease makes it very difficult to give statistical support to the clinical impressions. In fact most of the studies proposing the relationship of gallstone disease to possible pathogenetic factors concern mainly data obtained from clinical observations, necroscopy series or surgical records.

Because gallstone disease can be ignored throughout life by many of the patients[1], all these epidemiological approaches have many biases which can account for the differences found in different studies.

The Framingham study[2] was the first prospective approach to gallstone disease based on a random sample of a normal population. This study, however, confirmed many of the clinical impressions coming from previous reports, but failed to confirm others.

We carried out a longitudinal prospective study on the epidemiology of gallstone disease in the town of Sirmione. The study protocol is expressed in detail in Chapter 5 of this book. Briefly, the study protocol included a physical examination, an ultrasonographic examination of the upper abdomen, and a blood test for glucose, urea nitrogen, total and HDL cholesterol, triglycerides, GOT, GPT and GGT. The first part of the study concerning the prevalence of the disease has been completed.

In order to evaluate the possible factors associated with gallstone disease, the subjects participating in the study (1930 out of 2732 inhabitants, aged 18–65 years) have been interviewed on the basis of the outcoming literature information[6] regarding the natural history of the disease.

* *Progetto Sirmione:* L. Barbara, D. Festi, A. M. Morselli Labate, A. G. Rusticali, C. Sama, C. Sapio, F. Taroni (Clinica Medica III – Università di Bologna)

C. Banterle, S. Colasanti, G. Formentini, F. Nardin, G. Panzolato, A. Puci (Divisione di Medicina Generale – Ospedale di Desenzano)

To evaluate the relation between possible factors associated with gallstone disease, data were analysed by means of a cross-sectional procedure. The relative prevalence of gallstone disease in the population in which the factor was present vs. that of the control population was standardized for age, sex and other confounding factors using the procedure proposed by Mantel–Haenszel[3,4] and Miettinen[5].

AGE AND SEX

Both age and sex were found to be strongly correlated with the prevalence of cholelithiasis. In fact gallstone disease was revealed only in 2.1 % of the younger population (18–29 years) and increased progressively with age (30–39 years: 7.0 %; 40–49 years: 12.9 %; 50–56 years: 19.8 %). Moreover gallstone disease was more frequent in women (14.6 %) than in men (6.7 %) ($RR_{MH} = 2.16$; c.l.$_{0.001}$: 1.37, 3.41; standardized for age).

PREGNANCY

828 out of 1045 women attending the study have had one or more pregnancies. The prevalence of gallstone disease increased with the number of pregnancies. After standardization for age the prevalence of the disease was significantly higher in women who have been pregnant ($RR_{MH} = 1.60$; c.l.$_{0.05} = 1.01, 2.57$).

USE OF OESTROPROGESTINIC DRUGS

A lower prevalence of gallstone disease was observed in the 283 women (27.2 %) who had used oestroprogestinic drugs. It should be noted that oestroprogestinic drugs were mainly used by women belonging to the lower age groups (18–29 and 30–39 years). Standardizing for age we did not find any statistical difference between users and non-users ($RR_{MH} = 0.75$; c.l.$_{0.05}$: 0.49, 1.14).

DIABETES

In our study we have defined as diabetics those subjects who had fasting glucose levels higher than 140 mg/dl and/or those subjects who were using antidiabetic drugs.

The prevalence of this disease in our population was 2.5 % (42 subjects). The presence of diabetes was detected mainly in the subjects aged 40–65 years (37/980, 3.8 %).

The prevalence of gallstone disease in diabetics was not statistically significant when compared with non-diabetic subjects ($RR_{MH} = 1.10$; c.l.$_{0.05}$: 0.53, 2.32).

OBESITY

In our study we have defined as obese those subjects with a body mass index greater than 3 g/cm^2. The frequency of obesity accounted for 9.5 %. Obesity has been found to be highly correlated with age. In fact 2.6 % of the subjects studied were obese in the 18–29-year subgroup; whereas in the class aged 50–65 years obesity reached the value of 16.9 %. We did not find any correlation of this condition with sex.

In the obese population the prevalence of gallstone disease (22.9 %) was significantly higher than in non-obese subjects ($RR_{MH}=1.64$; $c.l._{0.01}$: 1.02, 2.61). This correlation was significantly evident in the younger subjects (18–29 years: $RR_{MH}=4.77$; $c.l._{0.001}$: 1.51, 15.09).

SERUM LIPIDS

In order to define hypertriglyceridaemic and hypercholesterolaemic subjects, the 70th sex- and age-specific percentile was defined as cut-off point for defining risk. No significant increase in the prevalence of gallstone disease has been observed in hypercholesterolaemic subjects ($RR_{MH}=1.10$; $c.l._{0.05}$: 0.84, 1.46). Gallstone disease was, however, found associated with hypertriglyceridaemia ($RR_{MH}=1.65$; $c.l._{0.001}$: 1.07, 2.54).

Since obesity was found to be higher in hypertriglyceridaemic subjects we carried out a bivariate analysis to evaluate the specific influence of each of these factors. Both of them were found to be significantly associated with gallstone disease (hypertriglyceridaemia: $RR_{MH}=1.56$; $c.l._{0.001}$: 1.00, 2.44; obesity: $RR_{MH}=1.48$; $c.l._{0.05}$: 1.07, 2.04).

CONCLUSIONS

We have designed a cohort study in order to better understand the epidemiology and the natural history of gallstone disease in a northern Italian town. The knowledge of the risk factors connected with the disease will probably aid prevention of gallstone formation. In the first part of the study we have evaluated some factors associated with gallstone disease that will be the basis of the identification of the risk factors, which will be possible in the next phases of the study.

References

1. Gracie, W. A. and Ransohoff, D. F. (1982). The natural history of silent gallstones. *N. Engl. J. Med.*, **307**, 798–800
2. Friedman, G. D., Kannel, W. B. and Dawber, T. R. (1966). The epidemiology of gallbladder disease: observations in the Framingham Study. *J. Chron. Dis.*, **19**, 273–292
3. Mantel, N. and Haenszel, W. (1959). Statistical aspects of the analysis of data from retrospective studies of disease. *J. Natl. Cancer Inst.*, **22**, 719–748
4. Mantel, N. (1963). Chi-square test with one degree of freedom: extension of the Mantel–Haenszel procedure. *Am. Stat. Assoc. J.*, **58**, 690–700
5. Miettinen, O. S. (1976). Stratification by a multivariate confounding score. *Am. J. Epidemiol.*, **104**, 609–620
6. Bennion, L. J. and Grundy, S. M. (1978). Risk factors for the development of cholelithiasis in man – part 2. *N. Engl. J. Med.*, **299**, 1221–7

28
Prevention of cholelithiasis: intervention on risk factors

C. N. WILLIAMS

ABSTRACT

Prevention of cholelithiasis is in its infancy and depends largely on a clear understanding of events during pathogenesis. Nucleation and stone growth-inhibiting factors are new areas. Abnormal bile composition resulting in excess cholesterol in bile is believed to be the precursor of cholesterol gallstone formation and intervention is directed against this hypothesis. Several populations have been identified with a high prevalence of gallstones and a high prevalence of cholesterol-saturated bile. Lithogenic bile is associated with (a) obesity, morbid or mild; (b) Crohn's disease, ileal resection or bypass and cystic fibrosis with pancreatic insufficiency; (c) clofibrate or oral contraceptives; (d) female relatives of patients with gallstones; (e) becoming worse on fasting in women compared to men. The factors documented for cholesterol saturation are also associated with an increased prevalence of cholesterol gallstones. Dietary constituents have been proposed as risk factors. We have performed prevalence studies, looked at dietary factors and with age-controlled discriminant stepwise analysis have found obesity; the presence of relatives with gallstones; reduced intakes of dietary fibre and iron as significant risk factors in patients who were found to have gallstones at the time of study and had not yet had time to change their diet. This is contrasted with the usual group of reported patients (which includes prior cholecystectomy, presence of gallstones in functioning gallbladders or otherwise), where obesity; relatives with cholecystectomy; reduced calcium or protein intake and duration of oral contraceptive use are significant factors.

We have tested these prospectively and find that (a) a high-protein diet protects against cholesterol-saturated bile, (b) a diet high in carbohydrate and high in refined carbohydrate promotes lithogenic bile and (c) duration of fasting and obesity are associated with lithogenic bile; we have established a modified diet, based on these findings. This modified diet includes reducing to ideal body weight and maintaining this; regular meals with a late-night snack with sufficient protein or fat to contract the gallbladder; a reduced duration of overnight fast; more protein (20–25 %); less carbohydrate (< 50 %); less refined carbohydrate (< 30 %); and 30 % dietary fibre.

Using this diet compared to the regular diet, and chenodeoxycholic acid to dissolve cholesterol gallstones, we have found that patients taking a modified diet dissolve gallstones quicker and more of them do so. On follow-up of these patients with 6-monthly bile analysis and repeated gallbladder ultrasounds, recurrences are predominantly in the second year of follow-up; lithogenic bile is seen more frequently in those maintaining their regular diet during the follow-up period.

There are several general measures we can take to prevent cholesterol gallstone disease; reduce and maintain ideal body weight, avoid repetitive and prolonged fasting, use an oral contraceptive of low oestrogen content or an alternative method of birth control, and reduce bile cholesterol saturation by diet changes. In addition, we may add cholelithic agents, such as chenodeoxycholic acid or ursodeoxycholic acid, particularly for ileal resection or bypass or where clofibrate is necessary. Diet should be of benefit in the most common form of gallstones; that seen in the situation of mild to moderate obesity and in the situation where ethnic groups are predisposed to gallstone formation.

INTRODUCTION: THE PROBLEM

There has been a tremendous surge of new knowledge concerning the pathogensis of cholesterol gallstones, particularly in the last decade or so. There is much less information available concerning the problem of pigment stones. Consequently, the emphasis will be placed on risk factors for cholesterol gallstones and intervention and prevention measures on these risk factors.

There are several gallbladder factors culminating in cholesterol gallstone formation[1]. These include nucleation factors; stone growth-inhibiting factors where knowledge is not yet in the intervention stage; bile lipid composition; stratification of bile and abnormal gallbladder motility.

Gallbladder motility is known to be altered in such conditions as pregnancy, diabetes, coeliac disease and following truncal vagotomy. The postulated increased cholesterol saturation seen in these conditions is largely offset by the increased bile acid pool, filling the enlarged gallbladder. The net result appears to be micellar bile. The congenital abnormality, Phrygian cap, predisposes to abnormal motility[2] and increased gallstone formation.

RISK FACTORS FOR CHOLESTEROL-SATURATED BILE

The current dogma is that cholesterol saturation occurs in bile prior to cholesterol gallstone formation. There are many factors which are known to predispose to cholesterol-saturated bile (Table 1). There are several ethnic groups characterized by high prevalence of gallstones and each presumably has increased cholesterol-saturated bile[3–5]. One such group is the Micmac Indian population living in Nova Scotia[6] where there is a high prevalence of cholesterol-saturated bile (54.3 %) in women without gallstones[7] (Table 2).

Table 1 Micmac Indian women (Nova Scotia, 1981)

	Gallstones	*No gallstones*
No.	13	46
Age, median range	29 (15–47)	23 (15–52)
Normal bile	0	21
Lithogenic bile		
Metastable	4	15
Above	9	10
Percentage	100 %	54.3 %

Table 2 Predisposing factors for cholesterol-saturated bile

Ethnic	Micmac Indian women
Sex	Puberty
Familial	Older sisters
Weight	Morbid obesity
	Relative obesity
Bile acid malabsorption	Crohn's disease
	Ileal resection
	Cystic fibrosis
	Pancreatic insufficiency
Drugs	Clofibrate
	Oral contraceptives
	Cholestyramine
Diet	High refined carbohydrate
	Low fibre
	High cholesterol
	High calorie
Fasting	Women > men

There is an increased predominance of cholesterol-saturated bile occurring at puberty in females[1] and in one study from the Mayo Clinic[8], half a group of older sisters of patients having cholesterol gallstones had cholesterol-saturated bile.

The main overriding factor that seems to predispose to the presence of cholesterol-saturated bile is excess weight[1,9]. This is exemplified by morbid obesity where typically the average molar percent cholesterol was 13, compared to a normal of 6.6; all having cholesterol-saturated bile of labile type[10]. This is also seen in the usual type of obesity; 30 % of more above ideal body weight, and also, importantly, in normal-weight women. Relative obesity, represented by the body mass index, correlates significantly with the ranked lithogenic index[7].

Situations where bile acid malabsorption is present are associated with bile with increased cholesterol saturation. Examples are Crohn's disease[11], ileal resection or bypass[12], and cystic fibrosis with pancreatic insufficiency[13]. There are several drugs which promote cholesterol-saturated bile. These include clofibrate[14], oral contraceptives[15] and probably cholestyramine[16]. There are several dietary factors which are found in association with cholesterol-saturated bile. These include diets with a high content of refined carbohydrate[17], cholesterol[18] and calories, and low in fibre[19].

In one reported study from our own laboratory[7], the following factors were found to correlate the presence of cholesterol-saturated bile: calorie range/calorie intake; iron and calcium intake; the duration of overnight fast and two factors in bile: the proportions of deoxycholic acid and chenodeoxycholic acid, the latter being an inverse relationship.

Fasting is known to be associated with increased cholesterol saturation of bile[20]. There is a sex difference in this regard; healthy women appear to tolerate 16 h of fasting more poorly than men, and have a significantly greater proportion with lithogenic bile at this time[21].

RISK FACTORS FOR CHOLESTEROL GALLSTONES

Similarly, factors which predispose to cholesterol gallstone formation are similar to those previously described for cholesterol-saturated bile. There are increased prevalences noted in specific ethnic groups[1]; American Indians, Northern Europe and western countries more than the Orient. Pregnancy is reportedly associated with an increased presentation of gallstones. With rapid weight loss, there is increased cholesterol secretion in bile and resultant gallstone formation[9].

In morbid obesity there is an increased prevalence of gallstones[10]. In Iowa 82 of 238 patients were found to have gallstones at surgery; an incidence of 34.4 %. In our own institution we found gallstones in 33 out of the first 100 operations for morbid obesity. During the phase of rapid weight loss a further 10 patients developed symptomatic gallstones.

Figure 1(a) shows the typical appearance of gallstones during the phase of

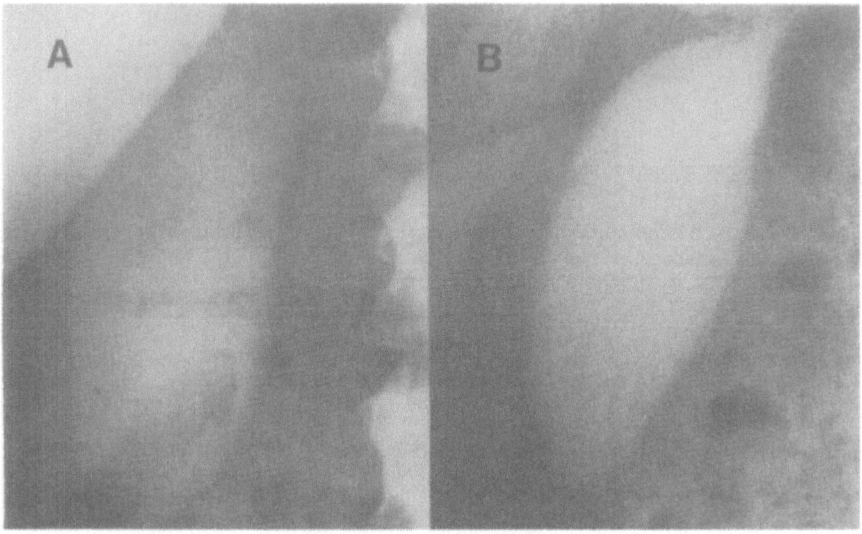

Figure 1 **a:** This oral cholecystogram from a patient with recent gastric bypass operation shows multiple radiolucent gallstones which 'float'. A cholecystogram prior to surgery was normal. **b:** The gallstones have dissolved after 3 months of chenodeoxycholic acid treatment

rapid weight loss. They always appear to be multiple tiny stones and dissolve very quickly after the use of chenodeoxycholic acid, shown in Fig. 1(b) in such a patient after 3 months' treatment.

The factors associated with cholesterol gallstones (Table 3) are the same as those associated with cholesterol-saturated bile with the exception of polyunsaturated fat. A diet containing polyunsaturated fat has been shown to be associated with a 2–3-fold increased risk of gallstones. No data are available concerning bile composition during this type of diet.

There are epidemiological data from Nova Scotia to suggest factors in diet associated with the presence of gallstones[6,22,23]. We have performed studies to substantiate particular factors and type of diet[21–25]. We have used this diet in interventional studies[24] and are now using this diet in preventional studies, after gallstone dissolution[24].

The epidemiological evidence from out institution is summarized here (Table 4). We have studied three populations – two rural[6,23], one urban[25] – of

Table 3 Factors associated with the presence of gallstones

Ethnic	American Indians
	Northern Europe
	West > Orient
Sex	Women
	Pregnancy
Familial	
Weight	Obesity
	Rapid weight loss
Bile acid malabsorption	Distal ileal disease, resection or bypass
	Cystic fibrosis with pancreatic insufficiency
Drugs	Clofibrate
	Oral contraceptives
Diet	High refined carbohydrate
	Low fibre
	High cholesterol
	High calorie
	Polyunsaturated fats
Fasting	

Table 4 Diet – Halifax studies; epidemiological: gallstone prevalence and pathogenesis in Nova Scotia, Canada

	Rural		*Urban:*
	Micmac Indian women	*Caucasian women*	*Caucasian women*
Gallstone prevalence/1000	211 (n=132)	167 (n=133)	183 (n=300)
Age-controlled factors	Obesity Parity	Obesity Narrow calorie range Reduced calcium Limited activity	Obesity Relatives with cholecystectomy Reduced calcium Limited activity Duration of oral contraceptive use

women all having a high prevalence of cholesterol gallstones. Using regression analysis we have reported the following to be age-controlled factors: obesity seen in all groups, parity only in the Indian women; reduced calcium and limited activity in both groups of Caucasian women; narrow calorie range in the rural women, with other factors in the urban group of relatives with cholecystectomy and the duration of oral contraceptive use. Further analysis of these data, using more precise analysis of the Wilks discriminant stepwise type, has revealed additional information. We have found the ratio of carbohydrate to crude fibre, and each alone, to be significant discriminating factors in the Micmac Indian women[23]. We have found that reduced calcium intake can be interchanged with reduced protein intake without losing any discrimination[25], and that oral contraceptive use becomes significant with this type of analysis, as does having relatives with a previous history of cholecystectomy, also found in the urban group.

In the literature there are many types of analysis used in reports concerning diet and risk factors for gallstones[26–28], which give rise to markedly different results. Most analyses are concerned with either a *t*-test or a chi-square for each variable. Discriminant analysis detects interactions between the variables and, when age-controlled and stepwise, becomes a very accurate tool. There is, however, a problem with distribution of these normal variables; the analyses assume a normal distribution which is often not present. Statistical advice (B. Garner) is that we need non-parametric distribution analysis which is not currently available on main-frame computers.

Table 5 shows factors detected by the *t*-test in a group of 55 patients who have either undergone prior cholecystectomy or were found to have stones or non-visualized gallbladders at the time of the study. This includes most significant factors described in the literature by others. Note that the inverse of the square of the body mass index gives the best distribution for obesity. The log of the calcium, the square root of fat, calories and protein are necessary

Table 5 Risk factors for gallstones in 300 Halifax Caucasian women (*t*-test, each variable, 55* vs. 245)

	p
IS body mass index	<0.0001
Relatives with gallstones	<0.0001
Relatives with cholecystectomy	<0.0001
Amount of alcohol	<0.001
L calcium	<0.002
S fat	<0.004
S calories	<0.005
L saturated fat	<0.01
S protein	<0.017
Number of pregnancies	<0.021
S cholesterol	<0.05
Age, chi-square, 16.0	<0.013

* Includes 55 patients with gallstones or prior cholecystectomy vs. 245 subjects without gallstones. IS represents the inverse of the square root, S square root, L logarithm

transformations to normalize the distribution. With discriminant analysis body mass index, age, calcium, ascorbic acid, iron, riboflavin, and refined carbohydrate intakes are significant.

Our working hypothesis was that if any factor was significantly contributing to the formation of cholesterol gallstones, then this factor would be present at the time of diagnosis before the diet was altered. To this end we analysed 12 patients with gallstones who were asymptomatic and who had not altered their diets at the time of study. Similarly, analysis of *t*-tests shows age, obesity, inverse relationship with ulcers, ascorbic acid intake, and the association with relatives with either gallstones or cholecystectomy as single significant factors. Discriminant analysis of these 12 shows the body mass index, iron, age, dietary fibre, ascorbic acid, calcium, crude fibre, and the polyunsaturated/saturated fat ratio as being significant. However, with age-controlled, stepwise discriminant analysis, these 12 showed obesity, the presence of relatives with gallstones, the amount of dietary fibre, and the amount of iron intake as significant risk factors for the presence of gallstones. This is contrasted with the group of 55 patients previously mentioned. Here obesity, relatives with cholecystectomy, calcium (or protein) intake, and duration of oral contraceptive use were significant factors.

EXPERIMENTAL STUDIES

If any of these epidemiological data are really significant, they would have to be supported by specific experiments. We have performed a series of studies over the past few years, as follows: we studied the effect of fasting on bile lithogenicity in 22 healthy men and 19 healthy women without gallstones and reported that women tolerate this change much less than men[21]. We reported previous correlations between the bile of the Micmac Indian women and their diets[7]. We specifically modified diets in 42 healthy women to define the effect of either high-protein, high-fat or high-carbohydrate and regular diet on bile lithogenicity. We have found that increasing protein intake decreases bile lithogenicity, increasing refined and total carbohydrate increases bile lithogenicity in those taking oral contraceptives and that fat modification has no measurable effect. Finally, we noted in one of our epidemiological studies in 1975 that the use of alcohol appeared to be helpful in reducing the risk for cholesterol gallstones (unpublished data). We have tested this effect directly using beer, as this was the beverage most commonly ingested in this epidemiological study[6].

There does not appear to be any significant difference in bile lithogenicity in the group of 15 healthy Caucasian women who are not normally beer drinkers, who consumed two beers a day for a period of 10 days (0.79 ± 0.04 vs. 0.86 ± 0.05, $p > 0.07$). However, the glycine:taurine bile acid ratio significantly increases (2.72 ± 0.6 vs. 3.4 ± 0.7, $p < 0.015$).

After the original epidemiological studies we used the diet found in association with the Micmac Indian women, who were demonstrated to have normal bile, as a starting point, and prescribed this diet to patients with gallstones to help reduce cholesterol saturation. This diet includes 15%

protein, 45 % carbohydrate, and 40 % fat in three meals and a late-night snack; crude fibre of 10 g; cholesterol of 400 mg and a p:s ratio of 0.17 with a calorie range of 1300.

In the mid-1970s our trial diet for gallstone dissolution was: reducing to ideal body weight; regular meals; wide range of calorie intake; a little more fat and less carbohydrate with a p:s ratio of about 0.15 and increase in fibre. We modified this diet after our intervention study in the 42 healthy women and showed that increased protein intake decreased the cholesterol present in bile, as well as the carbohydrate effects.

The design of the 1-month study is as follows: 30 healthy women were assigned at random to follow a different diet order. Diet A was 60 % high carbohydrate, of which 65 % was refined; Diet B: 45 % protein; Diet C: 55 % fat. The cholesterol, p:s ratio and fibre intake were the same in all these three diets. Twelve healthy subjects maintained their regular diets. Over the 1-month period of study bile samples were obtained, after each diet period (10 days), after a standardized 10 h overnight fast, starting with a fatty snack. After the high-carbohydrate diet, Diet A, there was a significant increase in the molar percent cholesterol, only in the group that took oral contraceptives. In addition there was a significant decrease of the molar percent cholesterol in bile with Diet B, the high-protein diet, whether oral contraceptives were taken or not. There was no significant difference with the high-fat diet, Diet C.

Oral contraceptives did not appear to exert any direct influence on the lithogenic index in this particular study (0.8 ± 0.15 vs. 0.84 ± 0.19, $n = 11$ vs. 19) when these healthy women consumed their regular diets.

INTERVENTION ON RISK FACTORS

We are currently comparing our modified diet to see whether a snack taken late at night or in the afternoon affects cholesterol saturation and the rate of gallstone dissolution, in patients with gallstones taking ursodeoxycholic acid.

Our diet for gallstone dissolution, modified by these studies, is now as follows: reducing to ideal body weight and maintaining this; regular meals and late-night snack with sufficient protein or fat to contract the gallbladder; a reduced duration of overnight fast; more protein; less carbohydrate; less refined carbohydrate and the use of dietary fibre of 30 g (Table 6).

Our studies in the prevention of gallstone formation using diet are directed

Table 6 Diet for gallstone dissolution

1.	Reduce to ideal body weight
2.	Maintain at ideal body weight
3.	Regular meals and late snack with sufficient protein or fat to contract the gallbladder
4.	Reduced duration of overnight fast
5.	More protein, 20–25 %
6.	Less carbohydrate, 50 %
7.	Less refined carbohydrate, 30 %
8.	More dietary fibre to 30 g

initially to the problem of gallstone recurrence following drug dissolution. We are studying a group of patients randomized in pairs to one of two groups to continue either their regular diet or our modified diet, and taking the same dose of chenodeoxycholic acid. We are also studying the effect of our modified diet with the variations as mentioned previously, concerning the timing of the snacks, in another group of patients whose gallstones are being dissolved with ursodeoxycholic acid.

In the chenodeoxycholic acid study we have randomized 54 patients to these two groups. Group I follow their regular diet; Group II follow our modified diet. Four have dropped out from Group I and five from Group II; giving us 24 in one group and 21 in the second. Nine have dissolved their stones in Group I and 14 in Group II. The percentage obtaining gallstone dissolution with chenodeoxycholic acid, 15 mg kg^{-1} day^{-1}, is 37.5%; maintaining their regular diet and two-thirds taking our modified diet. The mean time for dissolution: 16 months with the regular diet; about 9 months with our modified diet (Table 7).

Table 7 Halifax gallstone dissolution study, November 1983

Randomized	54			
Groups	1		11	
	28		26	
Dropped out	4		5	
	19F	5M	19F	4M
Dissolved	5	4	12	2
Percentage dissolved taking 6 months medication	37.5%		66.7%	
Mean time for dissolution (months)	16.0		8.9	

Figure 2 shows the cumulative number of patients with gallstones dissolved. As can be seen, the modified diet appears to hasten gallstone dissolution.

These patients have been followed in Group I, a mean of 19½ months; range 4–33 months. In Group II the 14 patients have been followed a mean of 27.5 months; range 6–50 months. We have had one recurrence in Group I and five in Group II; the mean recurrence being 18 months for the one patient in Group I, and 22 months for Group II, range 6–42 months. When these patients have their gallstones dissolved and the medication stopped, we follow their progress, asking them to stay on the diet; we obtain bile samples at 6, 12 and 18 months post-dissolution. So far, 4 of 5 in Group I, the regular diet, have a return of lithogenic bile; whereas 4 of 13 in Group II have a return. There are several more gallstone recurrences than anticipated in Group II; all had normal bile cholesterol to 18 months. However, the period of follow-up is longer. There are, thus more people at risk and four of the five patients with recurrences freely admitted they had cheated on the diet, especially

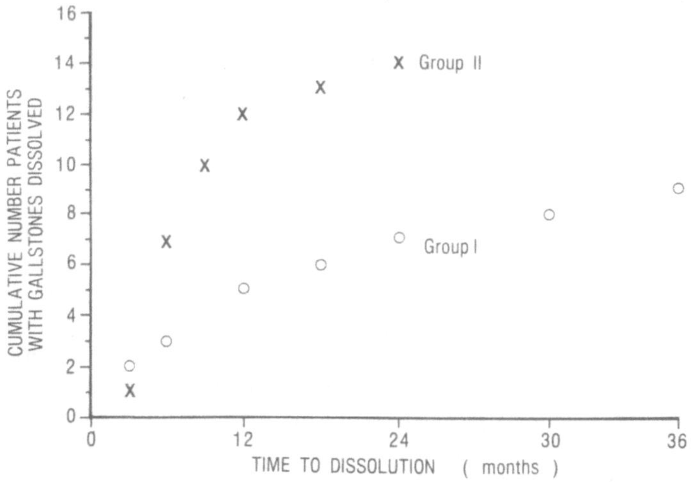

Figure 2 This shows the time of gallstone dissolution using chenodeoxycholic acid (15 mg kg^{-1} day^{-1}) in all patients. Group 1 ($n=9$) ate their regular diet and stones took longer to dissolve. Group 2 ($n=14$) ate the modified diet (Table 6) and more of them dissolved their gallstones in a shorter time

abandoning the late-night snack and indulging in foods rich in refined carbohydrate.

It is difficult to explain these five recurrences when the cholesterol content of bile was normal for 18 months; all were abnormal before treatment. However, in another study (Fig. 3), patients with radiolucent gallstones and

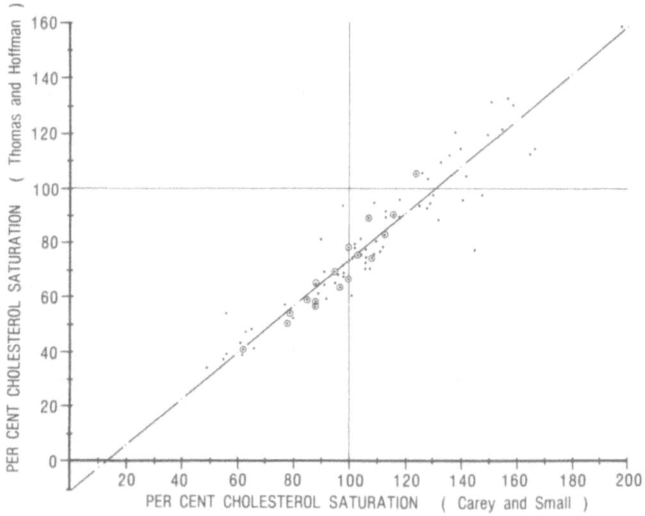

Figure 3 This shows the correlation between bile cholesterol saturation and gallstones, depicted as solid dots. Patients whose gallstones dissolved with chenodeoxycholic acid treatment are shown as dots within open circles. There are nine patients with normal bile and eight with lithogenic bile with gallstone dissolution; presumably all were cholesterol gallstones

normal bile dissolved their stones, presumably of cholesterol type. Other factors must be operative, perhaps gallbladder nucleating factors, as gallbladder motility is mostly normal (unpublished results).

PREVENTIVE MEASURES

What measures can we take to prevent cholesterol gallstone disease? There are several general measures: reduce and maintain ideal body weight; avoid repetitive prolonged fasting; use an oral contraceptive of low oestrogen content or an alternative method of birth control; and reduce bile cholesterol saturation by diet changes.

Diet alone may be useful in the following situations: the groups without particular high risk, that are most commonly in clinical practice; populations of high risk; possibly in patients whose gallstones have been dissolved by medication, especially if weight reduction is present and maintained, possibly to counteract the effects of certain drugs such as clofibrate.

Conversely, drugs alone are likely to be used in specific situations: e.g. ursodeoxycholic acid can be used in patients with ileal resection or bypass, during the catabolic phase of weight loss, especially following surgical

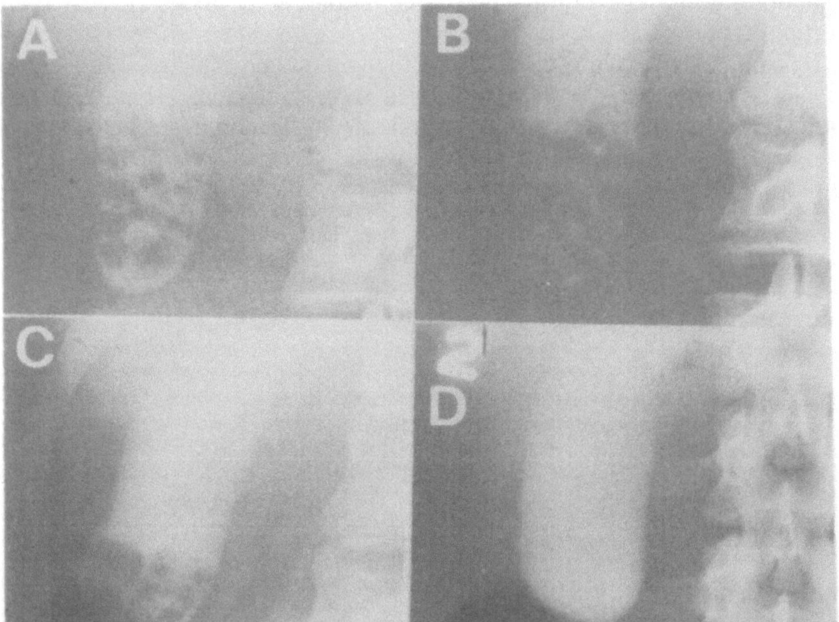

Figure 4 **a:** This oral cholecystogram contains multiple gallstones. **b:** After 6 months of diet there was no essential change. **c:** After a further 18 months of modified diet alone, there are less gallstones seen. **d:** After adding chenodeoxycholic acid while continuing the modified diet, complete gallstone dissolution has occurred; 3 years later the gallstones have not reoccurred while the modified diet is maintained

treatment of morbid obesity; where combined risk factors such as obesity, ileal disorder and oral contraceptives are present; and possibly to reduce the risk in patients requiring clofibrate. Lastly, ursodeoxycholic acid may be used in a situation we have seen with three patients who had acute pancreatitis; one with a small stone and others with cholesterol-saturated bile with no other cause present for the acute pancreatitis.

Treatment of these patients for 6 months with chenodeoxycholic acid, then maintenance on the modified diet, has resulted in the initial cholesterol-saturated bile returning to the normal micellar zone and remaining there without recurrent attacks of pancreatitis or gallstone formation.

Combinations of diet plus drugs may be used in high-risk populations, especially if weight loss is difficult to attain, and in the presence of ileal disease or any condition with a high risk of gallstones where high-fibre diet, especially, is not contraindicated.

The effect of diet alone on reducing the number of, and hence space occupied by, radiolucent gallstones in a patient on her regular diet without medical dissolution therapy is shown in Fig. 4. After 6 months of a modified diet gallbladder visualization appears better; half the gallbladder is full of radiolucent stones. After a further 18 months of modified diet alone the number of gallstones present was diminished by about a half. At this time she was given chenodeoxycholic acid (15 mg/kg bodyweight per day), and within 9 months these gallstones had all disappeared. This doctor's wife runs a lithogenic index of around 0.5 and 3 years later, while maintaining the modified diet, is still free of stones.

Acknowledgments

My grateful thanks to Ms Jan Johnstone, Mrs Sharon Scallion-George and Ms Kim Raine, three successive professional dietitians from 1973 to the present; to Mrs Sherry MacArthur and Mrs Annette Morris for their helpful bile lipid analyses; to B. Garner, Ph.D., for his excellent and ongoing statistical help, and to Ms Pat Wyman for her typing skills. This project was supported in part under the National Health Research and Development Project Number 603–1008–30 of Health and Welfare, Canada.

References

1. Bennion, L. J. and Grundy, S. M. (1978). Risk factors for the development of cholelithiasis in man (two parts). *N. Engl. J. Med.*, **299**, 1161–1221
2. Williams, C. N., Morse, J. W. I., Kotoor, R., Park-dincsoy, H. and Macdonald, I. A. (1976). Biliary pain, cholecystokinin cholecystography and lithogenic bile. *J. Gen.*, **31**, 91–100
3. Reid, J. M., Fullmer, S. D., Pettigrew, K. D. *et al.* (1971). Nutrient intake of Pima Indian women: relationships to diabetes mellitus and gallbladder disease. *Am. J. Clin. Nutr.*, **24**, 1281
4. Sampliner, R. E., Bennet, P. H., Comess, L. T. *et al.* Gallbladder disease in Pima Indians. *N. Engl. J. Med.* **283**, 1358
5. Brown, J. E. and Christensen, C. (1967). Biliary tract disease amongst the Navajos. *J. Am. Med. Assoc.*, **202**, 138

6. Williams, C. N., Johnston, J. L. and Weldon, K. L. M. (1977). Prevalence of gallstones and gallbladder disease in Canadian Micmac Indian women. *Can. Med. Assoc. J.*, **16**, 1356
7. Williams, C. N., Johnston, J. L., McCarthy, S. and Field, C. A. (1981). Biliary lipid bile acid composition and dietary correlations in Micmac Indian women. *Am. J. Dig. Dis.*, **26**, 42–49
8. Danzinger, R. G., Gordon, H., Schoenfield, L. J. and Thistle, J. L. (1972). Lithogenic bile in siblings of young women with cholelithiasis. *Mayo Clin. Proc.*, **47**, 762–766
9. Bennion, L. J. and Grundy, S. M. (1975). Effects of obesity and caloric intake on biliary lipid metabolism in man. *J. Clin. Invest.*, **56**, 996–1011
10. Freeman, J. B., Meyer, P. D., Printen, K. J., Mason, E. E. and DenBesten, L. (1975). Analysis of gallbladder bile in morbid obesity. *Am. J. Surg.*, **129**, 163–166
11. Cohen, S., Kaplan, M., Gottlieb, L. and Patterson, J. (1971). Liver disease and gallstones in regional enteritis. *Gastroenterology*, **60**, 237–244
12. Dowling, R. H., Bell, G. D. and White, J. (1972). Lithogenic bile in patients with ileal dysfunction. *Gut*, **13**, 415–420
13. Roy, C. C., Weber, A. M., Morin, C. L., *et al.* (1977). Abnormal biliary lipid composition in cystic fibrosis: effect of pancreatic enzymes. *N. Engl. J. Med.*, **297**, 1301–1305
14. Pertsemlidis, D., Panveliwalla, D. and Ahrens, E. H., Jr. (1971). Effects of clofibrate and of an estrogen-progestin combination on fasting biliary lipids and cholic acid kinetics in man. *Gastroenterology*, **61**, 488–496
15. Bennion, L. J., Ginsberg, R. L., Garnick, M. D. *et al.* (1976). Effects of oral contraceptives on the gallbladder bile of normal women. *N. Engl. J. Med.*, **294**, 189–192
16. Wood, P. D., Shioda, R., Estrich, El. *et al.* (1972). Effect of cholestyramine on composition of duodenal bile in obese human subjects. *Metabolism*, **21**, 107–116
17. Thornton, J. R., Emmet, P. M. and Heaton, K. W. (1973). Diet and gallstones: effect of refined and unrefined carbohydrate diets on bile cholesterol saturation and bile acid metabolisms. *Gut*, **24**, 2–6
18. DenBesten, L., Connor, W. C. and Bell, S. (1973). The effect of dietary cholesterol on the composition of human bile. *Surgery*, **73**, 266–273
19. McDougall, R. M., Yakymyshyn, L., Walker, K. and Thurston, O. G. (1978). Effect of wheat bran on serum lipoproteins and biliary lipids. *Can. J. Surg.*, **21**, 433–435
20. Metzger, A. L., Adler, R., Heymsfield, S. and Grundy, S. M. (1973). Diurnal variation in biliary lipid composition. *N. Engl. J. Med.*, **288**, 333–336
21. Williams, C. N., Morse, J. W. I., Macdonald, I. A., Katoor, R. and Riding, M. D. (1977). Increased lithogenicity of bile on fasting in normal subjects. *Am. J. Dig. Dis.*, **22**, 189–194
22. Johnston, J. L., Williams, C. N. and Weldon, K. L. M. (1977). Nutrient intake and meal patterns of Micmac Indian and Caucasian women in Shubenacadie, NS. *Can. Med. Assoc. J.*, **116**, 1356
23. Williams, C. N. and Johnston, J. L. (1980). Prevalence of gallstones and risk factors in Caucasian women in a rual Canadian community. *Can. Med. Assoc. J.*, **122**, 664–668
24. Williams, C. N. (1982). Diet changes enhance cholesterol gallstone dissolution. In Paumgarter, G., Stiehl, A. and Gerok, W. (eds.) *Bile Acids and Cholesterol in Health and Disease.* (Lancaster: MTP Press)
25. Williams, C. N. and Scallion-George, S. M. (1982). Prevalence of gallstones in urban Canadian Caucasian women: comparison with rural Caucasian and Indian women. *Ann. Roy. Coll. Phys. Surg. Can.*, **15**, 296A
26. Hesse, F. G. (1959). A dietary study of the Pima Indian. *Am. J. Clin. Nutr.*, **7**, 532–537
27. Sarles, H., Gerolami, A. and Cross, R. C. (1978). Diet and cholesterol gallstones, a multicentre study. *Digestion*, **17**, 121–127
28. Sarles, H., Gerolami, A. and Bord, A. (1978). Diet and cholesterol, a further study. *Digestion*, **17**, 128–134

Appendix
Logistic regression analysis in epidemiological research

R. CAPOCACCIA and the GREPCO Group*

FOREWORD

Logistic regression has been widely used as a statistical tool, beside the classical techniques of univariate analysis in several of the papers presented by GREPCO. As the use of logistic regression in the epidemiology of the gastrointestinal diseases is relatively recent, it appeared worthwhile commenting in some details on the main features of the method without interfering with the results presented in other chapters.

INTRODUCTION

Logistic regression is a statistical model relating the probability of an event to a set of explanatory (regressor) variables. It takes its name from the fact that the logistic transformation of the probability is expressed by a linear function of the regressor variables. In epidemiology, the model is used to analyse the relationships between a disease and a number of risk factors.

Historically, the method, mainly used to detect and analyse the statistical associations between factors and diseases, concerns cross-classification. Its main advantage is that it is computationally and theoretically simple, thus allowing the investigator to work very closely with his data. Even in the computer era this is the best way to check for possible data errors, to detect trends, and to generate new hypotheses. Unfortunately, such a method becomes impracticable as the number of variables to be investigated increases. Thus, if 10 variables are under consideration and each variable is to be studied at two levels (which, in any case, would probably result in a considerable loss of information) there would be 1024 cells in the multiple cross-classification, which would require an excessive number of individual observations to be properly analysed. Even more important are the limitations of the classical

* For the composition of the Group see p. xi

methods in analysing complex risk patterns arising from interactions between risk factors. The logistic regression method overcomes these difficulties. The method was first used in the field of cardiovascular epidemiology[1,2]. The introduction of maximum likelihood estimation[3,4] and the availability of specific computer software has greatly contributed to the applicability and diffusion of the method.

THE MODEL

Let $X_1, X_2, \ldots, X_k$ be the variables obtained by measuring k individual characteristics, or risk factors, for each of N individuals belonging to a certain population sample. Let y be a dummy variable for the occurrence ($y=1$) or not ($y=0$) of a certain event in each individual's life. In our case, the considered event may be the presence of a particular disease, or its occurrence during the follow-up.

The probability of being a case can be related to the variables via the equation:

$$\log[\Pr(y=1)] = \log\left[\frac{\Pr(y=1)}{1+\Pr(y=1)}\right] = \alpha + \sum_{j=1}^{k} \beta_j X_j$$

or:

$$\Pr(y=1) = \frac{1}{1+\exp[-\alpha-\Sigma_j-\beta_j X_j]} \qquad (1)$$

where α and β_j are the model parameters to be estimated from the observations, and $\exp(t)$ is the inverse of the natural logarithm of t. If only one explanatory variable is present, the expression (1) is easily recognized as the logistic function. Figure 1 shows the general shape of the logistic function.

The general expression (1) is known as the 'multiple logistic regression'. It has several important properties. It is bounded between 0 and 1, and is therefore consistent with its probabilistic meaning. The coefficients can be easily interpreted in terms of relative risk. It allows computing of the relative risk given by a simultaneous increase of several risk factors as the product of the relative risks produced by an independent increase of each of the considered factors. It is what is called a multiplicative model.

Expression (1) may be used to model a large number of different situations. The independent variables can be both true risk factors and confounding or nuisance variables. These can be categorical (i.e. dummy variables) or quantitative, discrete or continuous, and expressed in the original measurement scale or by some suitable transformation.

From expression (1), the odds ratio for individuals having two different sets of explanatory variables $(a_1, a_2, \ldots, a_k)$ and $(b_1, b_2, \ldots, b_k)$, and corresponding conditional disease probability levels P_a and P_b, is given by:

$$\frac{P_a(1-P_b)}{(1-P_a)P_b} = \exp[\Sigma_j \beta_j (a_j - b_j)] \qquad (2)$$

The above expressions lead to some interesting considerations.

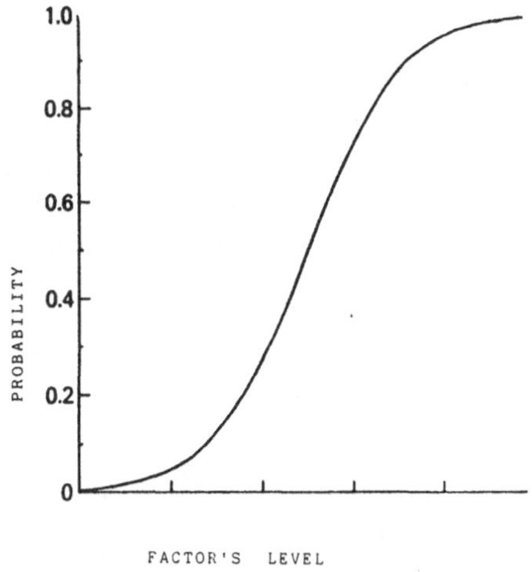

Figure 1 General shape of the logistic function: $P=1/(1+\exp(-X))$

(a) The value of α gives the odds for an individual having zero values for all the independent variables. When the variables are expressed as deviations from the mean, then α gives the odds for an individual with mean factor levels.

(b) If the disease frequency is small, the odds ratio given by expression (2) can be considered as a good approximation of the relative risk given to the different sets of values of the independent variables. The term, relative risk (RR), will be used here instead of the more correct odds ratio.

(c) The value of $\exp(\beta_j)$ gives the RR due to a unitary increase of the jth independent variable, all other variables being fixed. The RR due to an arbitrary increase ΔX_j of X_j is given by the expression:

$$RR=\exp(\beta_j \Delta X_j).$$

(d) The RR due to the simultaneous change of the k explanatory variables $X_1, X_2, \ldots, X_k$ is given by the product of the RRs due to the independent changes of each variable:

$$\exp(\beta_1 \Delta X_1) \cdot \exp(\beta_2 \Delta X_2) \ldots \exp(\beta_k \Delta X_k).$$

The easy interpretation of the parameters accounts for the wide use of multiple logistic regression for statistical analysis of epidemiological data. If the considered risk factors are acting on each other independently the independent contribution of each factor can be evaluated. Furthermore, confounding factors can be entered into the model as additional regressor variables, to be taken into account in the analysis.

STATISTICAL INFERENCE

The parameters α and β_j in expression (1) can be estimated from the sample observations by means of different methods. A full analysis, in this regard, of the whole matter is given in Cox's classical work *Analysis of Binary Data*[4]. Of the various methods available, unconditional maximum likelihood is the most suitable for epidemiological studies, since it is both computationally simple and has asymptotic (i.e. for large samples) good properties. Moreover, maximum likelihood estimation programs are now available in statistical computer packages, such as Biomedical Package (BMDP)[5] or General Linear Interactive Modelling (GLIM) system[6]. The key features of this method are briefly outlined below.

From expression (1), the joint probability of being a case for the observed cases, and a non-case for the observed non-cases is given by the product, computed over all the sample subjects:

$$L=\Pi_N\left[\frac{y}{1+\exp(-\alpha-\Sigma_j\beta_jX_j)}+(1-y)\frac{\exp(-\alpha-\Sigma_j\beta_jX_j)}{1+\exp(-\alpha-\Sigma_j\beta_jX_j)}\right] \quad (3)$$

The function L is known as the likelihood function of the sample. As the observed values of the outcome variable y and of the explanatory variables X_j are explicitly inserted into expression (3), L is a function of α and β_j parameters only. The estimates, $\hat{\alpha}$ and $\hat{\beta}_j$ are the set of values for which L or its logarithm is maximum. In some sense, maximum likelihood estimates are given by the parameter values which give maximum probability of having observed the true observed sample. It can be shown[7] that the estimates $\hat{\alpha}$ and $\hat{\beta}_j$ are normally distributed for large samples, and their covariance matrix can easily be computed from the second derivatives matrix of log L. The standard errors of the estimates are then given by the square root of the corresponding diagonal elements of the covariance matrix and are given by all available computer programs. BMDP or GLIM logistic regression programs also give the entire covariance matrix.

The hypothesis $H_0:\beta_j=0$ can then be tested by the statistic:

$$z=\frac{\hat{\beta}_j}{\text{standard error }(\hat{\beta}_j)} \quad (4)$$

If H_0 is true, the statistic (4) is (for large samples) normally distributed with zero mean and unit variance. Confidence limits for the value of the parameter β_j can be computed as:

$$\hat{\beta}_j \pm z_{\gamma/2}\text{ standard error }(\hat{\beta}_j) \quad (5)$$

where z_γ is the value cutting off a γ probability in the normal curve (for example, at the probability level $\gamma=0.05$, we have: $z_{\gamma/2}=1.96$). Expression (5) can be used to plot the confidence region of the relative risk against the level of a risk factor. Taking some arbitrary level $X_j=a$ as baseline, the confidence region is defined by the two lines:

$$\text{RR}(X_j)=\exp\{[\hat{\beta}_j \pm z_{\gamma/2}\text{ standard error }(\hat{\beta}_j)](X_j-a)\}$$

Some applications of this expression can be found in Chapters 12 and 24 in this volume.

Log likelihood statistic may also be used to test statistical hypotheses about parameter values. Once $\hat{\alpha}$ and $\hat{\beta}_j$ estimates are obtained, it is possible to compute, from expression (1) the estimated disease probability for each individual, and let us call it $\hat{P}_i$. Then the log likelihood statistic:

$$\text{LLS} = -2 \log L = -2 \sum_{i=1}^{N} [y_i \log \hat{P}_i + (1-y_i)\log(1-\hat{P}_i)] \qquad (6)$$

is a measure of how the estimated probabilities $\hat{P}_i$ approximate the observed quantities y_i. It is as small as the approximation is good, and has a theoretical minimum value of zero, which is reached when all the observed and estimated values coincide. If we consider two models, the first with k factors, the second with the same factors plus one additional factor, and compute the quantity (6) for each model, then the statistic

$$G = \text{LLS}_{(k\text{ factors})} - \text{LLS}_{(k+1\text{ factors})} \qquad (7)$$

can be used to test the contribution of the additional factor. Under the null hypothesis $\beta_{k+1} = 0$, the statistic expression (7) has (in large samples) an approximated chi-squared distribution with one degree of freedom. In general, if the two models contain k and $k+h$ factors respectively, then the difference of their log likelihoods, has, under the null hypothesis:

$$H_0\colon\ \beta_{k+1} = \beta_{k+2} = \ldots = \beta_{k+h} = 0$$

a (large sample) chi-squared distribution with h degrees of freedom. This statistic has the advantage of reliably testing the significance of the additional contribution of the factor(s) added to the equation *given the contribution of all other factors already in the model*. Then it is possible to build up the model step by step, starting from an equation with only the constant α parameter (and possibly the more relevant confounding factors), and adding, at each step, the factor giving the best decrease of the log likelihood statistic, until that decrease reaches a prefixed significance level. This is the so-called forward stepwise procedure. Conversely, a backward procedure consists in starting from the full model, containing all the considered factors, and removing them one by one until a significant increase of the log likelihood is found. The general stepwise procedure allows factors either to be entered into, or to be removed from, the model equation. The general technique and the problems in using a stepwise procedure for a logistic regression are similar to those arising in the linear case. Further details in this regard will be found in textbooks on linear regression[8,9]. The use of a statistical package such as, for example, BMDP, allows such procedures to be performed very easily by entering only a few lines of computer instructions.

Besides statistical testing of the model parameters it is useful to consider the problem of assessing the goodness of fit of the final model. This is quite a different matter. The former concerns the strength of the observed relationships between the disease and the risk factors, the latter how well the model can be considered a good description of the facts. Log likelihood statistic given by expression (6) can be considered a goodness of fit measure. However, it has neither an intuitive meaning nor, by itself, any known distributional properties. A very common procedure for assessing the goodness of fit of a given logistic regression model is to rank the individuals from the lowest estimated probability, let us call it 'risk', to the highest one, and defining deciles of risk. The first decile contains the individuals with the lowest risk values, and so on. If the model has a good fit it is reasonable to suppose that the number of observed cases in each decile will be close to the number of the expected ones. This number can be computed as the sum of the individual risks of all the subjects belonging to the considered decile. A global measure of the agreement between the expected and the observed values can be given by the chi-squared-like expression:

$$X^2 = \sum_{h=1}^{10} \frac{(o_h - e_h)^2}{e_h}$$

where e_h and o_h are the expected and observed cases in the hth decile of risk. This statistic is intuitively simple but its distribution is not known. It is only possible to state that a small value is better than a large value. The problem of assessing goodness of fit for logistic regression models has been studied by many authors, and a number of different statistics, with known distributional properties, have been proposed. Lemenshow and Hosmer[10] have recently published a comprehensive review of the main results obtained in this field.

NON-LINEARITIES AND INTERACTIONS

The logistic regression model, as formulated by expression (1), is based on the assumption of a logistic relationship between the disease probability and a linear combination of the explanatory variables. This hypothesis has two important implications that may, in some instances, be in disagreement with the actual features of the phenomenon under study.

(a) From expression (1), it follows that the RR given by an increase in the level of a risk factor is independent of its baseline value. This is not always true. A case has been reported (Chapter 24 in this volume) in which the risk for gallstone disease appears to be nearly constant for low values, but decreases significantly for high values of serum cholesterol.

(b) The RR given by each factor should be independent of the level of the other risk factors. When this is not true, an 'interaction' is said to exist between the factors. Interactions often occur between various factors and age, which can be a measure for the duration of exposure, or for the time elapsing since exposure.

In both cases the logistic regression model can be used, by introducing some higher-degree terms. In the first case an attempt can be made to enter, as an additional independent variable, the square of the factor for which a non-linear relationship is suspected. If the log likelihood statistic decreases significantly, the second-order term can be incorporated into the final model. In principle, also third- or higher-order terms can be tested, but in most cases they will be unnecessary. The second case can be clarified by considering that the dependence of the effect of some factor, say X_1, by the level of another, say

X_2, can be accounted for by considering the coefficient β_1 as a linear function of X_2. Thus:

$$\beta_1 X_1 = (\beta_1{}' 6 \beta_{12} X_2) X_1 = \beta_1{}' X_1 + \beta_{12} X_1 X_2$$

Interaction between the two factors can be taken into account by introducing into the model the additional variable given by the product X_1X_2.

In using higher-order terms some general considerations hold.

(a) All the lower-order terms must be present in the model. Thus, if a second-degree term is tested, the linear term cannot be removed. If an interaction term is present in the equation, the two main effects must also be present.

(b) There is little sense in interpreting the single high-order coefficient. Once their statistical significance has been ascertained, a plot of the RR vs. the independent variable level gives a more reliable and informative description of the actual relationship with the disease.

CONCLUSIONS

The logistic regression technique has several important advantages for the analysis of the relationships between factors and disease. It is powerful, easy to carry out, interpretation is simple but informative, and experience has generally shown that it fits the data well. Thus, in the analysis of binary outcome data, it plays the role that linear regression plays for continuous responses. However, it is not without problems.

If the regressor variables are closely correlated to each other, interpretation of the results may be difficult[11,12]. Indeed, the estimated value of the parameters which play a central role in interpreting the model in terms of relative risk may change, even drastically, according to which other variables are included in the equation. If a disease is associated with a certain factor it tends to be associated also with other factors closely correlated with the first one. This does not necessarily mean that an independent relationship holds between the disease and each of the factors, but only that the disease is more frequent in individuals with high levels of the considered factors. For example, if a disease is associated with socioeconomic conditions, each factor from a large varied set (income, educational level, ownership of different items, etc.) can well represent such an association. If the disease has a true direct relationship with only, say, education, in a multiple regression the coefficients of the other factors will be small and not significant. However, if the educational factor is not present in the equation, each one of the other factors can be used as a proxy, and the corresponding coefficient will probably increase and be found to be highly significant. When the independent variable values are correlated to each other in the sample, collinearity is said to exist between them. The problems arising from such a situation are common to all regression techniques, and no simple solution exists, except greater care should be exerted in performing the analysis and interpreting the results.

Below, some general rules are given to correctly build a logistic regression model. These should not, however, be considered as general laws.

Furthermore, a wide scope for the subjective judgment of the investigator still remains. The best guarantee for correct analysis is experience and skill.

(a) Simultaneous use of a stepwise procedure and test (expression (7)) is strongly recommended for the statistical testing of unstable coefficients, when a high degree of collinearity between the explanatory variables exists.
(b) Only those factors with a statistically significant contribution should be included in the model.
(c) On the other hand, the model should consider all the known confounding factors, regardless of the statistical significance. A factor can act as a confounder in the analysis even if its association with the disease or the risk factors is not statistically significant.
(d) If two or more factors are very closely correlated, only one, or only one combination of them, should be tested for inclusion in the model. This situation is frequent when factors arising from different measurements of the same phenomenon are considered (as, for example, systolic and diastolic blood pressure).
(e) Artificial collinearities should be avoided since they give rise to computational problems. For example, it is impossible to consider the total and the HDL, LDL and VLDL serum cholesterol levels in the same equation, because the exact relationship between them makes the estimated covariance matrix of the parameters singular.
(f) To reduce collinearities with linear terms, mean or modal values can be subtracted from the component parts of the second-order terms before multiplying.

A different kind of problem arises since the model does not incorporate, in longitudinal studies, any information about the time of occurrence of the event. When such information is known this causes some loss of power in the analysis. Further, in long-term longitudinal studies, the value of the estimated coefficients becomes dependent upon the time of follow-up[12,13]. This fact leads to some difficulty when comparing results obtained in different studies. These problems may be overcome by using the so-called 'proportional hazard model'[14]. This model generalizes the life table analysis method by expressing the logarithm of the instantaneous risk as a linear combination of the regressor variables. For statistical comparisons with the logistic regression model, several papers[13,15] can be consulted.

References

1. Truett, J., Cornfield, J. and Kannel, W. (1967). A multivariate analysis of the risk of coronary heart disease in Framingham. *J. Chron. Dis.*, **20**, 511–524
2. Keys, A. *et al.* (1972). Probability of middle-aged men developing coronary heart disease in five years. *Circulation*, **45**, 815–828
3. Walker, S. H. and Duncan, D. B. (1967). Estimation of the probability of an event as a function of several independent variables. *Biometrika*, **54**, 167–179
4. Cox, D. R. (1970). *The Analysis of Binary Data.* (London: Methuen)
5. Baker, R. J. and Nedler, J. A. (1978). *The GLIM System. Release* 3 (Oxford: Numerical Algorithm Group)

6. Dixon, W. J. and Brown, M. B. (eds.) (1981). *BMDP Statistical Software 1981*. (Berkeley, Calif.: University of California Press)
7. Kendall, M. G. and Stuart, A. (1961). *The Advanced Theory of Statistics*, Vol. 2. (London: Griffin)
8. Draper, W. and Smith, H. (1966). *Applied Regression Analysis*. (New York: Wiley)
9. Kerlinger, F. N. and Pedhazur, F. J. (1973). *Multiple Regression in Behavioral Research*. (New York: Holt, Rinehart & Winston)
10. Lemeshow, S. and Hosmer, D. W. (1982). A review of goodness of fit statistics for use in the development of logistic regression models. *Am. J. Epidemiol.*, **115**, 92–106
11. Breslow, N. E. and Day, N. E. (1980). *Statistical Methods in Cancer Research*. (Lyon: International Agency of Research on Cancer)
12. Woodbury, M. A., Manton, K. G. and Stallard, E. (1981). Longitudinal models for chronic disease risk: an evaluation of logistic multiple regression and alternative. *Int. J. Epidemiol.*, **10**, 187–197
13. Green, M. S. and Symons, M. J. (1983). A comparison of the logistic risk function and the proportional hazard model in prospective epidemiologic studies. *J. Chron. Dis.*, **36**, 715–724
14. Cox, D. R. (1972). Regression model and life tables. *J. R. Stat. Soc.*, **B34**, 187–220
15. Thomas, W. A. Jr. (1977). On the treatment of grouped observations in life studies. *Biometrics*, **33**, 463–470

Index